T0211101

Lecture Notes of the Institute for Computer Sciences, Social Informatics and Telecommunications Engineering 484

The LNICST series publishes ICST's conferences, symposia and workshops.
LNICST reports state-of-the-art results in areas related to the scope of the Institute.
The type of material published includes

- Proceedings (published in time for the respective event)
- Other edited monographs (such as project reports or invited volumes)

LNICST topics span the following areas:

- General Computer Science
- E-Economy
- E-Medicine
- Knowledge Management
- Multimedia
- Operations, Management and Policy
- Social Informatics
- Systems

António Cunha · Nuno M. Garcia ·
Jorge Marx Gómez · Sandra Pereira
Editors

Wireless Mobile Communication and Healthcare

11th EAI International Conference, MobiHealth 2022
Virtual Event, November 30 – December 2, 2022
Proceedings

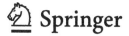 Springer

Editors
António Cunha ⓘ
University of Trás-os-Montes and Alto Douro
Vila Real, Portugal

Nuno M. Garcia ⓘ
University of Beira Interior
Covilha, Portugal

Jorge Marx Gómez ⓘ
Ossietzky Universität Oldenburg
Oldenburg, Niedersachsen, Germany

Sandra Pereira ⓘ
University of Trás-os-Montes and Alto Douro
Vila Real, Portugal

ISSN 1867-8211   ISSN 1867-822X (electronic)
Lecture Notes of the Institute for Computer Sciences, Social Informatics
and Telecommunications Engineering
ISBN 978-3-031-32028-6   ISBN 978-3-031-32029-3 (eBook)
https://doi.org/10.1007/978-3-031-32029-3

This Springer imprint is published by the registered company Springer Nature Switzerland AG
The registered company address is: Gewerbestrasse 11, 6330 Cham, Switzerland

Preface

We are delighted to introduce the proceedings of the second edition of the European Alliance for Innovation (EAI) International Conference on Wireless Mobile Communication and Healthcare (MobiHealth 2022). This conference, which was held online November 30 – December 2, 2022, brought together researchers, developers and practitioners worldwide who are leveraging and developing wireless communications, mobile computing and the healthcare application field.

The technical program of MobiHealth 2022 consisted of 28 full papers with oral presentation sessions at the main conference track and 1 Demo paper, and 1 Poster paper. Aside from the high-quality technical paper presentations, the technical program also featured two keynote speeches. The two keynote speeches were Emilio Luque from Universitat Autònoma de Barcelona, Spain and Hélder Oliveira from Institute for Systems and Computer Engineering, Technology and Science, Portugal.

Coordination with the steering chair, Imrich Chlamtac, was essential for the conference's success. We sincerely appreciate his support and guidance. It was also a great pleasure to work with such an excellent organizing committee team for their hard work in organizing and supporting the conference.

In particular, the Technical Program Committee, led by our TPC Co-Chairs, Anselmo Paiva, María Vanessa Villasana, Susanna Spinsante, Francesco Renna, and Paulo Salgado completed the peer-review process of technical papers and made a high-quality technical program. We are also grateful to all other organizing committee members for their support and all the authors who submitted their papers to the MobiHealth 2022 conference and workshops.

We strongly believe that the MobiHealth conference provides a good forum for all researchers, developers and practitioners to discuss all science and technology aspects that are relevant to the fields of wireless communications, mobile computing and healthcare applications. We also expect that the future MobiHealth conferences will be as successful and stimulating as indicated by the contributions presented in this volume.

May 2023

António Cunha
Nuno M. Garcia
Jorge Marx Gómez
Sandra Pereira

Organization

Steering Committee

Imrich Chlamtac   University of Trento, Italy

Organizing Committee

General Chair

António Cunha   Universidade de Trás-os-Montes e Alto Douro, Portugal

General Co-chair

Ivan Miguel Pires   Universidade da Beira Interior, Portugal

TPC Chair and Co-chairs

Nuno M. Garcia	Universidade da Beira Interior, Portugal
Jorge Marx Gómez	Carl von Ossietzky University of Oldenburg, Germany
María Vanessa Villasana	Centro Hospitalar Universitário da Cova da Beira, Portugal
Susanna Spinsante	Marche Polytechnic University, Italy
Francesco Renna	Universidade do Porto, Portugal
Anselmo Paiva	Universidade Federal do Maranhão, Brazil
Paulo Salgado	Universidade de Trás-os-Montes e Alto Douro, Portugal

Sponsorship and Exhibit Chair

Joaquim João Sousa   Universidade de Trás-os-Montes e Alto Douro, Portugal

Local Chair

Emanuel Peres   Universidade de Trás-os-Montes e Alto Douro,
                                 Portugal

Workshops Chair

Paulo Coelho   Instituto Politécnico de Leiria, Portugal

Publicity and Social Media Chairs

Miguel Coimbra   Universidade do Porto, Portugal
Pedro Mestre   Universidade de Trás-os-Montes e Alto Douro,
                                 Portugal

Publications Chair

Carlos Ferreira   INESC/TEC, Portugal

Web Chair

António Jorge Gouveia   Universidade de Trás-os-Montes e Alto Douro,
                                 Portugal

Posters and PhD Track Chair

Sandra Pereira   Universidade de Trás-os-Montes e Alto Douro,
                                 Portugal

Panels Chair

João Rodrigues   Univerisade do Algarve, Portugal

Demos Chair

Norberto Gonçalves   Universidade de Trás-os-Montes e Alto Douro,
                                 Portugal

Tutorials Chair

Eftim Zdravevski   Ss. Cyril and Methodius University in Skopje,
                                     Macedonia

Technical Program Committee

Abbas Aljuboori   University of Information Technology and
                                     Communications, Iraq
Alberto Taboada-Crispi   Universidad Central "Marta Abreu" de Las Villas,
                                     Cuba
Alessio Vecchio   University of Pisa, Italy
Ali Ghaffari   Islamic Azad University, Iran
Ali Hassan Sodhro   Kristianstad University, Sweden
Ana Maria Mendonça   Universidade do Porto, Portugal
Ana Paula Rocha   Universidade do Porto, Portugal
Ana Paula Silva   Instituto Politécnico de Castelo Branco, Portugal
Ana Sequeira   INESC TEC – Institute for Systems and
                                     Computer Engineering, Technology and
                                     Science, Portugal
André Moraes   Universidade Federal de Santa Catarina, Brasil
Anna Sandak   University of Primorska, Slovenia
Argentina Leite   Universidade de Trás-os-Montes e Alto Douro,
                                     Portugal
Aykut Karakaya   Zonguldak Bulent Ecevit University, Turkey
Carlos Albuquerque   Instituto Politécnico de Viseu, Portugal
Carlos Thomaz   FEI University, Brazil
Catarina I. Reis   Instituto Politécnico de Leiria, Portugal
Celia Ramos   University of the Algarve, Portugal
Cláudio Baptista   Federal University of Campina Grande, Brazil
Constandinos Mavromoustakis   University of Nicosia, Cyprus
Danilo Leite   Universidade Federal de Paraíba, Brasil
Diogo Marques   Universidade da Beira Interior, Portugal
Emmanuel Conchon   University of Limoges, France
Faisal Hussain   University of Engineering and Technology,
                                     Pakistan
Farhan Riaz   National University of Sciences and Technology,
                                     Islamabad, Pakistan
Fernando Ribeiro   Instituto Politécnico de Castelo Branco, Portugal
Filipe Caldeira   Instituto Politécnico de Viseu, Portugal
Francesco Renna   Universidade do Porto, Portugal
Francisco Florez-Revuelta   Universidad de Alicante, Spain

Gabriel Pires	Instituto Politécnico de Tomar, Portugal
Geraldo Braz Junior	Universidade Federal do Maranhão, Brazil
Hélder Oliveira	Universidade do Porto, Portugal
Henrique Neiva	Universidade da Beira Interior, Portugal
Inês Domingues	ISEC, Portugal
Isabel Bentes	Universidade de Trás-os-Montes e Alto Douro, Portugal
Ivan Chorbev	Ss. Cyril and Methodius University in Skopje, Macedonia
Ivan Ganchev	University of Limerick, Ireland
Ivan Štajduhar	University of Rijeka, Croatia
Jânio Monteiro	University of the Algarve, Portugal
João Carlos Lanzinha	Universidade da Beira Interior, Portugal
João Dallyson Sousa de Almeida	Universidade Federal do Maranhão, Brazil
João Henriques	University of Coimbra, Portugal
João Otávio Bandeira Diniz	Federal Institute of Education, Science and Technology of Maranhão, Brazil
João Paulo Cunha	Universidade do Porto, Portugal
João Pedrosa	Universidade do Porto, Portugal
João Tavares	Universidade do Porto, Portugal
John Gialelis	University of Patras, Greece
Jonatan Lerga	University of Rijeka, Croatia
Jorge Oliveira	ISEP, Portugal
Jorge Semião	University of the Algarve, Portugal
Jorge Tiago Pinto	Universidade de Trás-os-Montes e Alto Douro, Portugal
José Carlos Meireles Metrôlho	Instituto Politécnico de Castelo Branco, Portugal
José Lousado	Instituto Politécnico de Viseu, Portugal
José Valente de Oliveira	University of the Algarve, Portugal
Juliana Sá	Centro Hospitalar Universitário do Oporto, Portugal
Kalle Tammemäe	Tallinn University of Technology, Estonia
Kelson Romulo Teixeira Aires	Federal University of Piaui, Brazil
Korhan Cengiz	University of Fujairah, United Arab Emirates
Lambros Lambrinos	Cyprus University of Technology, Cyprus
Leonel Morgado	Open University, Portugal
Luis Augusto Silva	University of Salamanca, Spain
Luis Teixeira	Universidade do Porto, Portugal
Mário Marques	Universidade da Beira Interior, Portugal
Marta Chinnici	ENEA, Italy
Miguel Velhote Correia	Universidade do Porto, Portugal
Mónica Costa	Instituto Politécnico de Castelo Branco, Portugal

Contents

Medical, Communications and Networking

Signal/Data Processing and Computing For Health Systems

Biomedical, and Health Informatics

Deep Learning Glaucoma Detection Models in Retinal Images Capture by Mobile Devices

Roberto Flavio Rezende[1], Ana Coelho[1], Rodrigo Fernandes[1], José Camara[3],
Alexandre Neto[1,2], and António Cunha[1,2(✉)]

[1] Escola de Ciências e Tecnologia, Universidade de Trás-os-Montes e Alto Douro, Quinta de Prados, 5001-801 Vila Real, Portugal
acunha@utad.pt
[2] Instituto de Engenharia de Sistemas e Computadores, Tecnologia e Ciência, 3200-465 Porto, Portugal
[3] Departamento de Ciências e Tecnologia, Universidade Aberta, 1250-100 Lisbon, Portugal

Abstract. Glaucoma is a disease that arises from increased intraocular pressure and leads to irreversible partial or total loss of vision. Due to the lack of symptoms, this disease often progresses to more advanced stages, not being detected in the early phase. The screening of glaucoma can be made through visualization of the retina, through retinal images captured by medical equipment or mobile devices with an attached lens to the camera. Deep learning can enhance and increase mass glaucoma screening. In this study, domain transfer learning technique is important to better weight initialization and for understanding features more related to the problem. For this, classic convolutional neural networks, such as ResNet50 will be compared with Vision Transformers, in high and low-resolution images. The high-resolution retinal image will be used to pre-trained the network and use that knowledge for detecting glaucoma in retinal images captured by mobile devices. The ResNet50 model reached the highest values of AUC in the high-resolution dataset, being the more consistent model in all the experiments. However, the Vision Transformer proved to be a promising technique, especially in low-resolution retinal images.

Keywords: Glaucoma Screening · Deep Learning · Transfer Learning

1 Introduction

Glaucoma is a silent disease that arises from increased intraocular pressure and consequently leads to irreversible partial or total loss of vision. This loss of vision occurs due to the destruction of the ganglion cells, which belong to the optic nerve, a structure that connects the eye to the occipital brain and which is responsible for conducting images from the retina to the brain [1, 2]. Aqueous humor is a transparent liquid composed of water and dissolved salts. Its function is to nourish the cornea and the crystalline lens, besides regulating intraocular pressure. The liquid is located in the anterior and posterior chamber of the eyeball [1, 3]. The reason why aqueous humor production is so important

A. Cunha et al. (Eds.): MobiHealth 2022, LNICST 484, pp. 3–13, 2023.
https://doi.org/10.1007/978-3-031-32029-3_1

is that if this liquid is not drained in the same quantities as it is produced, the ocular pressures increases and irreversible damages the optic nerve, leading to the development of glaucoma. After all, in glaucoma patients, these fibers are atrophied, making it impossible to conduct images to the brain. Secondarily, there is the appearance of scotomas in the visual field and with the evolution of the disease, glaucoma causes progressive loss of vision [1, 3, 4]. Figure 1 show the effects of high intraocular pressure and the visual consequences.

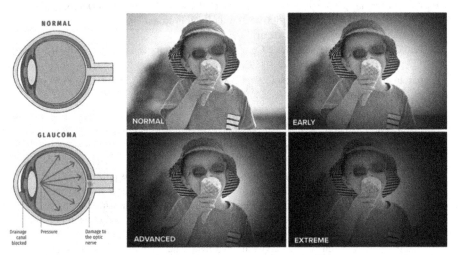

Fig. 1. Normal and glaucomatous eye. Consequences of glaucoma in vision loss (adapted from Hagiwara et al. [4]).

The retina can be directly examined by using an ophthalmoscope or can be examined indirectly through retinal fundus images. The retinal fundus images allow for the detection of indicators and parameters normally correlated to the appearance and development of cupping, such as disc diameter, peripapillary atrophy notching and cup-to-disc ratio (CDR). Retinal images turn the process very easy to access the data, duplication, archiving and delivery, which help in more immediate results in medical centers where is performed automatic or manual screening [5].

Since ophthalmology in general, and particularly the screening of glaucomatous diseases, is heavily based on image analysis, one of the emerging research areas in recent years is the interpretation of images using automated computational methods. In this field of visual analysis by computers for the identification of ophthalmic diseases the use of deep learning (DL) algorithms has stood out [6].

The use of deep learning in the identification of pathologies, especially those that are diagnosed through a visual pattern, offers the potential to improve the accuracy and speed of exam interpretation in addition to lowering their costs [7].

This study intends to compare the performance of two deep learning models in glaucoma classification, namely the ViT and ResNet50 architecture, and evaluate if this technique be beneficial to models created for glaucoma classification in low-resolution images.

2   Related Work

2.1   Convolutional Neural Network

In fields of investigation where information is collected more rapidly than analyzed and require experienced individuals to perform these investigations, DL strategies show up as tools for handling and analyzing a great amount of information. A typical method of DL for image processing is the convolutional neural network (CNN) [8, 9].

There is available a large variety of CNNs and in this section, some will be explained according to the ones that will be used in this work. One type of CNN is the residual network (ResNet) which was created with shortcut connections to increase the depth of CNN without gradient degradation. The shortcuts assist the gradient flowing easily during the backpropagation, leading to accuracy gains during the training. Normally this type of network is composed of 4 blocks, with convolutional blocks inside being the difference among the different versions of ResNet (50, 101 and 152) the number of consecutive convolutional blocks. With the use of residual blocks the gradient gradation problem is resolved [10].

Recently, a new type of neural network emerged as an alternative to CNNs, relying on self-attention mechanisms, called Vision Transformers (ViT). The ViT model, when compared to a traditional CNN, has a weaker inductive bias leading to greater reliance on the model regularization or data augmentation when training on smaller datasets. The training phase of ViT depends on measuring the relation among pairs of input tokens. The tokens, in the computer vision field, can be made by using image patches. The relation between these patches is learned through providing attention to the network [11].

Since classification DL models can be black boxes, explainable artificial intelligence (XAI) methods were created to provide transparency and explainability explainable to assist experts and non-experts in understanding which features are related and influence the models' decisions [12]. One of the methods that can be used for XAI is the Grad-CAM which uses the specific gradient information for each class from the last convolutional layer, to design a coarse location map of the important areas in the image [13]. The other method, designed for explainability in attention models is the attention rollout mechanism that quantifies how the information flows through in transformer blocks, doing the average of weights across all the heads [14].

2.2   Deep Learning for Glaucoma Detection

Machine learning techniques have become indispensable in many areas. With these techniques, computers are increasingly equipped with the capability to act without the need of explicitly being programmed, building models which can train from data and make decisions based on that data.

Chen [15] proposed a CNN-based DL algorithm to detect glaucoma presence in retinal fundus images, these images being present in the ORIGIN and SCES datasets. This CNN is composed of six layers comprising four convolutional layers and two fully connected layers. A dropout layer was added, and data augmentation was implemented to further increase the results of glaucoma detection. An area under the curve (AUC) of 0.831 and 0.887 for each of the databases was achieved, respectively.

In Raghavendra [16] study a CNN (18 convolution layers) was used for the same purpose of detecting glaucoma in retinal fundus images. For this were collected 1426 retinal fundus images composed of 589 normal cases and 837 with glaucoma train the network.

Chai [17] designed a multivariate neural network model, which was inspired by domain knowledge, to extract hidden features from the retinal images simultaneously while extracting important areas of images. The performance of the algorithm was quite high, as they achieved an accuracy of 0.9151, sensitivity of 0.9233 and specificity of 0.9090. Benzebouchi [18], used two DL models with multimodal data (RGB and grayscale images). The two models are composed of two convolutional layers and one fully convolutional layer. It turned out that it would be better if the two models were combined.

In Suguna [19], the authors used a pre-trained model called EyeNet, which was originally trained on fundus images for the classification of a different eye disease, to detect glaucoma presence in retinal fundus images. The contribution is that the model is more suited to the problem since the EyeNet model was trained to classify diabetic retinopathy, which is a very related problem. The similarities between the two disease domains largely influence the amount of knowledge transfer. Using pre-trained models of similar domains outperforms pre-trained models that used generic datasets, unrelated to the glaucoma classification. The proposed method reached better results when compared to pre-trained models based on generic datasets.

Alghamdi [20] proposes a framework for automatic glaucoma diagnosis based on three CNN models, each one with different methods for learning, comparing the results with ophthalmologists. In the first phase, the authors start with a pre-trained model which was trained in unrelated data and fine-tunes with the glaucoma data. Then, a semi-supervised model is developed to train using label and unlabeled data. This method demonstrates the effectiveness in glaucoma detection from the CNN models when tested in two different datasets (RIM-ONE and RIGA). All the models reached better performance when compared to the two ophthalmologists.

3   Materials and Methodologies

This project intends to compare the performance of two models in glaucoma classification, namely the ViT and ResNet50 architecture. These models will be first pre-trained in public high-resolution retinal images, with and without PCA color augmentation. After this, the weights of these models were used to pre-trained the same models in the private dataset of low-resolution retinal images (collected by mobile devices), with and without PCA color augmentation. In the end, both the glaucoma assessment in public and private databases will be evaluated and will be concluded if this transfer learning technique can benefit the models created for glaucoma classification in low-resolution images. To further explained the results, XAI techniques will be implemented as well. In this section, will be described the datasets used for this work (public and private), the pre-processing methods and the evaluation metrics to test the glaucoma assessment of each model.

3.1 Public Dataset

RIM-ONE consists of 169 optic nerve head (ONH) images obtained from 169 complete retinal fundus images of different patients (10 images were discarded because were not directly related to glaucoma) [21].

DRISHTI-GS is composed of a total of 101 images of which 50 images are for training and 51 images are for testing [22].

REFUGE is composed of 1200 retinal fundus images, acquired by ophthalmologists or technicians, from patients sitting upright (only 400 images are available for training) [23].

In Table 1 are described the proprieties of the three public databases used.

Table 1. Public retinal image datasets.

Database	RIM-ONE	Drishti-GS	REFUGE
Normal	85	31	360
Glaucoma	74	70	40

In the model developed for the training, the set consists of 128 images classified as glaucoma and 332 images classified as normal. For the testing set, 28 images are glaucoma and 72 normal, for validation the same number of images with same glaucoma/normal ratio. The percentage is then 70% training, 15% test and 15% validation.

3.2 Private Dataset

The "Private Dataset" is a dataset consisting of 491 images (356 normal and 135 with glaucoma). This dataset was provided by an ophthalmologist to help this study, given that the images used in this work must contain low quality examples and this is exactly what this dataset provides. Figure 2 illustrates some examples of low-resolution retinal images captured by mobile devices.

For training, testing and validation the percentages were the same as for the public dataset, so for training 260 normal and 95 glaucoma images were used, for testing 46 normal and 20 glaucoma images, and finally for validation 50 normal and 20 glaucoma images, making a percentage of about 70%, 15% and 15% respectively.

3.3 Image Pre-processing

Resize Images: Since the selected images did not all have the same resolution, a filter was applied to these same images, and all images were resized to a resolution of 512 × 512 pixels.

PCA Color Augmentation

Color augmentation principal components analysis (PCA), changes RGB channel intensities, using PCA of the pixel colors [24]. Specifically, PCA is performed on RGB pixel

NORMAL   **GLAUCOMA**

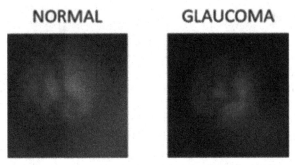

Fig. 2. Examples of normal and glaucoma images in private retinal images collected by mobile devices.

values in the entire data set. The principal component multiples are added to each image, with proportional to the corresponding eigenvalues times a random variable drawn from a Gaussian distribution with mean = 0 and standard deviation = 0.1.

3.4 Evaluation Metrics

Evaluation of a classification model is done by comparing the classes predicted by the model with the true classes of each example. All classification metrics have the common goal of measuring how far the model is from perfect classification, but they do this in different ways.

The accuracy (1) tells how many examples were classified correctly, regardless of class. Follows the accuracy equation:

$$Acc = \frac{TP + TN}{TP + TN + FP + FN} \tag{1}$$

Sensitivity (2) is also known as recall. This metric evaluates the method's ability to successfully detect results classified as positive. It can be obtained by the equation:

$$Sensitivity = \frac{TP}{TP + FN} \tag{2}$$

Specificity (3), on the other hand, evaluates the ability of the method to detect negative results. We can calculate it using the equation:

$$Specificity = \frac{TN}{FP + TN} \tag{3}$$

Precision (4) is a metric that evaluates the number of true positives over the sum of all positive values. It is calculated by the following formula:

$$Precision = \frac{TP}{TP + FP} \tag{4}$$

F-measure, F-score or F1 score (5) is a harmonic mean calculated based on precision and revocation. It can be obtained from the equation:

$$F1 \; Score = 2 \times \frac{precision \times sensitivity}{precision + sensitivity} \tag{5}$$

4 Results and Discussion

Deep learning models can help to increase the speed of mass glaucoma screening and maintain the performance between exams and examiners. The models' results in the high-resolution dataset are described in Table 2. Using deep learning algorithms for glaucoma detection in high-resolution images demonstrates high performance, with AUCs above 0.70. The standard CNN model (ResNet50) reached the highest performance among the models selected. The use of PCA pre-processing increased considerably the ResNet50 performance, thus, this pre-processing technique enhances the feature visualization related to glaucoma presence. Regarding the ViT models, the results did not reach the same standards as the ResNet50. Despite the high values of specificity and precision, the sensitivity was below 0.5. In this case, instead of enhancing the effectiveness of the ViT, the pre-processing using the PCA method downgraded the results.

Table 2. Model results in high-resolution retinal images with or without PCA pre-processing.

Models	Acc	Sen	Spec	Prec	F1	AUC
ViT	0.60	0.49	0.89	0.92	0.64	0.72
ViT PCA	0.58	0.42	**1.00**	**1.00**	0.59	0.70
ResNet50	0.80	**0.86**	0.64	0.86	**0.86**	0.78
ResNet50 PCA	**0.81**	0.82	0.79	0.86	**0.86**	**0.82**

After training and testing in high-resolution datasets, the weights of these models were used to initialize the training with low-resolution retinal images collected from mobile devices. The purpose is to use transfer learning techniques from a close and similar domain problem instead of using generic datasets. The results of the models in the images from mobile devices are presented in Table 3.

Table 3. Model results in low-resolution retinal images with or without PCA pre-processing.

Models	Acc	Sen	Spec	Prec	F1	AUC
ViT	0.67	0.25	0.85	0.42	0.31	0.58
ViT PCA	**0.76**	**0.40**	**0.90**	**0.62**	**0.48**	**0.83**
ResNet50	0.62	0.20	0.80	0.31	0.24	0.78
ResNet50 PCA	0.63	0.30	0.84	0.55	0.39	0.82

In this case, the PCA technique proved to be a good method for improving feature visualization in low-resolution retinal images. Both the ViT and ResNet50 with PCA pre-processing reached AUCs above 0.8. The ViT model in this dataset was the one reaching better results due to the fact of pair-wise pixel relations processing of the self-attention mechanisms which can detect more important features in low-resolution images. However, the ResNet50 showed consistency either in the high-resolution and low-resolution images, always with AUC above 0.75 with or without the PCA pre-processing. After testing the models, explainability methods were implemented to highlight important features related to the model decision. In Fig. 3 are some examples of ResNet50 predictions with Grad-CAM activation maps for low-resolution images and in Fig. 4 some examples of ViT predictions with attention rollouts activation maps in low-resolution retinal images as well. As can be seen in Fig. 3, the main features highlighted are within the optic disc, especially in the region with veins.

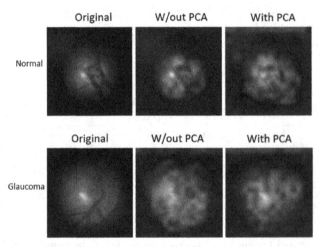

Fig. 3. Examples of Grad-CAM explainability in normal and glaucoma cases for ResNet50 model.

In Fig. 3, in the bottom row, in the case without the PCA, the model focus on the region corresponding to the optic cup. The correlation between a large optic cup and glaucoma presence is big. Thus, the ResNet50 model focus on an important feature to predict glaucoma presence.

Regarding the attention maps from the ViT models, the same can be concluded in Fig. 4. In both examples, either in normal or glaucoma cases, can be seen that the model highlights the optic disc region. In this case, in the normal case is possible to see that the model highlights the optic cup. The optic cup, in the normal case, is small, which does not demonstrate signs of glaucoma presence. Compared to the same example in Fig. 3 is possible to see that the models focus on similar features in the same image.

These recent ViT methods which rely on the self-attention mechanism prove to have promising results. However, the ResNet50 reached more stable results throughout the different experiments made, reaching at least 0.75 of AUC with or without PCA pre-processing in high and low-resolution retinal images. Despite this, the ViT model has shown great potential in detecting glaucoma in retinal images collected by mobile devices due to the process of pixel relation of the model. The domain transfer learning uses more similar datasets, inserted in the same type of problem, allowing the transfer of more related knowledge to another model for a better weight initialization. The PCA

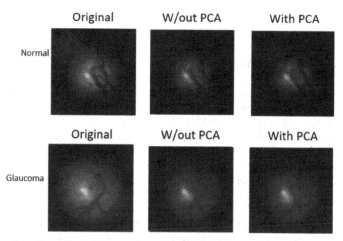

Fig. 4. Examples of attention rollout explainability in normal and glaucoma cases for ViT model.

pre-processing technique shows more relevance in the low-resolution dataset, where the models using this pre-processing method reached higher values of AUC, thus, this technique can enhance feature visualization in the retinal image.

5 Conclusions

The purposed methods in this study proved to be promising since the knowledge transfer of datasets related to the same domain can improve the model training, enabling to detect glaucoma in low-resolution images collected by mobile devices. The emerging techniques of transformers and self-attention mechanisms in ViT models reveal to have promising performance, especially in the low-resolution retinal images, where the model reached the highest results due to the process of the relation between pixels. In this specific case for the mobile retinal images, the PCA pre-processing reveal to have importance, enhancing feature visualization and improving the model results. The explainability methods, in the end, highlighted correlated features to the corresponding class of the image.

Future works could verify if adaptations in ViT models could increase the effectiveness of glaucoma detection by using shifted patch tokenization or/and locality self-attention are very useful, especially in small datasets. Also, more suitable local explainability methods will be explored such as local interpretable model-agnostic explanations.

Acknowledgements. This work is financed by National Funds through the Portuguese funding agency, FCT - Fundação para a Ciência e a Tecnologia, within project LA/P/0063/2020.

References

1. Claro, M.L., Veras, R., Santos, L., Frazão, M., Carvalho Filho, A., Leite, D.: Métodos computacionais para segmentação do disco óptico em imagens de retina: uma revisão. Rev. Bras. Comput. Apl. **10**(2), 29–43 (2018). https://doi.org/10.5335/rbca.v10i2.7661
2. Bajwa, M.N., et al.: Two-stage framework for optic disc localization and glaucoma classification in retinal fundus images using deep learning. BMC Med. Inform. Decis. Mak. **19**(1), 136 (2019). https://doi.org/10.1186/s12911-019-0842-8
3. Stella Mary, M.C.V., Rajsingh, E.B., Naik, G.R.: Retinal fundus image analysis for diagnosis of glaucoma: a comprehensive survey. IEEE Access **4**, 4327–4354 (2016). https://doi.org/10.1109/ACCESS.2016.2596761
4. Hagiwara, Y., et al.: Computer-aided diagnosis of glaucoma using fundus images: a review. Comput. Methods Programs Biomed. **165**, 1–12 (2018). https://doi.org/10.1016/j.cmpb.2018.07.012
5. Camara, J., Neto, A., Pires, I.M., Villasana, M.V., Zdravevski, E., Cunha, A.: A comprehensive review of methods and equipment for aiding automatic glaucoma tracking. Diagnostics **12**(4), 935 (2022). https://doi.org/10.3390/diagnostics12040935
6. Mayro, E.L., Wang, M., Elze, T., Pasquale, L.R.: The impact of artificial intelligence in the diagnosis and management of glaucoma. Eye **34**(1), 1–11 (2019). https://doi.org/10.1038/s41433-019-0577-x
7. Litjens, G., et al.: A survey on deep learning in medical image analysis. Med. Image Anal. **42**, 60–88 (2017). https://doi.org/10.1016/j.media.2017.07.005
8. Yamashita, R., Nishio, M., Do, R.K.G., Togashi, K.: Convolutional neural networks: an overview and application in radiology. Insights Imaging **9**(4), 611–629 (2018). https://doi.org/10.1007/s13244-018-0639-9
9. Zhao, R., Yan, R., Chen, Z., Mao, K., Wang, P., Gao, R.X.: Deep learning and its applications to machine health monitoring. Mech. Syst. Signal Process. **115**, 213–237 (2019). https://doi.org/10.1016/j.ymssp.2018.05.050
10. He, K., Zhang, X., Ren, S., Sun, J.: Deep residual learning for image recognition arXiv, arXiv:1512.03385 (2015). Accessed 05 June 2022
11. Dosovitskiy, A., et al.: An image is worth 16×16 words: transformers for image recognition at scale. arXiv, arXiv:2010.11929 (2021). Accessed 02 June 2022
12. Neto, A., Camara, J., Cunha, A.: Evaluations of deep learning approaches for glaucoma screening using retinal images from mobile device. Sensors **22**(4), 1449 (2022). https://doi.org/10.3390/s22041449
13. Linardatos, P., Papastefanopoulos, V., Kotsiantis, S.: Explainable AI: a review of machine learning interpretability methods. Entropy **23**(1), 1–45 (2021). https://doi.org/10.3390/e23010018
14. Abnar, S., Zuidema, W.: Quantifying attention flow in transformers (2020). http://arxiv.org/abs/2005.00928. Accessed 18 July 2022
15. Chen, X., Xu, Y., Kee Wong, D.W., Wong, T.Y., Liu, J.: Glaucoma detection based on deep convolutional neural network. In: 2015 37th Annual International Conference of the IEEE Engineering in Medicine and Biology Society (EMBC), Milan, pp. 715–718 (2015). https://doi.org/10.1109/EMBC.2015.7318462
16. Raghavendra, U., Fujita, H., Bhandary, S.V., Gudigar, A., Tan, J.H., Acharya, U.R.: Deep convolution neural network for accurate diagnosis of glaucoma using digital fundus images. Inf. Sci. **441**, 41–49 (2018). https://doi.org/10.1016/j.ins.2018.01.051
17. Chai, Y., Liu, H., Xu, J.: Glaucoma diagnosis based on both hidden features and domain knowledge through deep learning models. Knowl.-Based Syst. **161**, 147–156 (2018). https://doi.org/10.1016/j.knosys.2018.07.043

18. Benzebouchi, N.E., Azizi, N., Bouziane, S.E.: Glaucoma diagnosis using cooperative convolutional neural networks. Int. J. Adv. Electron. Comput. Sci. **5**(1), 31–36 (2018)
19. Suguna, G., Lavanya, R.: Performance assessment of EyeNet model in glaucoma diagnosis. Pattern Recogn. Image Anal. **31**(2), 334–344 (2021). https://doi.org/10.1134/S1054661821020164
20. Alghamdi, M., Abdel-Mottaleb, M.: A Comparative study of deep learning models for diagnosing glaucoma from fundus images. IEEE Access **9**, 23894–23906 (2021). https://doi.org/10.1109/ACCESS.2021.3056641
21. Fumero Batista, F.J., Diaz-Aleman, T., Sigut, J., Alayon, S., Arnay, R., Angel-Pereira, D.: RIM-ONE DL: a unified retinal image database for assessing glaucoma using deep learning. Image Anal. Stereol. **39**(3), Article no. 3 (2020). https://doi.org/10.5566/ias.2346
22. Sivaswamy, J., Krishnadas, S.R., Datt Joshi, G., Jain, M., Syed Tabish, A.U.: Drishti-GS: retinal image dataset for optic nerve head (ONH) segmentation. Presented at the 2014 IEEE 11th International Symposium on Biomedical Imaging (ISBI), pp. 53–56 (2014). https://doi.org/10.1109/ISBI.2014.6867807
23. Fu, H.: REFUGE: Retinal Fundus Glaucoma Challenge. IEEE (2019). https://ieee-dataport.org/documents/refuge-retinal-fundus-glaucoma-challenge. Accessed 16 Nov 2022
24. Bargoti, S., Underwood, J.: Deep fruit detection in orchards (2017). http://arxiv.org/abs/1610.03677. Accessed 28 July 2022

Diabetic Retinopathy Detection Using Convolutional Neural Networks for Mobile Use

Meltem Esengönül[1,2], Anselmo Cardoso de Paiva[3], João Rodrigues[4], and António Cunha[1,5(✉)]

[1] Escola de Ciências e Tecnologia, University of Trás-os-Montes e Alto Douro, 5000-801 Vila Real, Portugal
acunha@utad.pt
[2] University of Applied Sciences Technikum Wien, Vienna, Austria
[3] Applied Computing Group NCA-UFMA Federal University of Maranhão, Sao Luis, MA 65072-561, Brazil
[4] LARSyS and ISE, Universidade de Algarve, 8005-139 Faro, Portugal
[5] Instituto de Engenharia de Sistemas e Computadores, Tecnologia e Ciência, 4200-465 Porto, Portugal

Abstract. Diabetes has significant effects on the human body, one of which is the increase in the blood pressure and when not diagnosed early, can cause severe vision complications and even lead to blindness. Early screening is the key to overcoming such issues which can have a significant impact on rural areas and overcrowded regions. Mobile systems can help bring the technology to those in need. Transfer learning based Deep Learning algorithms combined with mobile retinal imaging systems can significantly reduce the screening time and lower the burden on healthcare workers. In this paper, several efficiency factors of Diabetic Retinopathy detection systems based on Convolutional Neural Networks are tested and evaluated for mobile applications. Two main techniques are used to measure the efficiency of DL based DR detection systems. The first method evaluates the effect of dataset change, where the base architecture of the DL model remains the same. The second method measures the effect of base architecture variation, where the dataset remains unchanged. The results suggest that the inclusivity of the datasets, and the dataset size significantly impact the DR detection accuracy and sensitivity. Amongst the five chosen lightweight architectures, EfficientNet-based DR detection algorithms outperformed the other transfer learning models along with APTOS Blindness Detection dataset.

Keywords: Diabetic Retinopathy · Deep Learning · Transfer Learning · Convolutional Neural Networks · Mobile Use

1 Introduction

Diabetes mellitus is a set of metabolic illnesses distinguished by hyperglycemia caused by abnormalities in insulin production, insulin action, or perhaps both [1]. Diabetes

A. Cunha et al. (Eds.): MobiHealth 2022, LNICST 484, pp. 14–23, 2023.
https://doi.org/10.1007/978-3-031-32029-3_2

causes long-term significant harm, malfunction, and breakdown of multiple organ systems, including the eyes, kidneys, nerves, heart, and blood vessels [1]. One of the most common types of eye complications associated with Diabetes Mellitus is Diabetic Retinopathy (DR), and it is considered a major cause of visual loss worldwide [2]. Early detection/screening is the key to preventing blindness from DR, since this illness in its early stages is asymptomatic [3]. With the growth of Deep Learning (DL) methods such as Convolutional Neural Networks (CNNs), various stages of DR can be detected automatically, assisting in detecting more cases in mass screenings. There are several challenges in regions with restricted eye health services access, like underdeveloped and overcrowded regions. A mobile-based automatic DR detection system can be used to overcome these challenges. In this paper, several different CNN-based models are investigated, and their efficiency is compared for mobile DR detection systems.

2 Related Work

There are several state-of-the-art techniques to detect DR for mobile use. In 2018, a CNN method based on a pre-trained MobileNet model was trained on Kaggle DR Detection Dataset with 16,798 fundus images and tested to detect the presence of DR, which did not need an internet connection [4–6]. By using this system, authors were able to achieve approx. 0.73 accuracy score, and their results suggest that their model compared to earlier Inception and VGGNet counterparts was 4 times lighter [6–8]. In the same year, as another essential indicator of DR, researchers applied Optic Nerve Head (ONH) detection method based on Radon Transform for the Android smartphone application with the use of images taken with D-EYE lenses attached to a smartphone [9, 10]. This method was able to reach approx. 0.96 and 1.00 accuracy scores for STARE and DRIVE datasets, respectively [10–12]. An automated mobile DR diagnosis system was introduced in 2019 based on the pre-trained Inception CNN model and a decision tree-based binary ensemble classifier [7, 13]. The method proposed was trained on Kaggle DR Detection Dataset with 1000 images and was able to classify DR into 5 different classes with an accuracy score of 0.99 [5, 13]. In another study, cloud computing and big data analytics are employed aside from mobile DR detection with AI [14]. The authors used a Deep Convolutional Neural Network (DCNN) for training, followed by a Support Vector Machine (SVM) for classification. Also, they created their mobile application called "Deep Retina" to use with a handheld ophthalmoscope [14]. Results depict that, for binary classification the system's accuracy was higher than the multi-class classification technique with approx. 0.91 and 0.86, respectively [14]. In a 2020 study, authors explored the fine-tuning effects after the CNN architecture with MobileNetV2 for DR detection [15, 16]. Their outcomes resulted in an increase of 0.21 in training and 0.31 in validation accuracy (from 0.7 to 0.91 and from 0.5 to 0.81 correspondingly).]. Another effective mobile application implementation was using the EfficientNet-B5 based CNN model for DR detection and classification into 5 labels, where the authors achieved a training accuracy value of approx. 0.94 and Quadratic Weighted Kappa value of 0.93 [17, 18]. In 2021, researchers introduced a new DL-based software called VeriSee™ for image analysis and validated its use for DR severity classification [19, 20]. The VeriSee™ software achieved higher sensitivity and specificity than the ophthalmologists [19, 20].

These results indicated that it could be viable for clinical use in ophthalmology. Around this time, another team tested the use of Phelcom Eyer Technology, a smartphone-based DR detection system, integrated with CNN based software algorithm PhelcomNet was also able to achieve high sensitivity and specificity results and an Area Under Curve (AUC) score of 0.89 [21, 22]. Their research gave a real-life example of portable retinal imaging systems combined with DL algorithms for patients enrolled in the Itabuna Diabetes Campaign in Brazil [22]. In a recent study, a Diabetic Retinopathy Graph Neural Network, in other words, the DRG-NET model was introduced for DR grading and trained with public datasets such as APTOS 2019 Blindness Detection and MESSIDOR datasets [23–25]. In this network, the input images are given as nodes, which are 3D graphs, and Scale Invariant Feature Transform methods feature extraction is performed [25]. Using this technique, the authors reached accuracy scores of 0.9954 and 0.9984, respectively, according to the datasets [25]. Another approach in 2022 was to test the efficiency of the NasnetMobile network with a multi-layer perceptron (MLP) classifier on 440 fundus images taken with smartphone-based systems [26, 27]. With this light algorithm, on low-quality images (compared to table-top fundus camera images), they achieved a high accuracy value of around 0.96 in a fast mobile execution time of less than a minute [27].

3   Methods

In this paper, two different methods were applied to test the smartphone-based applications of DL methods for DR detection. The first three public DR detection datasets were pre-processed, and data augmentation was applied and later trained and tested with MobileNet pre-trained model [4]. The second method used the same preprocessing and data augmentation techniques; however, only one chosen dataset was trained with five different CNN-based transfer learning architectures and tested for mobile use.

3.1   Datasets

The datasets used in the paper are: APTOS 2019 Blindness Detection [23], IDRID [28], and MESSIDOR [24] datasets. From the APTOS dataset, a total of 3662 fundus images were used. Whereas, we used all images from the IDRID and MESSIDOR datasets, 516 and 1200 images respectively. The APTOS and IDRID datasets included similar image classes, which had five distinct labels such as: 0 - No DR, 1 - Mild DR, 2 - Moderate DR, 3 - Severe DR, and 4 - Proliferative DR [23, 28].

As per the MESSIDOR dataset, the classification labels did not include the proliferative DR (PDR), thus were labeled from 0–3 with the following distinction [24]:

- 0 - When both microaneurysm AND hemorrhage numbers are zero
- 1 - When microaneurysm numbers are between 0- 5 (including 5) AND hemorrhage numbers are zero
- 2 - When microaneurysm numbers are between 5–15 OR hemorrhage numbers are between 0–5 AND neovascularization is not found

- 3 - When microaneurysm numbers are equal or more than 15 OR hemorrhage numbers are equal or more than 5 OR neovascularization is found

3.2 Pre-processing and Data Augmentation

For pre-processing of several images and testing, first both training and validation images were resized to 224x224 pixels in order to fit into the MobileNet model, as the original dataset contained pictures with varying pixel sizes, later the images were changed to grayscale, and cropped. CLAHE, which stands for contrast limited adaptive histogram equalization, was also applied after cropping. As the dataset sizes are small on all three chosen public datasets, data augmentation was employed to avoid overfitting, which utilized a zooming factor of 0.035 and rotation range of 0.025. In order to keep a similar appearance to fundus images they were not flipped. For training and testing all datasets were split with 80–20 split percentage.

3.3 CNN Architectures

Transfer learning is the use of prior knowledge from another task to apply it to a newer problem. Here five different pre-trained models were employed as part of transfer learning to increase the accuracy of DR detection methods. These pre-trained models were MobileNet [4], MobileNetV2 [15], EfficientNetB0 [17], EfficientNetV2B0 [29], and NasNetMobile [26]. The reason behind this selection is that according to Keras applications, these models have the least model size, meaning they are lighter weight compared to other pre-trained models, which was taken as an indicator of faster mobile applications.

All the models were tested three times. First, without fine-tuning and a smaller added dense layer structure where on top of the pre-trained MobileNet model several sequential dense layers were added. The first two layers are *global_average_pooling2d, flatten,* Then two *dense* layers are added with *(None, 32)* output shape and *ReLU* activation function, followed by a *dropout* layer, and finally a *dense* layer with *(None, 5)* output shape with *sigmoid* activation function since there were 5 different DR classes. Except for the MESSIDOR dataset, where there are four different DR classes, thus the last layer had *(None, 4)* output shape with a sigmoid activation function. As an optimizer, *adam* was chosen and for the loss function several were employed such as *mse, categorical_crossentropy,* and *binary_crossentropy.* This model was denoted as Model-1.

The second model, Model-2, has a slightly bigger architecture for dense. In this model, similar to Model-1, sequential layers were added on top of the MobileNet. These layers start with global_average_pooling2d, flatten and then continues with dense layers starting from (None, 256) output shape and ReLU activation function, followed by a dropout layer, continually adding dense layers that has the output shape halved in each layer until to the last dense layer with (None, 5) output shape with sigmoid, as before.

The third model, named Model-FT, first applied fine-tuning by setting the trainable layer true and after the same model structure as Model-1 was used, which had MobileNet as a pre-trained model.

3.4 Evaluation Metrics

This paper utilizes AUC score, and Receiver Operator Characteristic (ROC) values, Training time in addition to the basic DL evaluation metrics like Accuracy, Loss, Sensitivity, and Specificity.

The ratio of true predictions to total outputs is known as accuracy, and it may be expressed as [30]:

$$\frac{TP + TN}{TP + TN + FP + FN} \tag{1}$$

Sensitivity is also known as Recall or True Positive Rate, and it has the following formula [30]:

$$\frac{TP}{TP + FN} \tag{2}$$

The True Negative Rate is also known as Specificity, and it contains the following formula [30]:

$$\frac{TN}{TN + FP} \tag{3}$$

Loss value comes from the loss function, or in other words, the cost function, which boils down all of the positive and negative characteristics of a potentially complicated system to a scalar value, between 0–1, that can be used to rank and compare viable solutions [31].

ROC plots are 2D graphs with the true positive (TP) rate on the Y axis and the false positive (FP) rate on the X [32]. The relative tradeoffs between gains (TP) and costs (FP) are depicted on a ROC plot [32].

AUC Score, or area under a ROC curve, is a numerical value that quantifies a binary classifier's current effectiveness and ranges between 0.5–1.0 [33].

4   Results

As explained above, there are two main methods used to detect the effectiveness of DR detection algorithms. First, the dataset used to train the algorithm influences the evaluation metrics; second, the pre-trained model is based on architecture, and that has a different impact on the results. Lastly, the added layers on the model or whether the model include fine-tuning or not can change the effectiveness of the DL method used.

In Table 1 below, it is possible to see that the highest mean values for accuracy, sensitivity, specificity, and AUC were with the use of the APTOS dataset. In fact, in terms of sensitivity and AUC values, there is a notable drop for the MESSIDOR dataset. This drop might be due to the difference in the number of training images and the representation of different classes. The APTOS dataset included more than triple the number of images of the MESSIDOR dataset and more than 7 times higher than the IDRID dataset. Thus, we can see that the average training time is also higher compared

Table 1. Comparison of mean evaluation metrics by dataset types

	APTOS	IDRID	MESSIDOR
Accuracy	0.880	0.803	0.750
Loss	0.084	0.147	0.174
Sensitivity	0.966	0.909	0.511
Specificity	0.994	0.849	0.815
AUC	0.894	0.700	0.649
Time (min)	62.633	8.056	14.250

to other dataset types. The loss value of APTOS is considerably lower than IDRID and MESSIDOR models, which means that the average loss over time is smaller.

Table 2 depicts that, in general, EfficientNets perform higher than MobileNets, followed by NasNetMobile for the APTOS dataset. However, on the contrary, the mean training time is much lower for MobileNets compared to EfficientNets. In terms of sensitivity and AUC scores, there was a significant decrease in NasNetMobile models. The explanation is that fine-tuning did not perform well with this network, thus decreasing the average values.

Table 2. Comparison of mean evaluation metrics by architecture types.

	EfficientNetB0	EfficientNetV2B0	MobileNet	MobileNetV2	NasNetMobile
Acc.	0.903	0.902	0.880	0.850	0.841
Loss	0.072	0.074	0.084	0.124	0.126
Sens.	0.987	0.979	0.966	0.829	0.668
Spec.	0.997	0.995	0.994	0.958	0.946
AUC	0.933	0.929	0.894	0.824	0.753
T (min)	96.589	70.228	62.633	67.745	123.378

Acc. is short for Accuracy, Sens. is short for Sensitivity, Spec. is short for Specificity, AUC stands for Area Under Curve, and T (min) is to express the training time given in minutes.

Effects of different model testing are given in Table 3, where models with the Model-1 structure, which had a smaller structure on top of MobileNet and did not include fine-tuning, overall achieved the highest sensitivity values. However, there was generally no significant difference in terms of accuracy, loss, and AUC scores. As per the specificity, Model-2, where a larger model was used on top of MobileNet and did not include fine-tuning, showed the highest average value with being slightly more than Model-1. As well as, mean training time was the least with the Model-2. In this metric, the mean values are highly variable depending on the dataset size as well, however in terms of models, fine-tuning significantly increases the training time, more than triple that of Model-2, which shows the fastest method.

Table 3. Comparison of mean evaluation metrics by model types.

	Model-1	Model-2	Model-FT
Accuracy	0.811	0.810	0.811
Loss	0.135	0.136	0.134
Sensitivity	0.853	0.790	0.744
Specificity	0.887	0.892	0.879
AUC	0.748	0.747	0.748
Time (min)	25.244	13.000	46.695

Overall, the highest ROC values were achieved with the APTOS dataset. For the EfficientNet-based models, the Model-1 structure achieved the highest ROC values shown in Fig. 1, given below.

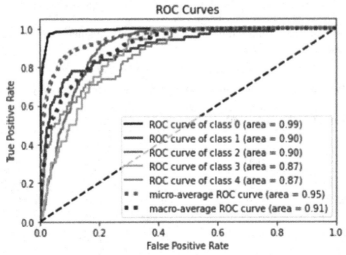

Fig. 1. ROC values achieved with APTOS 2019 Blindness Detection Dataset with EfficientNetB0 base, Model-1.

The second best results were achieved with MobileNet based architecture with the APTOS dataset and fine-tuning model (Model-FT), which can be seen in Fig. 2. Compared to the MobileNet, EfficientNetB0 was able to identify all the classes effectively, whereas the MobileNet did not perform at a similar level for Class 1, Class 3 and Class 4. In comparison, EfficientNetV2B0, a lighter version of EffficientNets, did not perform higher than EfficientNetB0.

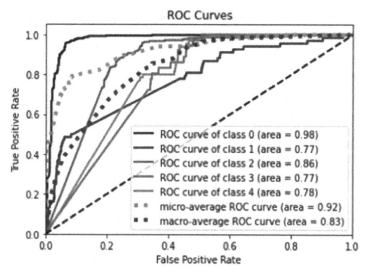

Fig. 2. ROC values achieved with APTOS 2019 Blindness Detection Dataset with MobileNet, Model-FT.

5   Conclusion

Overall, testing results show that EfficientNet-based DR detection algorithms perform better in terms of DR severity detection along with APTOS 2019 Blindness Detection dataset, even though this dataset was not distributed equally. However, they significantly take more time to train compared to MobileNets. For comparison of various models, fine-tuning might contribute to higher outcomes although significantly increasing the training time.

Acknowledgment. This work is financed by National Funds through the Portuguese funding agency, FCT - Fundação para a Ciência e a Tecnologia, within project LA/P/0063/2020. Furthermore, this paper is a part of the Master's thesis titled "Deep Learning Methods for Diabetic Eye Disease Screening and Smartphone based Applications" by M.E.

References

1. American Diabetes Association: Diagnosis and classification of diabetes mellitus. Diabetes Care **27**(Suppl_1), s5–s10 (2004). https://doi.org/10.2337/diacare.27.2007.S5
2. The progress in understanding and treatment of diabetic retinopathy. Prog. Retin. Eye Res. **51**, 156–186 (2016). https://doi.org/10.1016/j.preteyeres.2015.08.001
3. Detection and classification of retinal lesions for grading of diabetic retinopathy. Comput. Biol. Med. **45**, 161–171 (2014). https://doi.org/10.1016/j.compbiomed.2013.11.014
4. Howard, A.G., et al.: MobileNets: efficient convolutional neural networks for mobile vision applications (2017). https://doi.org/10.48550/arXiv.1704.04861
5. Diabetic Retinopathy Detection. https://kaggle.com/competitions/diabetic-retinopathy-det ection. Accessed 10 May 2022

6. Mobile assisted diabetic retinopathy detection using deep neural network. https://ieeexplore.ieee.org/document/8400760. Accessed 10 May 2022
7. Szegedy, C., et al.: Going deeper with convolutions (2014). https://doi.org/10.48550/arXiv.1409.4842
8. Simonyan, K., Zisserman, A.: Very deep convolutional networks for large-scale image recognition (2014). http://arxiv.org/abs/1409.1556. Accessed 10 May 2022
9. Website. https://www.d-eyecare.com/en_US/product
10. A mobile computer aided system for optic nerve head detection. Comput. Methods Programs Biomed. **162**, 139–148 (2018). https://doi.org/10.1016/j.cmpb.2018.05.004
11. The STARE Project. https://cecas.clemson.edu/~ahoover/stare/. Accessed 10 May 2022
12. DRIVE - Grand Challenge, grand-challenge.org. https://drive.grand-challenge.org/. Accessed 10 May 2022
13. Automated Smartphone Based System for Diagnosis of Diabetic Retinopathy. https://ieeexplore.ieee.org/document/8974492. Accessed 10 May 2022
14. Li, Y.-H., Yeh, N.-N., Chen, S.-J., Chung, Y.-C.: Computer-assisted diagnosis for diabetic retinopathy based on fundus images using deep convolutional neural network. Mob. Inf. Syst. **2019** (2019). https://doi.org/10.1155/2019/6142839
15. Sandler, M., Howard, A., Zhu, M., Zhmoginov, A., Chen, L.-C.: MobileNetV2: inverted residuals and linear bottlenecks (2018). https://doi.org/10.48550/arXiv.1801.04381
16. Transfer Learning with Fine-Tuned MobileNetV2 for Diabetic Retinopathy. https://ieeexplore.ieee.org/abstract/document/9154014. Accessed 10 May 2022
17. Tan, M., Le, Q.V.: EfficientNet: rethinking model scaling for convolutional neural networks (2019). https://doi.org/10.48550/arXiv.1905.11946
18. CNN Based Detection of the Severity of Diabetic Retinopathy from the Fundus Photography using EfficientNet-B5. https://ieeexplore.ieee.org/document/9284944. Accessed 10 May 2022
19. VeriSee DR. Acer Medical (2021). https://www.acer-medical.com/solutions/verisee-dr/. Accessed 10 May 2022
20. Application of deep learning image assessment software VeriSee^{TM} for diabetic retinopathy screening. J. Formos. Med. Assoc. **120**(1), 165–171 (2021). https://doi.org/10.1016/j.jfma.2020.03.024
21. PHELCOM Technologies. PHELCOM Technologies (2019). https://phelcom.com/en/. Accessed 10 May 2022
22. Malerbi, F.K., et al.: Diabetic retinopathy screening using artificial intelligence and handheld smartphone-based retinal camera. J. Diabetes Sci. Technol. (2021). https://doi.org/10.1177/1932296820985567
23. APTOS 2019 Blindness Detection. https://kaggle.com/competitions/aptos2019-blindness-detection. Accessed 10 May 2022
24. Patry, G., et al.: Messidor. ADCIS (2019). https://www.adcis.net/en/third-party/messidor/. Accessed 10 May 2022
25. Salam, A.A., Mahadevappa, M., Das, A., Nair, M.S.: DRG-NET: a graph neural network for computer-aided grading of diabetic retinopathy. J. VLSI Signal Process. Syst. Signal Image Video Technol. 1–7 (2022). https://doi.org/10.1007/s11760-022-02146-x
26. Zoph, B., Vasudevan, V., Shlens, J., Le, Q.V.: Learning transferable architectures for scalable image recognition (2017). http://arxiv.org/abs/1707.07012. Accessed 10 May 2022
27. Elloumi, Y., Abroug, N., Bedoui, M.H.: End-to-end mobile system for diabetic retinopathy screening based on lightweight deep neural network. In: Bouadi, T., Fromont, E., Hüllermeier, E. (eds.) IDA 2022. LNCS, vol. 13205, pp. 66–77. Springer, Cham (2022). https://doi.org/10.1007/978-3-031-01333-1_6
28. IDRiD - Grand Challenge. grand-challenge.org. https://idrid.grand-challenge.org/. Accessed 10 May 2022

29. Tan, M., Le, Q.V.: EfficientNetV2: smaller models and faster training (2021). https://doi.org/10.48550/arXiv.2104.00298
30. Tharwat, A.: Classification assessment methods. Appl. Comput. Inform. **17**(1), 168–192 (2020). https://doi.org/10.1016/j.aci.2018.08.003
31. The MIT Press. Neural Smithing. The MIT Press. https://mitpress.mit.edu/books/neural-smithing. Accessed 10 May 2022
32. An introduction to ROC analysis. Pattern Recogn. Lett. **27**(8), 861–874 (2006). https://doi.org/10.1016/j.patrec.2005.10.010
33. Melo, F.: Area under the ROC curve. In: Dubitzky, W., Wolkenhauer, O., Cho, K.-H., Yokota, H. (eds.) Encyclopedia of Systems Biology, pp. 38–39. Springer, New York (2013). https://doi.org/10.1007/978-1-4419-9863-7_209

Evaluating Rotation Invariant Strategies for Mitosis Detection Through YOLO Algorithms

Dibet Garcia Gonzalez[1]([✉]) [iD], João Carias[1] [iD], Yusbel Chávez Castilla[1] [iD],
José Rodrigues[1] [iD], Telmo Adão[1,2] [iD], Rui Jesus[3],
Luís Gonzaga Mendes Magalhães[2] [iD], Vitor Manuel Leitão de Sousa[4] [iD],
Lina Carvalho[4] [iD], Rui Almeida[4] [iD], and António Cunha[5] [iD]

[1] Center for Computer Graphics, Guimarães, Portugal
dibet.gonzalez@ccg.pt
[2] Algoritmi Center, Minho University, Guimarães, Portugal
[3] University of A Coruña, BMD Software, A Coruña, Spain
[4] Institute of Anatomical and Molecular Pathology, Faculty of Medicine, University of Coimbra, Coimbra, Portugal
[5] Universidade de Trás-os-Montes e Alto Douro, Vila Real, Portugal

Abstract. Cancer diagnosis is of major importance in the field of human medical pathology, wherein a cell division process known as mitosis constitutes a relevant biological pattern analyzed by professional experts, who seek for such occurrence in presence and number through visual observation of microscopic imagery. This is a time-consuming and exhausting task that can benefit from modern artificial intelligence approaches, namely those handling object detection through deep learning, from which YOLO can be highlighted as one of the most successful, and, as such, a good candidate for performing automatic mitoses detection. Considering that low sensibility for rotation/flip variations is of high importance to ensure mitosis deep detection robustness, in this work, we propose an offline augmentation procedure focusing rotation operations, to address the impact of lost/clipped mitoses induced by online augmentation. YOLOv4 and YOLOv5 were compared, using an augmented test dataset with an exhaustive set of rotation angles, to investigate their performance. YOLOv5 with a mixture of offline and online rotation augmentation methods presented the best averaged F1-score results over three runs.

Keywords: Rotation invariance · deep learning · YOLO · mitosis counting

1 Introduction

Cancer is of great interest to medical specialists and pathologists because of its consequences on people's health. This disease affects populations everywhere and can be fatal if not treated on time. Nowadays, there are several ways to diagnose this pathology, involving the presence of several specialists (clinicians, pathologists) with a high level

A. Cunha et al. (Eds.): MobiHealth 2022, LNICST 484, pp. 24–33, 2023.
https://doi.org/10.1007/978-3-031-32029-3_3

of expertise. For example, there are strategies to characterize certain cancers, such as the Nottingham Grading System [1], which aids in the determination of breast cancer grade, resorting to three biomarkers: nuclear atypia, tubule formation and the mitotic cell count.

One of the known ways to assess tumor proliferation is mitotic counting, widely used by pathologists, who manually perform this task by analyzing biopsy Hematoxylin and Eosin (H&E) stained samples, from high-resolution microscope imagery. This process refers to the number of dividing cells visible in H&E stained histopathology [2], and it is an established step in cancer diagnosis and prognosis procedures [3]. In [4] authors note that *"the mitotic cell count is an important biomarker for predicting the aggressiveness, prognosis, and grade of breast cancer"*.

Diagnosis can be influenced by multiple factors intrinsic to the biomaterial under analysis (e.g., small differences between mitotic and normal cells) or by the lack or absence of qualified professionals. Also, it is time-consuming, tiresome and subjective [4] which encourages the search for new diagnosis procedures. Digital decision support systems can help to overcome these problems. Advances in various domains such as image capture, image storage, image visualizing and deep learning algorithms allow the development of more robust and reliable decision support systems, speeding up the diagnosis, reducing the workload and supplying an opportunity to improve diagnosis and patient outcome [5].

Moreover, Whole Slide Images technology known as WSI, which allows scanning of conventional glass slides to produce digital image with high resolution [6], has been providing significant contributes for the development of digital pathology. Today, it is paving the way for DL algorithms (e.g. classification, object detection, segmentation) by capturing the required data (images).

Although deep learning-based algorithms have achieved superior results in recent years, there are challenges to overcome. For example, the digitalization methods output cell with assorted rotation angles but, generally, pathologists are successful at classifying independently of this condition. Thus, it is expected that any ideal mitosis detector would be robust to disturbances such as rotation or flip.

In this work, we present an evaluation of the You Only Look Once (YOLOv4 [7] and YOLOv5 [8]) algorithms in relation with rotation and/or flip transformations for the mitoses detection use-case. We consider the mitotic detection process useful for mitotic counting task, and, thereby, we trained several YOLO models, and evaluated their performances on an exhaustive rotated test dataset. Afterwards, according to our experiments, we proposed a suitable procedure to obtain a performant mitosis detection model regarding rotation invariance.

The main contributions of this work are:

- a rotation invariant strategy for mitosis detection for object detection algorithms, and
- a direct comparison between YOLOv4 and YOLOv5 considering the proposed strategy in the training stage.

The rest of this work is organized as follows: Sect. 2 includes background about the application of deep learning methods for mitotic counting; Sect. 3 presents the strategy used to train the YOLO models and the creation of datasets from two public set of images; Sect. 4 shows some results; Sect. 5 elaborates on these results and conclusions are drawn in Sect. 6.

2 Previous Work

According to mitosis detection reviews [3, 9], there are three ways to address this problem:

1) using hand-crafted features: where morphology, color and texture features are provided, as input, to machine learning algorithms for pattern recognition or classification (e.g., Support Vector Machine, Artificial Neural Networks);
2) using deep learning methods: which is able to learn sub-visual image features that may not be easily discernible by the human eye [5]. Convolutional Neural Networks (CNN) are the most popular algorithms; and
3) using a combination of previous methods: where this strategy combines the speed of hand-crafted methods and the accuracy of CNN.

In [10], the authors explain how they carry out digital image processing and deep learning techniques in some use cases under the context of Digital Pathology (DP). One of these is mitosis detection, where they apply a blue-ratio segmentation technique combined with morphological operations (e.g., dilate using a 20 pixels disk radial mask) and deep learning for the classification task. In [11], the combination of hand-crafted features (morphology, color, and texture features) and CNN-derived features maximize the performance by leveraging the disconnected feature sets.

In [12], a framework for the analysis and prediction of tumor proliferation from histological images is proposed. The framework includes three modules: i) Whole Slide Image Handling, ii) Deep Convolutional Neural Networks based Mitosis Detection, and iii) Tumor Proliferation Score Prediction. The first module applies the Otsu thresholding and binary dilation method to extract the Region of Interest (ROI). The second uses a pre-trained ResNet model (128×128) to classify into two classes (mitosis or normal). The last includes a Support Vector Machine (SVM) with radial basis function (RBF) kernel using an RBF kernel for tumor proliferation prediction.

You Only Look Once, also known as YOLO, was created in 2015 [13] as an approach for object detection task and over the years it has continued to evolve, constantly improving its performance. This architecture identifies bounding boxes in a single shot regression approach. Version 4 includes improved feature aggregation, mish activation, bag of freebies with augmentation, and other improvements. Version 5 is faster and smaller than version 4, allowing it to be embedded in devices more easily. In training stage, YOLOv5 combines auto learning bounding box anchors with a data loader that make online augmentation (e.g., scaling, color space adjustments and mosaic augmentation).

YOLOv3 [14] was applied for mitosis detection reaching a F1-score equal to 0.8924. YOLOv4 was proposed in [15] to evaluate the efficacy of training a deep learning model. The authors used a private dataset which include 778 images of breast carcinoma slides from Sunshine Coast University Hospital. The model has a sensitivity of 0.92 and a positive predictive value of 0.64 but is frequently wrong for pyknotic cells.

3   Materials and Methods

In this article, the process of mitosis cell detection is considered as object detection task. In this sense, we present a multi-resolution pipeline including: i) a tissue detection step combining the Otsu thresholding technique and mathematical morphology on low resolution image, ii) a slide window approach with size 640 × 640 pixels on high resolution, and iii) application of object detection strategy over each patch on images containing tissue. Next, we present the image dataset used in this work and the experiments carried out to compare the deep learning models.

3.1   Initial Dataset

In this work, we use a dataset annotated at tiled patch level with dimension 640 × 640 pixels. We adjusted two datasets of breast cancer histological images mitos-atypia-14 [16] and TUPAC16 [17] for object detection tasks containing images that include at least one cell undergoing mitosis (See Fig. 1).

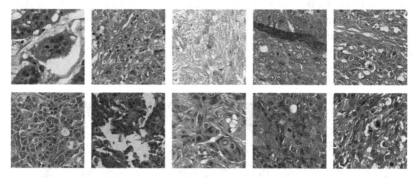

Fig. 1. Dataset samples of breast cancer histological images for object detection tasks. Image dimensions: 640 × 640 pixels. Five top images belongs to mitos-atypia-14 [16]. Five bottom images belongs to TUPAC16 [17].

Both datasets include images from 22 and 500 WSI respectively, which are scanned using two different scanners (Aperio and Hamamatsu). They were previously annotated using the center of the mitotic events. To adapt this dataset for object detection task, it was necessary to transform the center into a rectangular region in a manually way. Finally, the **base** dataset contains a total of 2502 images including one or more cells in mitotic events. The dataset was randomly partitioned into three sets: train (70%), validation (15%) and test (15%).

3.2   Rotation and Flip Augmentation Experiment

The application of automatic algorithms to detect mitosis should be rotation/flip invariant (i.e., the same mitosis should be detected independently from image rotation angle). Generally, to tackle the rotation/flip invariant object detection problems, the training dataset is augmented with random rotations and flips. In this section, we make experiments to evaluate the rotation and flip response of the YOLOv4 and YOLOv5 algorithms.

The horizontal flip augmentation is a simple procedure that mirrors the pixels along a centered **y** axis. Depending on the object of interest (its symmetry), it may look entirely different to most object detection models so it's a very useful strategy to increase the dataset.

The rotation augmentation, while simple in itself, introduces some challenges. For the image rotation, either the size is changed or it remains the same but with clipping part of it. This means some mitotic events may be clipped or lost altogether. To keep all the identified mitosis and avoid its duplication, for each image and corresponding annotations, we apply the following procedure:

1. According to the dataset specification, apply a horizontal flip transformation and add to the initial dataset;
2. Rotate images by the objective rotation maintaining its original size;
3. If mitosis annotations fit inside the (possibly clipped) rotated image, insert this image into the dataset;
4. Else try to re-center the image fitting annotations considering its bounding boxes;
5. If all annotations are fitted inside the image, add the image and annotations to dataset;
6. Else, different pairs of images/annotations are created in order to have represented all the original mitosis; duplicated mitoses are erased (see Fig. 2).

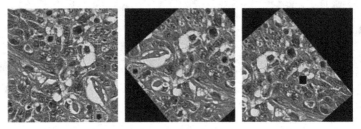

Fig. 2. Rotation augmentation example.

With the application of this procedure, an increase of the performance is expected since the augmentations allow the models to train on complete mitosis events, i.e. without clipping.

According with Fig. 2, the image on the left was flipped and rotated 50°, clockwise. Since a single image wasn't able to contain all the annotations, two images were generated. On the right image, since the left mitosis was already contained in the previous image, a black box was applied over the mitosis bounding box.

To apply the rotation in the previously mentioned step 2, three strategies for the rotation of annotated bounding boxes were considered (see Fig. 3). In the first strategy, the new bounding box is calculated by finding the minimums and maximums x and y coordinates of the corners of the rotated bounding box; in the second one, only the center point of each side is considered; while in the third, each side is divided by 3 and only the midsection is considered for the new bounding box.

For the first strategy, the area of the bounding box (in some cases) increase significantly. For the second one, the inverse was observed, often clipping relevant areas of the target object. A reasonable middle ground was found in the third strategy keeping the relevant parts of the mitosis inside the new bounding box while minimizing the increase of its area size. In this work, we used the third strategy.

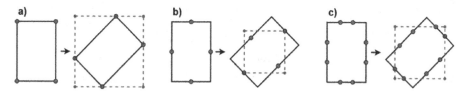

Fig. 3. New bounding box (red) for a 45° angle rotation. a) first strategy, b) second strategy and c) third strategy. (Color figure online)

The training and validation subsets of the dataset were augmented, in a case-by-case basis, with 2 different transformations: horizontal flip (referred as flip) and a set of rotations (see Table 1) following the third strategy. Concretely, for the "**16rots**" dataset, each image in the **base** dataset was rotated by a multiple of 22.5°, completing a 360° turn. For the "**flip/04rots**", each image was flipped and, for both flipped and un-flipped images, a set of a multiple of a 90° rotation was applied; the latter procedure was also applied to create the "**flip/36rots**" dataset but a multiple of 10° was used instead. Finally, the test subset, is transformed according with the "**flip/360rots**" parameters, i.e., flip and an extensive rotation of 1°, containing 270440 images occupying 170 GB.

Table 1. Details of the created datasets.

Dataset	Flip	Angle	Images Count	Goal
base	no	Not apply	1751	Train/Validation
16rots	no	22.5°	28036	Train/Validation
flip/04rots	yes	90°	14008	Train/Validation
flip/36rots	yes	10°	126168	Train/Validation
flip/360rots	yes	1°	270440	Test

3.3 Object Detection Models

From two object detection architectures, YOLOv4 and YOLOv5, we apply transfer learning technique using the pre-trained models: *yolov4-custom* and *yolov5x* respectively. Models trained on several datasets (see Table 1) with different online (i.e., during training) data augmentation strategies (see Table 2). As the original YOLOv4 framework doesn't have the online rotation augmentation capability, we implement this feature in the context of this paper.

Table 2. Trained models.

Name	Architecture	Dataset	Online Flip	Online Rotation
v4	YOLOv4	**Base**	Not apply	Not apply
v5	YOLOv5	**Base**	Not apply	Not apply
v4/tf/tr180	YOLOv4	**Base**	Yes	180°
v5/tf/tr180	YOLOv5	**Base**	Yes	180°
v4/f/36	YOLOv4	**flip/36rots**	Not apply	Not apply
v5/f/36	YOLOv5	**flip/36rots**	Not apply	Not apply
v4/16/tf	YOLOv4	**16rots**	Yes	Not apply
v5/16/tf	YOLOv5	**16rots**	Yes	Not apply
v4/16/tf/tr11	YOLOv4	**16rots**	Yes	11°
v5/16/tf/tr11	YOLOv5	**16rots**	Yes	11°

When using flip during training, there's a 50% probability of the image being flipped. For both architectures, when online rotation is active, the model trains on a rotated image by a random angle of a given interval - possibly clipping or removing some cells in mitosis. The rotation intervals were chosen in order to cover, approximately, the entire circumference.

All models were trained on a single GPU (RTX 3080, with 10 GB) and thus, their batch and model size were constrained by the graphics card memory. For each architecture, the best training settings were found empirically and, from there, the only variations were the target dataset and the online data augmentations. For YOLOv4, the model weights were saved every 100 training steps; after training, the best version was found by comparing the F1-score calculated on the validation set (augmented the same way as the training set). In YOLOv5, the framework already saves, at every epoch, the best weights of a fitness function that targets the validation set, therefore the fitness function was changed to output the F1-score. Finally, the models were compared by calculating their F1-Score against the "**flip/360rots**" test subset. Each model comprised three instantiations (the same settings trained three times on the same dataset) and the final F1-Score resulting from their average.

4   Results

Table 3 shows a summary of the experiments results where we can observe a direct comparison between YOLOv4 and YOLOv5 considering previously defined datasets (Table 1) and training configurations (Table 2). Throughout the results, YOLOv5 shows better performance than YOLOv4, often requiring more time to train.

Table 3. Models results, inferenced on the "**flip/360rots**" test subset, averaged after 3 runs. The last column in the table (timestamp) represents the time to reach the best model, avoiding overfitting, considering the maximum F1-score on the validation subset.

Name	F1-score	Recall	Precision	mAP@0.50	Timestamp
v4	0.809	0.794	0.824	0.787	7h
v5	0.825	0.829	0.822	0.810	5h
v4/tf/tr180	0.844	0.832	0.857	0.855	4h
v5/tf/tr180	0.883	0.875	0.892	0.891	5h
v4/f/36	0.882	0.904	0.861	0.924	4h
v5/f/36	0.900	0.889	0.912	0.922	13h
v4/16/tf	0.883	0.908	0.860	0.927	4h
v5/16/tf	0.901	0.910	0.893	0.909	8h
v4/16/tf/tr11	0.876	0.870	0.882	0.917	6h
v5/16/tf/tr11	0.907	0.905	0.909	0.921	14h

From the comparison between the models **v4** vs **v4/tf/tr180** and **v5** vs **v5/tf/tr180** we observe that using online data augmentations lead to a better performance when used on a baseline dataset. Also, to evaluate the proposed offline augmentation procedure, we compare the results of the **v4/tf/tr180** vs **v4/f/36** and **v5/tf/tr180** vs **v5/f/36** where models trained on **flip/36rots** dataset show better F1-score results.

In addition, the comparisons between **v4/f/36** vs **v4/16/tf** and **v5/f/36** vs **v5/16/tf** show that a decrease in the offline augmentations (and the corresponding reduction in train dataset size) didn't affect the performance of both models.

Finally, **v5/t16/tf/tr11** achieved the top performance among all the models tested, this being a YOLOv5 model with online flip and ±11° rotation interval trained on offline augmented dataset with 16 multiples rotations of 22.5°, reaching a good balance between precision (0.909) and recall (0.905).

5   Discussion

YOLOv5, when compared with YOLOv4, has the benefits of having online augmented rotations, a valuable tool for a better performance in mitosis detection. Considering that both algorithms are open source, we decided to implement this functionality to guarantee an impartial comparison between them.

In our experiments, YOLOv5 usually needs more training time than YOLOv4. However, it performs better than YOLOv4 and can be considered a good choice for the mitosis detection use case.

Analyzing the results of applying offline and online data augmentation strategies, we demonstrate that both are beneficial for the use case of this work. An increasing number of offline rotation augmentations usually led to a higher performance on any model, except for YOLOv4 when changing the number of rotations from 16 to 36.

Our proposed offline rotation augmentation procedure is beneficial for mitosis detection, mainly because, otherwise, some mitoses may be clipped or disappear when the training process applies a large enough online random rotation augmentation, as in the cases of **v4/tf/tr180** and **v5/tf/tr180**. As the number of mitotic events that are localized in the periphery increase, the importance of this strategy also increases. On the other hand, having an increase amount of augmented offline training data directly leads to an increasing amount of occupied memory which, for big enough datasets, could be a challenge or even not practical. Moreover, the results obtained with datasets **flip/36rots** and **16rots** shows that a significant reduction in data size (from 126168 to 28036 images) doesn't translate to a relevant decrease in the model's performance (F1-score).

For YOLOv5, combining offline and online rotation augmentations, as in **v5/16/tf/tr11**, showed the best performance from all the models tested.

6 Conclusions

From these experiments, we conclude that the proposed offline augmentation procedure helps YOLO algorithms achieve a better detection response in presence of mitotic events. Moreover, a reasonably small amount of offline rotation augmentations and the complementing online default augmentations are a good combination for maximizing the F1-score. Considering the memory limitations of our system, we conclude, according to our experiments, that YOLOv5 offers the best performance for mitosis detection.

As future work and taking in consideration the best result of our experiments, we will explore if a better compromise of data size and performance can be achieved by combining other offline and online rotations augmentations.

Acknowledgements. This work was financed by the project "iPATH, An Intelligent Network Center for Digital Pathology" (N° POCI-01-0247-FEDER-047069 and CENTRO-01-0247-FEDER-047069), financed by Portugal 2020, under the Competitiveness and Internationalization Operational Program, the Lisbon Regional Operational Program, and by the European Regional Development Fund (ERDF).

References

1. Elston, C.W., Ellis, I.O.: Pathological prognostic factors in breast cancer. I. the value of histological grade in breast cancer: experience from a large study with long-term follow-up. Histopathology **19**(5), 403–410 (1991). https://doi.org/10.1111/j.1365-2559.1991.tb00229.x
2. Cree, I.A., et al.: Counting mitoses: SI (ze) matters! Mod. Pathol. **34**, 1651–1657 (2021)
3. Mathew, T., Kini, J.R., Rajan, J.: Computational methods for automated mitosis detection in histopathology images: a review. Biocybern. Biomed. Eng. **41**(1), 64–82 (Jan.2021). https://doi.org/10.1016/J.BBE.2020.11.005
4. Mahmood, T., Arsalan, M., Owais, M., Lee, M.B., Park, K.R.: Artificial intelligence-based mitosis detection in breast cancer histopathology images using faster R-CNN and Deep CNNs. J. Clin. Med. **9**(3), 749 (2020). https://doi.org/10.3390/jcm9030749
5. Pati, P., Foncubierta-Rodríguez, A., Goksel, O., Gabrani, M.: Reducing annotation effort in digital pathology: A Co-Representation learning framework for classification tasks. Med. Image Anal. **67**, 101859 (2021). https://doi.org/10.1016/j.media.2020.101859

6. Jahn, S.W., Plass, M., Moinfar, F.: Digital pathology: advantages, limitations and emerging perspectives. J. Clin. Med. **9**(11), 3697 (2020). https://doi.org/10.3390/jcm9113697

7. Bochkovskiy, A., Wang, C.-Y., Liao, H.-Y.M.: YOLOv4: optimal speed and accuracy of object detection (2020)

8. Jocher, G., et. al.: ultralytics/yolov5: v6.0 - YOLOv5n 'Nano' models, Roboflow integration, TensorFlow export, OpenCVDNN support. Zenodo (2021). https://doi.org/10.5281/zenodo.5563715

9. Pan, X., et al.: Mitosis detection techniques in H&E stained breast cancer pathological images: a comprehensive review. Comput. Electr. Eng. **91**, 107038 (2021). https://doi.org/10.1016/j.compeleceng.2021.107038

10. Janowczyk, A., Madabhushi, A.: Deep learning for digital pathology image analysis: a comprehensive tutorial with selected use cases. J. Pathol. Inform. **7**(1), 29 (2016). https://doi.org/10.4103/2153-3539.186902

11. Wang, H., et al.: Mitosis detection in breast cancer pathology images by combining hand-crafted and convolutional neural network features. J. Med. Imaging **1**(3), 34003 (2014). https://doi.org/10.1117/1.jmi.1.3.034003

12. Paeng, K., Hwang, S., Park, S., Kim, M., Kim, S.: A unified framework for tumor proliferation score prediction in BreastHistopathology. CoRR, vol. abs/1612.07180 (2016). http://arxiv.org/abs/1612.07180

13. Redmon, J., Divvala, S.K., Girshick, R.B., Farhadi, A.: You only look once: unified, real-time object detection. CoRR, vol. abs/1506.0, 2015. http://arxiv.org/abs/1506.02640

14. Sreeraj, M., Joy, J.: A machine learning based framework for assisting pathologists in grading and counting of breast cancer cells. ICT Express, **7**(4), 440–444 (2021). https://doi.org/10.1016/j.icte.2021.02.005

15. Clarke, N., Dettrick, A., Armes, J.: Efficacy of training a deep learning model for mitotic count in breast carcinoma using opensource software. Pathology **53**, S23–S24 (2021). https://doi.org/10.1016/j.pathol.2021.06.019

16. Ludovic, R.: Mitos & Atypia 14 Contest (2014). https://mitos-atypia-14.grand-challenge.org/Home/. Accessed 28 Dec 2021

17. Veta, M., et al.: Predicting breast tumor proliferation from whole-slide images: the TUPAC16 challenge. Med. Image Anal. **54**, 111–121 (2019). https://doi.org/10.1016/j.media.2019.02.012

Preliminary Study of Deep Learning Algorithms for Metaplasia Detection in Upper Gastrointestinal Endoscopy

Alexandre Neto[1,2], Sofia Ferreira[2], Diogo Libânio[3], Mário Dinis-Ribeiro[3], Miguel Coimbra[1,4], and António Cunha[1,2(✉)]

[1] Instituto de Engenharia de Sistemas e Computadores, Tecnologia e Ciência, 3200-465 Porto, Portugal
acunha@utad.pt
[2] Escola de Ciências e Tecnologia, Universidade de Trás-os-Montes e Alto Douro, Quinta de Prados, 5001-801 Vila Real, Portugal
[3] Departamento de Ciências da Informação e da Decisão em Saúde/Centro de Investigação em Tecnologias e Serviços de Saúde (CIDES/CINTESIS), Faculdade de Medicina, Universidade do Porto, 4200-319 Porto, Portugal
[4] Faculdade de Ciências, Universidade do Porto, 4169-007 Porto, Portugal

Abstract. Precancerous conditions such as intestinal metaplasia (IM) have a key role in gastric cancer development and can be detected during endoscopy. During upper gastrointestinal endoscopy (UGIE), misdiagnosis can occur due to technical and human factors or by the nature of the lesions, leading to a wrong diagnosis which can result in no surveillance/treatment and impairing the prevention of gastric cancer. Deep learning systems show great potential in detecting precancerous gastric conditions and lesions by using endoscopic images and thus improving and aiding physicians in this task, resulting in higher detection rates and fewer operation errors. This study aims to develop deep learning algorithms capable of detecting IM in UGIE images with a focus on model explainability and interpretability. In this work, white light and narrow-band imaging UGIE images collected in the Portuguese Institute of Oncology of Porto were used to train deep learning models for IM classification. Standard models such as ResNet50, VGG16 and InceptionV3 were compared to more recent algorithms that rely on attention mechanisms, namely the Vision Transformer (ViT), trained in 818 UGIE images (409 normal and 409 IM). All the models were trained using a 5-fold cross-validation technique and for validation, an external dataset will be tested with 100 UGIE images (50 normal and 50 IM). In the end, explainability methods (Grad-CAM and attention rollout) were used for more clear and more interpretable results. The model which performed better was ResNet50 with a sensitivity of 0.75 ($\pm$0.05), an accuracy of 0.79 ($\pm$0.01), and a specificity of 0.82 ($\pm$0.04). This model obtained an AUC of 0.83 ($\pm$0.01), where the standard deviation was 0.01, which means that all iterations of the 5-fold cross-validation have a more significant agreement in classifying the samples than the other models. The ViT model showed promising performance, reaching similar results compared to the remaining models.

A. Cunha et al. (Eds.): MobiHealth 2022, LNICST 484, pp. 34–50, 2023.
https://doi.org/10.1007/978-3-031-32029-3_4

Keywords: Deep Learning · Gastrointestinal Metaplasia · Computer Vision · Gastrointestinal Endoscopy

1   Introduction

1.1   Motivation

Upper gastrointestinal endoscopy (UGIE) is a medical procedure that is used to diagnose and treat multiple pathologies. UGIE consists of the introduction of an endoscope through the mouth, allowing the observation of the mucosa of the esophagus, stomach and duodenum, performing endoscopic diagnosis using visual characteristics that are complemented, when necessary, with biopsy and histopathological analysis. Regarding the stomach, endoscopy is used to detect premalignant conditions and to treat pre-malignant lesions and early neoplastic lesions. The pathogenesis of gastric cancer (GC) involves a series of events beginning with *Helicobacter pylori*-induced chronic inflammation (*H. pylori*), progressing to atrophic gastritis (AG), intestinal metaplasia (IM), dysplasia, and eventually GC [1–3]. In Fig. 1 are some examples of these lesions.

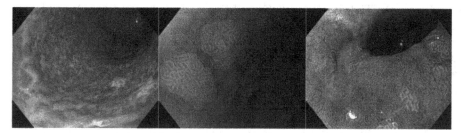

Fig. 1. Precancerous lesions from left to right from our private dataset: AG, IM and dysplasia.

Gastritis consists of inflammation of the stomach mucosa, which can be chronic, most of the time in the setting of *H. pylori* infection. Persistent inflammatory changes can result in gastric atrophy (loss of gastric glands and consequent reduction in the thickness of the gastric mucosa) and in intestinal metaplasia (substitution of gastric glands by intestinal-type glands formed by caliciform mucin-containing cells, paneth cells and absorptive cells). These conditions increase the risk of gastric cancer. Factors such as age, race/ethnicity, family history, environmental factors, and *H. pylori* strain are additional factors that can modify the risk of gastric cancer [3].

Endoscopy is important to detect these precancerous conditions (AG and IM) since patients with extensive precancerous conditions indicate periodical endoscopic surveillance [4]. One of the aims of endoscopic surveillance is the detection of these types of lesions, which can lead to early gastric cancer (EGC). Thus, the detection of AG and IM is a key role to increase the chances of survival since advanced GC has a poor long-term prognosis. However, training for the detection of precancerous conditions is suboptimal and these may be difficult to detect for the majority of endoscopists, even if virtual chromoendoscopy (a technique that uses light filters to increase the contrast of the image) is used [4]. Moreover, AG and IM show subtle alterations in the mucosa, which requires careful observation during the examination. Due to the nature of these lesions and lack of attention and tiredness, mistakes could be made by endoscopists, leading to missed diagnostics [5, 6].

1.2 State-of-the-Art

Deep learning (DL) in medical image analysis has provided comparable results to humans in multiple classification tasks. This machine learning paradigm, which is based on architectures made of multiple layers, is not intended to replace medical professionals in the diagnostic process but can be integrated into workflows to extract important information from images by recognizing patterns implicit to humans [7]. These DL systems are capable of real-time UGIE lesions detection in endoscopic videos, which can be helpful for endoscopists, pointing to suspicious areas during the examination. It can also be helpful for the endoscopist's learning process. It would allow less experienced endoscopists to learn visual patterns associated with GI lesions [8, 9]. Follows some examples of studies using DL for EGC lesion detection, such as IM and GA, in UGIE images.

The collected studies use well-known convolutional neural networks such as Xception, EfficientNETB4, ResNets, VGGs and DenseNets either to detect AG or IM or both. Of particular relevance, Hongyan Li and colleagues [10] proposed a multi-fusion method for metaplasia detection. First, three feature modules (ResNet50) are used for feature extraction in RGC, HSV and LBP images. The three types of features are fused into one representation based on attention mechanisms throughout an attention fusion module (AFM). The AFM is optimized by a regularization module which combines L1 regularization and label smoothing. Using this module can alleviate the overfitting more effectively and the model overconfidence caused by one hot encoding. Another example is the study of Tao Yan et al. [11] which a system was developed where the first model selects magnifying narrow-band imaging (M-NBI) and narrow-band imaging (NBI) images and then detects the presence of IM using two classifiers, one trained with M-NBI images and another trained with NBI images.

No specific image preprocessing methods are explicit in the described works [10, 12, 13]. Only in [11], after the images were classified as M-NBI or NBI, the black frames were cropped and the resulting image was resized to 224×224 pixels to then detect the IM presence.

To increase the interpretability of model predictions, explainable artificial intelligence (XAI) methods were applied in [11] by using Grad-CAMs for highlighting fine-grained features and in [12] by using class activation maps to indicate the features of the lesion that the CNNs focused on.

Transfer learning methods are usually applied in a variety of classification methods for a good initialization of weights and enhanced robustness against overfitting. All the mentioned works [10–13] used CNN architectures pre-trained using images from the ImageNet datasets.

All the considered works used private UGIE images to train and validate the models and performed 5-fold cross-validation methods, with exception of [13]. Tao Yan [11] used 1880 endoscopic images (1048 IM and 832 non-IM) to train the models. And 477 pathologically images (242 IM and 235 non-IM) to evaluate the models. Ming Xu [13] to train and evaluate these models collected 3 datasets composed of M-NBI and blue laser imaging (BLI) images: 1) collected from two institutions, split into a train (2439 AG and 2017 IM), validation and (internal) test (610 AG and 530 IM) set; 2) collected from 3 institutions, as an external test set (708 AG and 590 IM); 3) a prospective single-centre external test dataset containing 71 precancerous and 36 control images served as a benchmarking for the comparison of the algorithm with trained endoscopists. In the work of Ne Lin [12] 5,883 images were assigned (2,713 AG and 2,912 IM) for training, 606 images (199 AG and 201 IM) for validation and 548 images (180 AG and 188 IM) for testing. Hongyan Li [10] used 1050 UGIE NBI images (585 IM and 465 non-IM) to train and evaluate the models.

For the exclusion criteria, the images affected by artefacts created by mucus, poor focus and motion-blurring were excluded from the datasets used for training and evaluation [10–13]. Depending on the aim of the work, the authors used different types of image modalities. For example, Tao Yan [11] only used M-NBI and NBI images, Ming Xu [13] used M-NBI and BLI images, Ne Lin [12] only used WLI images and Hongyan Lin [10] only used NBI images.

In order to increase the amount of data, all the mentioned works used augmentation processes such as random rotations, flips, shifts and zooms, generating augmented data.

In Tao Yan work [11] it was possible to verify that M-NBI images help the model to achieve a better performance when compared to NBI images, for IM classification. The NBI and M-NBI classifiers achieved a sensitivity of 91%, a specificity of 71%, an accuracy of 83% and a sensitivity of 94%, a specificity of 84%, an accuracy of 89%, respectively.

In Ming Xu study [13], using the VGG16 model, the AG classification achieved 90% of accuracy, 90% of sensitivity and 91% of specificity in the internal test set, 86% of accuracy, 90% of sensitivity and 80% of specificity in the external test set and 88% of accuracy, 97% of sensitivity and 73% of specificity in the prospective video test set. For IM classification achieved 91% of accuracy, 89% of sensitivity and 93% of specificity in the internal test set, 86% of accuracy, 97% of sensitivity and 72% of specificity in the external test set and 90% of accuracy, 95% of sensitivity and 84% of specificity in the prospective video test set. The use of several datasets from different hospitals provides reliability in the robustness of the model since the select methodologies present good results when evaluated in unbiased data. Comparably, Ne Lin [12] used a TResNet achieving an area under the ROC curve (AUC) of 98%, the sensitivity of 96%, specificity of 96% and accuracy of 96% for AG classification and an AUC of 99%, the sensitivity of 98%, specificity of 98% and accuracy of 98% for IM classification. When comparing the results of Ming Xu [13] using M-NBI and BLI images and Ne Lin's [12] results using WLI, it is possible to conclude that a better performance can be achieved by using WLI images instead of using M-NBI and BLI. The TResNet reached better results when compared to the VGG16 using less data, however, in [13] was used more data from different hospitals, providing more robustness to the model for better generalization.

The proposed methodology made by Hongyan Li [10] for IM classification achieved 90% of accuracy, 90% of precision, 93% of recall and 92% of F1-Score.

Table 1 described the most important characteristics of the described works.

Table 1. Summary of the collected state-of-the-art studies.

Author	Year	Lesion	Datasets	Image Modality	Model	XAI	Results
Hongyan Li et al. [10]	2021	IM	(Private Dataset) Train and evaluation: 1050 UGIE images (585 IM and 465 non-IM)	NBI	ResNet50	-	Accuracy: 90% Precision: 90% Recall: 93% F1-Score: 92%
Tao Yan et al. [11]	2020	IM	(Private Dataset) Train: 1880 UGIE images (1048 IM and 832 non-IM) Evaluation: 477 UGIE images (242 IM and 235 non-IM)	M-NBI and NBI	Xception, NASNet and EfficientNetB4	Grad-CAM	IM in NBI Sensitivity: 91% Specificity: 71% Accuracy: 83% IM in M-NBI Sensitivity: 94% Specificity: 84% Accuracy: 89%,
Ne Lin et al. [12]	2021	AG and IM	(Private Dataset) Train: 5,883 images (2,713 AG and 2,912 IM) Validation: 606 images (199 AG and 201 IM) Test: 548 images (180 AG and 188 IM)	WLI	TResNet	Class Activation Maps	AG AUC: 98% Sensitivity: 96% Specificity: 96% Accuracy: 96% IM AUC: 99% Sensitivity: 98% Specificity: 98% Accuracy: 98%
Ming Xu et al. [13]	2021	AG and IM	(Private Dataset) 2149 GA images 3049 IM images	M-NBI and BLI	ResNet50, VGG16, DenseNet169 and EfficientNetB4	-	AG Accuracy: 90% Sensitivity: 90% Specificity: 91% IM Accuracy: 91% Sensitivity: 89% Specificity: 93%

1.3 Contributions

This work will compare the performance of DL models which achieved better results, based on the collected studies, to more recent approaches that rely on self-attention mechanisms, for IM classification. In the end, explainability methods for the models' predictions will be applied to verify if correlated features of the disease are highlighted.

For this, two research questions were formulated:

- **RQ1** - Can novel Vision Transformers (ViT) DL architectures outperform current DL architectures in the task of metaplasia detection in UGIE images?
- **RQ2** - Can explainable techniques highlight regions with clinical relevance and correlate to the metaplasia presence?

By answering these questions, the proposed study will contribute to understanding if these methods, which rely on attention mechanisms, can be applied to IM detection and reach similar performance or outperform the classic CNN architectures. After training and testing the models, in the end, explainability methods will be applied to understand if the features identified by the model have clinical relevance correlated to the output prediction.

This paper is organized into 5 sections, starting with this introduction, in Sect. 1, composed of the motivation, state-of-the-art and contributions. In Sect. 2, the DL architectures applied in this work will be described. In Sect. 3, the methodology used for the proposed study is explained in detail. In Sect. 4 the results will be described and in

Sect. 5 these results will be discussed. Finally, Sect. 6 will point out the conclusions of this work and future perspectives regarding the classification of IM using DL techniques.

2 Deep Learning Models

To select the methods to be used for this work, it was necessary to study in detail some architectures to achieve the initial objectives. Thus, DL models to be used for IM detection in endoscopy images will be analysed in detail, and then use XAI techniques in order to give interpretability and explainability to understand the predictions of the model.

ResNet50 is considered a deep network since it is 50 layers deep (Fig. 2). A residual layer in this stacked layers architecture in the residual block always contains 1×1, 3×3 and 1×1 convolution layers. The first 1×1 convolution will reduce the dimension and then the features will be calculated in the 3×3 bottleneck layer. In the next 1×1 layer, the dimension is increased again. The 1×1 filter is used in this architecture to reduce and increase the dimension of the feature maps before and after the bottleneck layer. Since there is no pooling layer within the residual block, the dimension is reduced in 1×1 convolutions with strides of 2 [14].

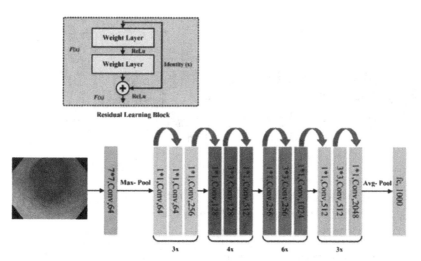

Fig. 2. Block diagram of the ResNet50 architecture, adapted from [15].

Visual Geometry Group (VGG), also known as VGGNet, was created to increase the depth of Convolutional Neural Networks (CNN), with the main goal of increasing model performance. Due to the number of convolutional layers, the VGG architecture is referred to as a deep architecture, i.e., VGG16 means that it has 16 layers (Fig. 3). This architecture is developed with very small convolutional filters. This has then 13 convolutional layers divided into five groups, and a max-pooling layer follows each group and 3 fully connected layers [15]. VGG16 has a 224×224 image as input. The convolution steps are fixed to keep the spatial resolution preserved after resolution.

When it comes to the hidden layers these use ReLu. As mentioned here VGG uses 3 fully connected layers, two of these layers with a size of 4096 neurons and the last one with a size of 1000 neurons [16].

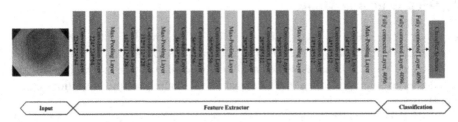

Fig. 3. Block diagram of the VGG16 architecture, adapted from [15].

The Inception V3 model involves more than 20 million parameters. This model includes symmetric and asymmetric building blocks, where each block is composed of various convolutional, average, and max pooling, concats, dropouts, and fully connected layers (Fig. 4). Batch normalization is usually used and applied in the activation layer in this model. This architecture has 42 layers of depth [17].

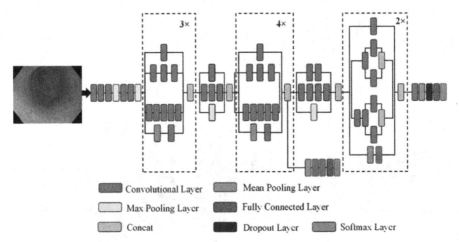

Fig. 4. Block diagram of the InceptionV3 architecture, adapted from [15].

Visual Transformers (ViT) have recently emerged as an alternative to CNN (Fig. 5). Compared to CNNs, it is generally found that the weaker inductive bias of the ViT leads to a greater reliance on model regularization or data augmentation when training on smaller training datasets. Internally, the transformer learns by measuring the relationship between pairs of input tokens. In computer vision, we can use image patches as a token. This relationship can be learned by providing attention to the network. This can be done in conjunction with a convolutional network or by replacing some components of convolutional networks. These network structures can be applied to image classification tasks [18].

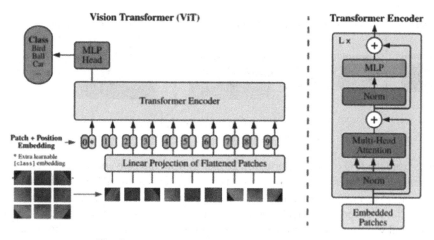

Fig. 5. Overview of ViT model, adapted from [18].

To better understand the model decisions, some XAI techniques were created to provide transparency, explainability and interpretability, helping non-experts to understand which features/attributes are responsible for the model's prediction.

Grad-CAM is a generalization of CAM, since it produces visual explanations for the CNN regardless of the architecture, thus overcoming one of the limitations of CAM. This method is a gradient-base, which uses the class-specific gradient information flowing into the last convolutional layer of a CNN, to design a coarse location map of the important regions in the image, in cases dealing with classification, thus making CNN-based models more transparent. This technique learns the information about the importance of the neurons in the decision process, using the gradient going to the last convolutional layer [19].

For ViT models Abnar and Zuidema [20] introduced the Attention Rollout mechanism which quantifies how the information flows through self-attention layers of transformer blocks. Is an average of the attention weights across all heads and then recursively multiplied by the weight matrices of all layers.

3 Materials and Methods

The workflow of this paper is illustrated in Fig. 6 which will be further explained in this section. Summarily, from the Portuguese Institute of Oncology (IPO) of Porto, a dataset with IM images and healthy gastric tissue was used. All the images suffered pre-processing before being split into the train, test, and validation sets to train and evaluate the different models.

3.1 IPO Dataset for IM Detection

The IPO Post-Map dataset is a private dataset of UGIE images obtained from a total of 170 different exams. The exams were performed in different health institutions: 20

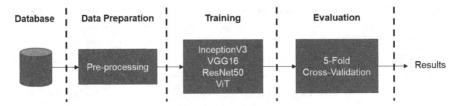

Fig. 6. Pipeline of the developed work.

exams from the IPO of Porto (Portugal), 28 exams from the University of Medicine and Pharmacy TG., Mures (Romania), 14 exams from Queen's Medical Centre, Nottingham (UK), and 75 exams from Hospital Sant 'Andrea, University Sapienza Roma (Italy). The dataset tries to cover various pathologies, allowing the diagnosis of various precancerous lesions and was created using images of three stomach locations (corpus, incisura, and antrum). Samples from patients without indication for biopsy, with significant comorbidities, anticoagulant therapy or coagulation disorders, previous gastric neoplasia or surgery and not being able to perform at least three biopsies during the endoscopy were excluded [21]. It contains a total number of 1355 images, Narrow-Band Imaging (NBI) and White Light Imaging (WLI), of which 499 are high resolution and 856 are low resolution, ranging between 1350 × 1080 to 514 × 476 resolution. It has four classes (AG, dysplasia, IM, and healthy tissue).

3.2 Data Preparation

The images used were resized for the respective input size of each model, for ResNet50, VGG16, and ViT the images were resized to 224 × 224, and for InceptionV3 the images were resized to 229 × 229. Aiming to classify images into one of two classes, only WLI and NBI images of IM and healthy stomach tissue, a total of 818 images, 409 of each class, were selected from the IPO Post-Map dataset. The UGIE images were annotated, by two interns of the IPO of Porto, image-wise using a design annotation tool for this purpose. For the image-based annotation, the UGIE images were classified as normal or IM. Some examples of images from the IPO Post-Map are illustrated in Fig. 7.

Due to the small amount of data a 5-fold cross-validation (CV) was performed to train and evaluate the models. An external dataset, in the end, was used to test the robustness of each model trained in each fold. Figure 8 is present the dataset split used to create and evaluate the four models.

Each network has a different preprocessing method. In the case of ResNet50 and VGG16, the images are converted from RGB to BGR, and then each colour channel is zero-centred concerning the ImageNet dataset, without scaling. For inceptionV3 and ViT the input pixel values are scaled between -1 and 1, sample-wise.

3.3 Training

To execute the binary classification task described previously, multiple state-of-the-art models were tested. VGG16, InceptionV3 and ResNet50 were selected based on their

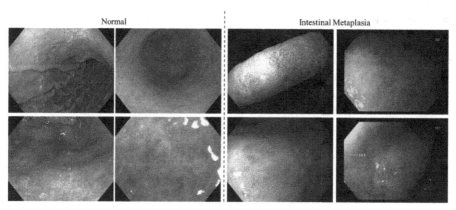

Fig. 7. Examples of WLI and NBI UGIE images of the Post-Map dataset, from normal or intestinal metaplasia samples.

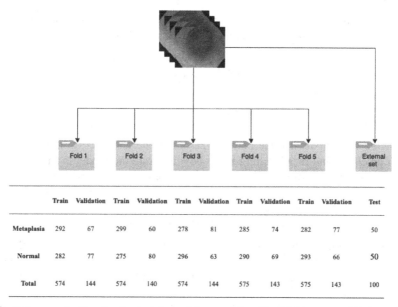

	Train	Validation	Train	Validation	Train	Validation	Train	Validation	Train	Validation	Test
Metaplasia	292	67	299	60	278	81	285	74	282	77	50
Normal	282	77	275	80	296	63	290	69	293	66	50
Total	574	144	574	140	574	144	575	143	575	143	100

Fig. 8. Data organization for the training of the models with 5-fold cross-validation with an external set.

performance in classification tasks related to the aim of this study. These models were compared to a more recent approach that relies on self-attention mechanisms, called Vision Transformers (ViT), which recently emerged as an alternative to CNNs. For this study the Keras API was used integrated into the Tensorflow framework running the different experiments in a Nvidia RTX 3060ti GPU. All the models were trained during 100 epochs, with a dropout layer of 0.3, a learning rate of $1e^{-4}$, Adam optimizer, binary focal loss as loss function and batch size of 16 with exception of ViT model which had a batch size of 8.

3.4 Evaluation

Considering the number of True Positives (TP), False Positives (FP), True Negatives (TN), and False Negatives (FN) produced by each one of the models in the test set, the following metrics were calculated aiming to evaluate their performance:

The accuracy (1) is the ratio between the number of correct predictions and the total number of input samples.

$$\text{Accuracy} = \frac{\text{TP} + \text{TN}}{\text{TP} + \text{FP} + \text{TN} + \text{FN}} \tag{1}$$

Precision (2) is the ratio of correct predictions to the number of positive results predicted by the classifier.

$$\text{Precision} = \frac{\text{TP}}{\text{TP} + \text{FP}} \tag{2}$$

Specificity (3) measures the proportion of the negative cases that were correctly classified. Recall or sensitivity (4) is the number of correctly predicted results divided by the number of all those that should have been classified as positive.

$$\text{Specificity} = \frac{\text{TN}}{\text{TN} + \text{FP}} \tag{3}$$

$$\text{Recall} = \frac{\text{TP}}{\text{TP} + \text{FN}} \tag{4}$$

F1-Score (5) outputs a value between zero and one and tries to find the balance between precision and recall, letting know how accurate the model is and how many samples it correctly classifies. The F1-Score is the harmonic mean of these two.

$$\text{F1-Score} = \frac{2 \times \text{TP}}{2 \times \text{TP} + \text{FN} + \text{FP}} \tag{5}$$

In addition to these measures, other measures were also used, such as rank-based performance measures. These measures rank predictions relative to the probability of an outcome. For this work, measures such as the Receptor Operating Characteristic (ROC) Curve were used.

The ROC curve is a performance measure for classification problems at various threshold parameters. ROC is a probability curve and AUC represents the degree or measure of separability. Essentially this is how well the model can distinguish between classes. It can be concluded that the higher the AUC the better the model distinguishes between patients with and without the disease. The ROC curve is plotted with TPR (sensitivity) against FPR (False Positive Rate).

4 Results

Throughout this project, several experiments were carried out to evaluate the different state-of-the-art architectures in the binary classification task.

The results will be discussed and compared with the study described in Sect. 1. In the end, will be performed a brief comparison of the standard methodologies and the ViT methodology.

Table 2 shows the average results obtained in each fold of the 5-fold CV validation set.

Overall, the model with the best performance was the InceptionV3 with 0.82 ($\pm$0.03) of accuracy, 0.82 ($\pm$0.07) of sensitivity, 0.80 ($\pm$0.11) of specificity, 0.82 ($\pm$0.04) of precision, 0.82 ($\pm$0.04) of F1-Score and 0.84 ($\pm$0.05) of AUC. The ResNet50 achieved very similar results, with slight changes, and all the models reached an AUC over 0.80.

The ViT model reached similar results when compared to the VGG16, with 0.77 ($\pm$0.03) of accuracy, 0.76 ($\pm$0.07) of sensitivity, 0.80 ($\pm$0.06) of specificity, 0.79 ($\pm$0.08) of precision, 0.77 ($\pm$0.03) of F1-Score and 0.82 ($\pm$0.03) of AUC.

Table 2. Results for the validation set in 5-fold CV. The higher results are highlighted in bold.

Metrics	ResNet50	VGG16	InceptionV3	ViT
Accuracy	0.80 ($\pm$0.02)	0.75 ($\pm$0.03)	**0.82 ($\pm$0.03)**	0.77 ($\pm$0.03)
Sensitivity	0.77 ($\pm$0.04)	0.75 ($\pm$0.10)	**0.82 ($\pm$0.07)**	0.76 ($\pm$0.07)
Specificity	**0.83 ($\pm$0.04)**	0.74 ($\pm$0.15)	0.80 ($\pm$0.11)	0.80 ($\pm$0.06)
Precision	**0.82 ($\pm$0.07)**	0.76 ($\pm$0.06)	**0.82 ($\pm$0.04)**	0.79 ($\pm$0.08)
F1-Score	0.79 ($\pm$0.03)	0.75 ($\pm$0.05)	**0.82 ($\pm$0.04)**	0.77 ($\pm$0.03)
AUC	**0.84 ($\pm$0.02)**	0.80 ($\pm$0.05)	**0.84 ($\pm$0.05)**	0.82 ($\pm$0.03)

Finally, to evaluate the robustness of these models was presented an external test set to further test the performance of these models in data never used for validation or training (Table 3). The ResNet50 model reached the best results, with 0.79 ($\pm$0.01) of accuracy, 0.75 ($\pm$0.05) of sensitivity, 0.82 ($\pm$0.04) of specificity, 0.81 ($\pm$0.03) of precision, 0.77 ($\pm$0.02) of F1-Score and 0.83 ($\pm$0.01) of AUC, followed by the InceptionV3, once again, with a very similar performance. The VGG16 and the ViT model achieved comparable performances between them, with an AUC of 0.79 when tested with the external dataset.

Table 3. Results for the external set in 5-fold CV. The higher results are highlighted in bold.

Metrics	ResNet50	VGG16	InceptionV3	ViT
Accuracy	**0.79 ($\pm$0.01)**	0.76 ($\pm$0.02)	0.77 ($\pm$0.01)	0.75 ($\pm$0.02)
Sensitivity	0.75 ($\pm$0.05)	0.76 ($\pm$0.04)	**0.78 ($\pm$0.04)**	0.66 ($\pm$0.04)
Specificity	0.82 ($\pm$0.04)	0.76 ($\pm$0.07)	0.76 ($\pm$0.04)	**0.85 ($\pm$0.04)**
Precision	**0.81 ($\pm$0.03)**	0.76 ($\pm$0.05)	0.77 ($\pm$0.02)	**0.81 ($\pm$0.03)**
F1-Score	**0.77 ($\pm$0.02)**	0.76 ($\pm$0.01)	**0.77 ($\pm$0.01)**	0.73 ($\pm$0.02)
AUC	**0.83 ($\pm$0.01)**	0.79 ($\pm$0.02)	0.81 ($\pm$0.01)	0.79 ($\pm$0.03)

5 Discussion

Overall the results are very similar between all the models. Generally, for the validation set, InceptionV3 achieved the best values in almost all used metrics with exception of the specificity. Either way, the results are very similar when compared to the ResNet50 model and both reached an AUC of 0.84 with a small standard deviation which proves the agreement in the different folds. Although the models did not reach comparable results with the studies presented in Sect. 1 mostly due to the huge gap in data that exists between this work and the described state-of-the-art works.

The ViT achieved comparable performance, especially when compared to the ResNet50 model, reaching an AUC of 0.82 and proving to have a better performance than the VGG16. In overall, the models show consistency in predicting either normal or IM images.

In Fig. 9 are illustrated the ROC curves with the respective AUC values of each model, with the mean ROC for the 5-fold for each model and, in grey, the standard deviation between all folds of each model.

Analysing the ROC curves can be seen that the ResNet50 and InceptionV3 curves are very similar but the ResNet50 presents less grey area, consequently a smaller standard deviation which represents a bigger agreement between the different folds of this model.

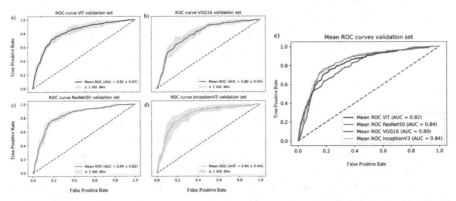

Fig. 9. ROC curves of the validation set of the models: (a) ViT, (b) VGG16, (c) ResNet50, (d) InceptionV3 and (e) is the mean of all ROC curves.

For the external test set, ResNet50 and InceptioV3 achieved overall better results, although this time, the ResNet50 has slightly better performance. As said before, the ResNet50 shows a bigger agreement between all the folds, reaching the best values for all the metrics except for the sensitivity and specificity.

The ViT proved one more time to be a reliable model with similar results to the VGG16. In Fig. 10 the ROC curves for the external test set are represented. The ROC curves follow the same pattern as seen in Fig. 9, where the InceptionV3 and ResNet50 achieved the best AUC values and have the best ROC curves shape. The ResNet50 has the smallest standard deviation, proving again the most agreement between the different folds, now to an external test set, reinforcing the best generalization and robustness of all models.

When comparing the state-of-the-art results it is possible to see that although the performance of these models is good, they did not achieve the results presented in the literature review, mostly due to the lack of data.

As far as transformers are concerned, so far no other studies were found using ViT models in the IM classification of UGIE images. The ViT model in this presented study proves to achieve similar results compared to the remaining models, even reaching a better performance than the VGG16 model. These self-attention models rely even more upon great amounts of data when compared to traditional CNN architectures, which could be the problem for not reaching even better results.

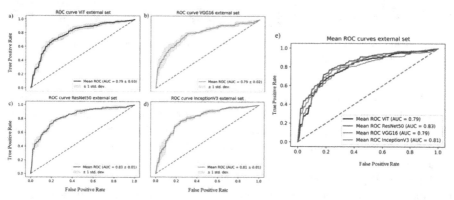

Fig. 10. ROC curves of the external set of the models: (a) ViT, (b) VGG16, (c) ResNet50, (d) InceptionV3 and (e) is the mean of all ROC curves.

CNNs can be extremely difficult for non-experts to explain and understand, so was decided to apply XAI methods, which help to create transparency, interpretability, and explainability as a basis for the output of the neural networks.

Figure 11 presents the activation maps for the different models, using Grad-CAMs for traditional CNNs and Attention Rollout for the ViT model.

The Grad-CAMs attention maps point to important areas that lead the model for predicting IM presence in the images, by using the gradient of the model of the final convolutional layer. The attention rollout uses the weights average across the different attention blocks to highlight the most important regions for the ViT decision.

In most cases, the highlighted areas are common for the different models and reveal IM-related characteristics. For example, the different models focus on flat and patchy regions with irregularities and in NBI images bluish-white appearance of the gastric mucosa is highlighted as well, which is a feature of IM presence. In other cases, the ViT model highlight more accurate regions, more correlated and indicative of IM presence. For instance, in Fig. 11 mid-row images, the ViT model points to more important regions with more clinical indications of IM presence, when compared to the regions highlighted by the CNN models, with no presence of IM characteristics.

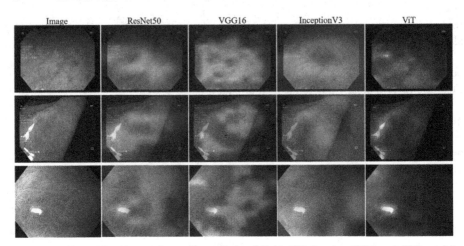

Fig. 11. Grad-CAM and attention rollout of the 5-Fold CV for the CNN and ViT model, respectively. All the UGIE images are IM examples.

This type of explainability is extremely important for trustworthy models so that the physicians can understand why is made certain predictions from the models and which features are related to that decision. More trustworthy models will understand which features are more indicative of IM presence, thus highlighting regions with these characteristics.

Regarding RQ1, the ViT models reached similar performance when compared to more traditional CNNs, however, did not outperform ResNet50 and InceptionV3 architectures. More adaptations can be applied for ViT performance enhancement, such as shifted patch tokenization or/and locality self-attention to tackle the problem of locality inductive bias present in ViTs. Nonetheless, regarding RQ2, the ViT activation maps highlight IM characteristic with more clinical relevance. Thus, despite not outperforming the ResNet50 and InceptionV3 models, the ViT architecture has promising applications in IM detection due to the relation process at the pixel level, understanding different features which are not identified by traditional CNNs.

6 Conclusions

This paper focuses on the evaluation of multiple state-of-the-art architectures in image classification in IM and normal gastric mucosa. The results achieved in the multiple experiments were satisfactory compared to the described works in Sect. 1, although not reaching the same performance mostly due to the gap of data between works. Additionally, self-attention models such as ViT were tested and reached comparable results to the standard CNNs. This type of architecture which relies on transformer blocks needs even more data than a CNN. However, with the data available, it was possible to achieve satisfactory results similar to the performance of the CNNs. For all the models activation maps were computed to give interpretability and explainability of the results.

This is a required step nowadays when DL models are applied especially to the healthcare field in order to justify the algorithmic results to non-experts and highlight which features/attributes are strongly related to the model decision.

In future works, increasing the data will be essential and this can be done using generative adversarial methods, creating synthetic UGIE images. Adaptation in ViT models can enhance the performance of IM detection, especially in small datasets, by using shifted patch tokenization or/and locality self-attention. Further explainability methods should be explored to provide even more transparency to DL models, such as local interpretable model-agnostic explanations which are more suitable for local explanations.

Acknowledgements. This work is financed by National Funds through the Portuguese funding agency, FCT - Fundação para a Ciência e a Tecnologia, within project PTDC/EEI-EEE/5557/2020.

References

1. ASGE Standards of Practice Committee, et al.: Appropriate use of GI endoscopy. Gastrointest. Endosc. **75**(6), 1127–1131 (2012). https://doi.org/10.1016/j.gie.2012.01.011
2. Evans, J.A., et al.: The role of endoscopy in the management of premalignant and malignant conditions of the stomach. Gastrointest. Endosc. **82**(1), 1–8 (2015). https://doi.org/10.1016/j.gie.2015.03.1967
3. Peixoto, A., Silva, M., Pereira, P., Macedo, G.: Biopsies in gastrointestinal endoscopy: when and how. GE Port. J. Gastroenterol. **23**(1), 19–27 (2016). https://doi.org/10.1016/j.jpge.2015.07.004
4. Pimentel-Nunes, P., et al.: Management of epithelial precancerous conditions and lesions in the stomach (MAPS II): European Society of Gastrointestinal Endoscopy (ESGE), European Helicobacter and Microbiota Study Group (EHMSG), European Society of Pathology (ESP), and Sociedade Portuguesa de Endoscopia Digestiva (SPED) guideline update 2019. Endoscopy **51**(04), 365–388 (2019). https://doi.org/10.1055/a-0859-1883
5. Sitarz, R., Skierucha, M., Mielko, J., Offerhaus, G.J.A., Maciejewski, R., Polkowski, W.P.: Gastric cancer: epidemiology, prevention, classification, and treatment. Cancer Manag. Res. **10**, 239–248 (2018). https://doi.org/10.2147/CMAR.S149619
6. Moon, H.S.: Improving the endoscopic detection rate in patients with early gastric cancer. Clin. Endosc. **48**(4), 291 (2015). https://doi.org/10.5946/ce.2015.48.4.291
7. e Gonçalves, W.G., Dos Santos, M.H.D.P., Lobato, F.M.F., Ribeiro-dos-Santos, Â., de Araújo, G.S.: Deep learning in gastric tissue diseases: a systematic review. BMJ Open Gastroenterol. **7**(1), e000371 (2020). https://doi.org/10.1136/bmjgast-2019-000371
8. Renna, F., et al.: Artificial intelligence for upper gastrointestinal endoscopy: a roadmap from technology development to clinical practice. Diagnostics **12**(5), 1278 (2022). https://doi.org/10.3390/diagnostics12051278
9. Arribas, J., et al.: Standalone performance of artificial intelligence for upper GI neoplasia: a meta-analysis. Gut **70**(8), 1458–1468 (2021). https://doi.org/10.1136/gutjnl-2020-321922
10. Li, H., et al.: A multi-feature fusion method for image recognition of gastrointestinal metaplasia (GIM). Biomed. Signal Process. Control **69**, 102909 (2021). https://doi.org/10.1016/j.bspc.2021.102909
11. Yan, T., Wong, P.K., Choi, I.C., Vong, C.M., Yu, H.H.: Intelligent diagnosis of gastric intestinal metaplasia based on convolutional neural network and limited number of endoscopic images. Comput. Biol. Med. **126**, 104026 (2020). https://doi.org/10.1016/j.compbiomed.2020.104026

12. Lin, N., et al.: Simultaneous recognition of atrophic gastritis and intestinal metaplasia on white light endoscopic images based on convolutional neural networks: a multicenter study. Clin. Transl. Gastroenterol. **12**(8), e00385 (2021). https://doi.org/10.14309/ctg.000000000 0000385

13. Xu, M., et al.: Artificial intelligence in the diagnosis of gastric precancerous conditions by image-enhanced endoscopy: a multicenter, diagnostic study (with video). Gastrointest. Endosc. **94**(3), 540–548 (2021). https://doi.org/10.1016/j.gie.2021.03.013

14. He, K., Zhang, X., Ren, S., Sun, J.: Deep residual learning for image recognition. arXiv: arXiv:1512.03385 (2015). http://arxiv.org/abs/1512.03385. Accessed 05 Jun 2022

15. Ali, L., Alnajjar, F., Jassmi, H.A., Gocho, M., Khan, W., Serhani, M.A.: Performance evaluation of deep CNN-based crack detection and localization techniques for concrete structures. Sensors **21**(5), 1688 (2021). https://doi.org/10.3390/s21051688

16. Simonyan, K., Zisserman, A.: Very deep convolutional networks for large-scale image recognition, p. 14 (2015)

17. Szegedy, C., Vanhoucke, V., Ioffe, S., Shlens, J., Wojna, Z.: Rethinking the inception architecture for computer vision. In: 2016 IEEE Conference on Computer Vision and Pattern Recognition (CVPR), pp. 2818–2826. Las Vegas, NV, USA (2016). https://doi.org/10.1109/CVPR.2016.308

18. Dosovitskiy, A., et al.: An image is worth 16x16 words: transformers for image recognition at scale. arXiv: arXiv:2010.11929 (2021). http://arxiv.org/abs/2010.11929. Accessed 02 Jun 2022

19. Linardatos, P., Papastefanopoulos, V., Kotsiantis, S.: Explainable AI: a review of machine learning interpretability methods. Entropy **23**(1), 1–45 (2021). https://doi.org/10.3390/e23 010018

20. Abnar, S., Zuidema, W.: Quantifying attention flow in transformers. arXiv (2020). http://arxiv.org/abs/2005.00928. Accessed 18 Jul 2022

21. Pimentel-Nunes, P., et al.: A multicenter prospective study of the real-time use of narrow-band imaging in the diagnosis of premalignant gastric conditions and lesions. Endoscopy **48**(08), 723–730 (2016). https://doi.org/10.1055/s-0042-108435

Prediction of Ventricular Tachyarrhythmia Using Deep Learning

Dalila Barbosa[1], E. J. Solteiro Pires[1,2]([✉])[iD], Argentina Leite[1,2][iD],
and P. B. de Moura Oliveira[1,2][iD]

[1] Escola de Ciências e Tecnologia Universidade de Trás-os-Montes e Alto Douro,
Vila Real, Portugal
al71375@utad.eu, {epires,tinucha,oliveira}@utad.pt
[2] INESC TEC, Porto, Portugal

Abstract. Ventricular tachyarrhythmia (VTA), mainly ventricular tachycardia (VT) and ventricular fibrillation (VF) are the major causes of sudden cardiac death in the world. This work uses deep learning, more precisely, LSTM and biLSTM networks to predict VTA events. The Spontaneous Ventricular Tachyarrhythmia Database from PhysioNET was chosen, which contains 78 patients, 135 VTA signals, and 135 control rhythms. After the pre-processing of these signals and feature extraction, the classifiers were able to predict whether a patient was going to suffer a VTA event or not. A better result using a biLSTM was obtained, with a 5-fold-cross-validation, reaching an accuracy of 96.30%, 94.07% of precision, 98.45% of sensibility, and 96.17% of F1-Score.

Keywords: Ventricular Tachyarrhythmia · Deep learning · Long Short Term Memory

1 Introduction

Ventricular tachycardia and Fibrillation are the primary ventricular tachyarrhythmias that cause sudden death. Ventricular tachycardia (VT) is mostly caused by a faulty heart signal that triggers a fast heart rate in the lower heart chambers, i.e., the ventricles. The fast heart rate does not allow the ventricles to completely fill and squeeze to pump the blood needed for the body. Ventricular fibrillation (VF) is also a type of abnormal heart rhythm that affects the heart's signals and causes the lower heart chambers to twitch uselessly. This result in the heart not pumping blood to the rest of the body. One solution to this problem is implanting cardioverter defibrillators. Implantable cardioverter defibrillators (ICDs) are the cornerstone of sudden cardiac death prevention by terminating ventricular tachyarrhythmias, such as ventricular tachycardia and ventricular fibrillation. Over the past four decades, ICDs have been used to reduce the risk

© ICST Institute for Computer Sciences, Social Informatics and Telecommunications Engineering 2023
Published by Springer Nature Switzerland AG 2023. All Rights Reserved
A. Cunha et al. (Eds.): MobiHealth 2022, LNICST 484, pp. 51–60, 2023.
https://doi.org/10.1007/978-3-031-32029-3_5

of cardiac arrest [7] by detecting arrhythmia and delivering electrical shocks to restore the heart rhythm [11]. It can be incorporated into the ICD, a reliable predictor of an imminent ventricular tachyarrhythmia, episode capable of preventive therapy, which would have important clinical utilities [10].

Several studies were made, considering signal features used to develop detection algorithms for anomalous cardiac signals. Oliver Faust *et al.* [2] proposed a deep learning system to identify irregularities in the heart signals, partitioning them into windows of 100 beats and feeding a Recurrent Neural Network with a Long Short-Term Memory. They obtained an accuracy in the range 95.51%-99.77% accurate. Atiye Riasi *et al.* [10] presented an technique using morphological features of an electrocardiogram (ECG). Also, the classification of selected features done by a Support Vector Machine (SVM) identified hidden patterns in the ECG before the occurrence of the episode, achieving 88% and 100% of sensitivity and specificity, respectively. Segyeong Joo *et al.* [4] proposed a classifier that could predict events recurring to artificial neural networks (ANNs) considering time-domain and non-linear parameters. It achieved 82.9% of sensitivity and 71.4% of specificity. Taye *et al.* [14] proposed a convolutional neural network, considering one dimension (1-D CNN) with signal features. Furthermore, comparing the obtained CNN prediction to other machine learning performances, such as ANN, SVM, and KNN, the higher accuracy value of 84.6% was reached.

Analyzing the aforementioned, this work uses a long short-term memory (LSTM) network, analyzing different features, which can help to predict the occurrence of abnormal episodes.

The paper is organized into more three sections. Section 2 describes the database used, the signals pre-processing, the features extracted, and neural networks. Next, Sect. 3 presents and discusses the results. Finally, Sect. 4, draws the conclusions.

2   Materials and Methods

2.1   Dataset

The dataset considered was collected from the PhysioNet database, known as the Spontaneous Ventricular Tachyarrhythmia Database [3]. The dataset consists of 135 RR interval pairs, recorded by ICD, of 78 patients (RR is the time elapsing between two consecutive R waves in the electrocardiogram). The patient dataset has different numbers for VF and VF events. Of the 135 pairs of RR intervals, 29 were VF and 106 VT, and every one of them had its corresponding normal sinus rhythm.

2.2   Pre-processing

Every signal collected from the Spontaneous Ventricular Tachyarrhythmia Database was initially filtered to reduce and smooth out high-frequency noise. The length of each signal has approximately 1024 beats. From every signal, we only use a specific section. Out of the normal sinus rhythm, we used the first 256 beats and the last 256 beats before the abnormal episode occurred.

2.3 Feature Extraction

Several methods can analyze variations in heart signals. The data analysis can be performed directly on the signals or indirectly, extracting characteristics in the first step and then analyzing these features. This work extracted some features from the time regions, the first 256 beats from the normal signal and the last 256 from the abnormal signal. Eight features were considered, three in the time domain, two in the frequency domain, and the last three are nonlinear features.

Time-Domain. The time-domain measures are the easiest to determine. In this category, the features used were the mean RR intervals (meanRR), the NN intervals standard deviation (SDNN), which comprises the cyclic components liable for variability in the recording period [1], and the proportion of successive RR interval differences greater than 50 ms (pNN50).

Frequency Domain. The frequency domain characteristics are obtained with the parametric power spectrum estimation from the RR intervals. The AutoRegressive (AR) model is the most widely used in this domain to characterize the data. [1]. This model eases the determination of the parameters by solving linear equations. Right below, it is represented the AR model in order of p, $AR(p)$:

$$x_t = \sum_{k=0}^{p} \alpha_k x_{t-k} + \varepsilon_t \tag{1}$$

with α_k representing the AR coefficients, ε_t the white noise with zero mean and σ_ε^2 variance. There is also the AR model a spectrum equation:

$$P_{AR}(\omega) = \frac{\sigma_\varepsilon^2}{|1 - \sum_{k=1}^{p} \alpha_k e^{(-iwk)}|^2} \tag{2}$$

Information quantification relative to different frequency bands is possible because of spectral analysis. In this case, the low frequency (LF) and high frequency (HF) bands are in between (0.04–0.15 Hz), and (0.15–0.4 Hz), respectively. Typically, HF characterizes parasympathetic nervous system activity, while LF is associated with sympathetic and parasympathetic systems. The evaluation between these two components generally is made from the determination of LF and HF areas [1].

Nonlinear-Domain. The nonlinear features were obtained through nonlinear methodologies, such as, Detrended Fluctuation Analysis (DFA) [8] and Approximate Entropy (ApEn) [9]. DFA can understand unique insights into the neural organization [12], identifying long-range correlations embedded in a nonstationary time series. The first step of this method has to do the first integration, using Eq. (3):

$$y(i) = \sum_{t=1}^{i} [u(t) - \overline{u}] \tag{3}$$

Then, it divides the signal into k segments, where the linear local trend $y_k(i)$ is calculated by a linear regression. DFA is summarized by Eq. (4), which gives the root-mean-square between a segment of the first integrated signal and $y_k(i)$.

$$DFA(k) = \sqrt{\frac{1}{N}\sum_{i=1}^{N}[y(i) - y_k(i)]^2} \tag{4}$$

Equation (4) is repeated for several segments of length k. This work considers two scaling exponents: $\alpha 1$ for $4 \leq k \leq 11$ and $\alpha 2$ for $12 \leq k \leq 32$, corresponding to the short memory correlation. For non correlated data, the scaling exponent adopted is $\alpha = 0.5$. On the other hand, values of $\alpha > 0.5$ for large scales k indicate data with long-range correlations [8].

ApEn is commonly used in short and noisy data. Being m and r an integer and real positive number, respectively. Given a signal $u(1), u(2), ..., u(N)$, form a sequence of vectors $x(1), x(2), ..., x(N - m + 1)$ in $\mathbb{R}^m$, defined by $x(i) = [u(i), u(i + 1), ..., u(i + m - 1)]$ [9].

Next, it is defined for each $i, 1 \leq i \leq N - m + 1$,

$$C_i^m(r) = \frac{\text{number of } j : d[x(i), x(j)] \leq r}{N - m + 1},$$

where $d[x(i), x(j)] = max(|u(i + k - 1) - u(j + k - 1)|)$, $k = 1, 2, ..., m$

Therefore, the *ApEn* feature is calculated by

$$ApEn(m, r, N) = \phi^m(r) - \phi^{m+1}(r)$$

where

$$\phi^m(r) = (N - m + 1)^{-1}\sum_{i=1}^{N-m+1}\log(C_i^m(r)).$$

In the present work, the *ApEn* uses $m = 2$ and $r = 0.2\sigma$, where σ is the data standard as recommended by [9]. Features were extracted from the RR intervals, and in Fig. 1, it can be seen the values of each class, the normal sinus rhythm, and the precedent of the abnormal episode.

Table 1 presents the mean values of the several features extracted. On the left are the values of the normal sinus rhythm, and on the right, we have the ones from the abnormal signal.

2.4 Neural Network

Artificial neural networks (ANNs) are a machine learning subset considered the heart of deep learning models. ANNs' structure is inspired by the human brain, imitating how biological neurons' signals spread between them. In the network, the neurons nodes are connected with links, enabling them to communicate and exchange information, conceiving them to store information.

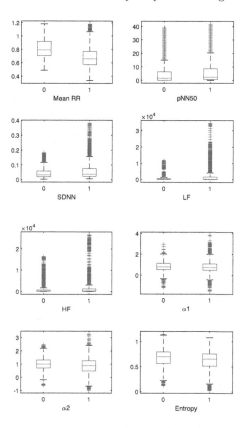

Fig. 1. Boxplot of HRV features for two groups: Normal Sinus Rhythm (0) and Signal before the VTA episode (1).

This work considers a long short-term memory (LSTM) and a biLSTM, which are a type of recurrent neural network (RNN). There is an architectural difference between RNN and LSTM, where the LSTM is a specialized form of RNN architecture. In practice, simple RNNs have limitations related to the capacity to learn longer-term dependencies. RNNs are commonly trained through backpropagation, in which they may experience either a 'vanishing', or 'exploding' gradient problem, causing the network to become very small or very large, affecting the effectiveness in applications using a network. That is where LSTMs come in. To overcome this problem by using additional gates to control the information exported from the hidden cells as output and to the next hidden state.

An LSTM unity has three gates: input, output, and forget. These gates control the information flow within the cell. The input gate updates the unit status and decides the relevant information to the current step. The output gate determines the next hidden state value. The forget gate has better control over the gradient flow than RNN and determines the important information from those that should be ignored. The choice to preserve or delete information is defined

Table 1. HRV features: Control and VTA dataset

Features	Control Sinus Rhythm	VTA
MeanRR (s)	0.81 ± 0.14	0.69 ± 0.16
pNN50 (%)	5.03 ± 7.71	5.92 ± 8.20
SDNN (s)	0.04 ± 0.03	0.05 ± 0.04
LF (s^2)	535.80 ± 1046.8	1455.20 ± 2759.60
HF (s^2)	766.21 ± 1684.1	1124.80 ± 2202.30
$\alpha 1$	0.84 ± 0.39	0.80 ± 0.44
$\alpha 2$	1.00 ± 0.42	0.89 ± 0.51
Entropy	0.67 ± 0.16	0.62 ± 0.20

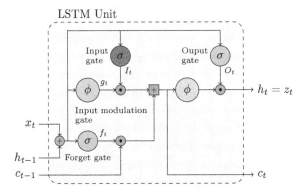

Fig. 2. Long short-term memory unit [6].

by weights determined during the training phase [13]. The advantage these gates bring is that they allow learning long-term relationships more effectively.

The Bidirectional LSTM (BiLSTM) consists of two hidden layers one after another. The additional LSTM layer allows the information flow to be routed in both directions, *i.e.*, the input sequence flows backward in the additional LSTM layer. Therefore, the network is able to learn long terms easier [13]. Figures 2 and 3 illustrates the LSTM unit and biLSTM architecture.

2.5 Classifier Performance

The classifiers performance is evaluated using four metrics. These are accuracy ACC (5) which determines how close a measurement is to the true or accepted value of being true, precision (PRE), referring to how close measurements are to each other, and sensibility (SEN) to evaluate how the parameters and states of the model influence the model output, and F1-Score (F1), measuring the model's accuracy on our dataset. These metrics were evaluated from the equations below:

$$ACC = \frac{TP + TN}{TP + TN + FP + FN} \tag{5}$$

$$PRE = \frac{TP}{TP + FP} \tag{6}$$

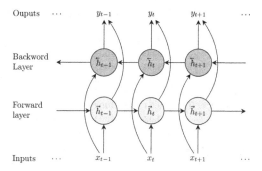

Fig. 3. Bidirectional long short-term memory [6].

$$SEN = \frac{TP}{TP + FN} \tag{7}$$

$$F1 = \frac{2PRE.SEN}{PRE + SEN} \tag{8}$$

The network performance evaluation is measured using four groups of results: TP, TN, FP, and FN. Where TP represents the true positive data, *i.e*, the correctly classified patients as positive; TN represents the true negative, also classified correctly but this time as negative; FP represents the false positive, classified patients improperly as positive; And lastly, FN represents the false negative data, this is, the incorrectly classified data as negative.

The technique used to evaluate the performance of the model, in particular the generalization ability, is k-fold cross-validation. This technique consists of dividing the data (signals) into k groups. Each group is separated to test the estimation obtained by training the other groups [5]. In this study, 5-fold cross-validation was used, meaning the signals are divided into five groups executing five iterations, one for each group.

3   Results and Discussion

In this study, two networks were trained and tested. We tried different quantity combinations of hidden units, epochs, and mini-batch size for better performance. The number of hidden units in an LSTM refers to the dimensionality of the 'hidden state' of the LSTM. The hyperparameter *Epochs* defines the number of times the entire training dataset is processed, and mini-batch size is used for a subset of the dataset to take another step in the learning process. The LSTM model used 30 hidden units, 30 epochs, and 20 mini-batch size were used. The biLSTM model used the same numbers except for the epochs, instead of 30, 20 was used.

Table 2. Training Set LSTM (Hidden Units - 30, maxEpochs - 30, miniBatchsize - 20)

It.	TP	TN	FP	FN	ACC (%)	PRE (%)	SEN (%)	$F1$ (%)
1.º	108	108	0	0	100.00	100.00	100.00	100.00
2.º	107	108	0	1	99.54	100.00	99.07	99.53
3.º	107	108	0	1	99.54	100.00	99.07	99.53
4.º	107	108	0	1	99.54	100.00	99.07	99.53
5.º	107	108	0	1	99.54	100.00	99.07	99.53
mean					99.63	100.00	99.26	99.63

Table 3. Testing Set LSTM (Hidden Units - 30, maxEpochs - 30, miniBatchsize - 20)

It.	TP	TN	FP	FN	ACC (%)	PRE (%)	SEN (%)	F1-Score (%)
1.º	25	26	1	2	94.44	96.15	92.59	94.34
2.º	26	26	1	1	96.30	96.30	96.30	96.30
3.º	27	27	0	0	100.00	100.00	100.00	100.00
4.º	26	25	2	1	94.44	92.86	96.30	94.55
5.º	25	26	1	2	94.44	96.15	92.59	94.34
mean					95.93	96.29	95.56	95.90

Table 4. Training Set biLSTM (Hidden Units - 30, maxEpochs - 20, miniBatchsize - 20)

It.	TP	TN	FP	FN	ACC (%)	PRE (%)	SEN (%)	F1-Score (%)
1.º	107	108	0	1	99.54	100.00	99.07	99.53
2.º	107	108	0	1	99.54	100.00	99.07	99.53
3.º	107	108	0	1	99.54	100.00	99.07	99.53
4.º	107	108	0	1	99.54	100.00	99.07	99.53
5.º	108	108	0	0	100.00	100.00	100.00	100.00
mean					99.63	100.00	99.26	99.63

We applied a 5-fold cross-validation using the 8 features extracted from the signals, such as meanRR, SDNN, pNN50, LF, HF, α_1, α_2, and entropy. The 270 signals were divided into 80% of the data for train, and the last 20% for the test classifier, then 216 signals train the model and the last 54 test it. From the 270 signals, 135 of them are from a normal sinus signal, more precisely, the first 256 beats from the normal signal. The other 135 signals are from a signal that precedes a ventricular tachyarrhythmia episode, and it was only used the last 256 beats before the abnormal episode happens.

Tables 2, 3, 4 and 5 presents the obtained results. The best result are achieved with the biLSTM with 30 hidden units, 20 epochs, and 20 mini-batch size, getting an accuracy of 95.93%, 96.29% of precision, 95.56% of sensibility, and lastly, 95.90% of F1-score. On the other hand, with the LSTM, the results were very similar, but slightly lower than the biLSTM. It used 30 hidden units and 20 mini-batch size, changing only the number of epochs to 30. It reached an accuracy of 96.30%, 94.07% of precision, 98.45% of sensibility and 96.17% of F1-Score.

Table 5. Testing Set biLSTM (Hidden Units - 30, maxEpochs - 20, miniBatchsize - 20)

It.	TP	TN	FP	FN	ACC (%)	PRE (%)	SEN (%)	F1-Score (%)
1.º	26	27	0	1	98.15	100.00	96.30	98.11
2.º	24	26	1	3	92.59	96.00	88.89	92.31
3.º	27	27	0	0	100.00	100.00	100.00	100.00
4.º	26	26	1	1	96.30	96.30	96.30	96.30
5.º	24	27	0	3	94.44	100.00	88.89	94.12
mean					96.30	94.07	98.46	96.17

4   Conclusion and Future Work

This work considered LSTM and BiLSTM networks to predict humans from having a ventricular tachyarrhythmia episode, *i.e.*, Ventricular Fibrillation or Ventricular Tachycardia, using a dataset retrieved from PhysioNET. Features were extracted from the RR intervals considering 270 signals from the RR intervals retrieved from the dataset. The data was separated in 80% and 20% for training and testing, respectively. The results indicate that using deep learning with features extraction from the RR intervals, it is possible to prevent with high accuracy a VTA event.

The BiLSTM network normally has higher accuracy than the LSTM network outperforming it by 0.4% in the mean accuracy. Thus by using this method it is possible to detect an episode of ventricular tachycardia or fibrillation and allow the patient to ask for quick assistance when needed. The best result of the BiLSTM was obtained using RR intervals features extraction obtaining 96.30% accuracy, 94.07% precision, 98.45% sensibility, and 96.17% F1-Score. Although the results between the two neural networks were really close, biLSTM got a slightly better outcome. Future work can be developed, focusing on trying a different group of features that could raise the accuracy.

References

1. Electrophysiology, task force of the European society of cardiology the north American society of pacing: heart rate variability: standards of measurement, physiological interpretation, and clinical use. Circulation **93**(5), 1043–1065 (1996)
2. Faust, O., Shenfield, A., Kareem, M., San, T.R., Fujita, H., Acharya, U.R.: Automated detection of atrial fibrillation using long short-term memory network with RR interval signals. Comput. Biol. Med. **102**, 327–335 (2018)
3. Goldberger, A.L., et al.: PhysioBank, PhysioToolkit, and PhysioNet: components of a new research resource for complex physiologic signals. Circulation **101**(23), e215–e220 (2000)
4. Joo, S., Choi, K.J., Huh, S.J.: Prediction of ventricular tachycardia by a neural network using parameters of heart rate variability. In: 2010 Computing in Cardiology, pp. 585–588. IEEE (2010)
5. Karal, Ö.: Performance comparison of different kernel functions in SVM for different k value in k-fold cross-validation. In: 2020 Innovations in Intelligent Systems and Applications Conference (ASYU), pp. 1–5. IEEE (2020)

6. Monteiro, S., Leite, A., Solteiro Pires, E.J.: Deep learning on automatic fall detection. In: 2021 IEEE Latin American Conference on Computational Intelligence (LA-CCI), pp. 1–6 (2021). https://doi.org/10.1109/LA-CCI48322.2021.9769783

7. Parsi, A., O'Loughlin, D., Glavin, M., Jones, E.: Prediction of sudden cardiac death in implantable cardioverter defibrillators: a review and comparative study of heart rate variability features. IEEE Rev. Biomed. Eng. **13**, 5–16 (2019)

8. Peng, C.K., Havlin, S., Stanley, H.E., Goldberger, A.L.: Quantification of scaling exponents and crossover phenomena in nonstationary heartbeat time series. Chaos: Interdisc. J. Nonlin. Sci. **5**(1), 82–87 (1995)

9. Pincus, S.M.: Approximate entropy as a measure of system complexity. Proc. Natl. Acad. Sci. **88**(6), 2297–2301 (1991)

10. Riasi, A., Mohebbi, M.: Prediction of ventricular tachycardia using morphological features of ECG signal. In: 2015 The International Symposium on Artificial Intelligence and Signal Processing (AISP), pp. 170–175. IEEE (2015)

11. Sanghera, R., Sanders, R., Husby, M., Bentsen, J.G.: Development of the subcutaneous implantable cardioverter-defibrillator for reducing sudden cardiac death. Ann. N. Y. Acad. Sci. **1329**(1), 1–17 (2014)

12. Sengupta, S., et al.: Emotion specification from musical stimuli: an EEG study with AFA and DFA. In: 2017 4th International Conference on Signal Processing and Integrated Networks (SPIN), pp. 596–600. IEEE (2017)

13. Siami-Namini, S., Tavakoli, N., Namin, A.S.: The performance of LSTM and BiLSTM in forecasting time series. In: 2019 IEEE International Conference on Big Data (Big Data), pp. 3285–3292. IEEE (2019)

14. Taye, G.T., Hwang, H.J., Lim, K.M.: Application of a convolutional neural network for predicting the occurrence of ventricular tachyarrhythmia using heart rate variability features. Sci. Rep. **10**(1), 1–7 (2020)

Development of a Wrist Rehabilitation Game with Haptic Feedback

Erik Lamprecht⬥, Alireza Abbasimoshaei(✉)⬥, and Thorsten A. Kern⬥

Institute for Mechatronics in Mechanics, Hamburg University of Technology,
21073 Hamburg, Germany
al.abbasimoshaei@tuhh.de

Abstract. Our hands are the primary body part to interact with objects around us and perform most daily activities. Consequently, a disability of the hand after a stroke or an injury is one of the most severe restrictions to an independent life. To regain the function of the hand, physical therapy is used. Since the resulting rehabilitation process is slow and exhausting, there is a demand to use technology to create a way for patients to train medical exercises independently.

In this paper, a rehabilitation system is presented that allows the patient to independently train medical wrist exercises while playing a serious video game. To identify the requirements, an analysis of previous systems is presented. The designed system consists of a haptic robot with a mechanical support structure that records the hand movements and inputs them into the rehabilitation game. The wrist and forearm movements of flexion & extension, radial & ulnar deviation and supination & pronation can be trained through this. To allow for the biggest possible usability throughout the therapy process, haptic feedback is used to either support the patient's movement or offer resistance, which especially allows the use of passive training in the early stages of therapy.

Keywords: Haptic robotics · Rehabilitation robotics · Serious video game

1 Introduction

A stroke is a drastic event in the life of everybody who had to undergo such an incident. 2.4% of the male and 2.6% of the female population in Germany survived a stroke [4]. In addition to the immediate medical consequences, strokes are also a major reason for disabilities of the upper extremities. 38.4% of male and 39.2% of female stroke victims experience hemiparesis as an acute stroke symptom [6].

While such an occurrence in itself already requires the patient to run through immediate serious medical interventions, the process of fully recovering to the former medical status can last for months or even years. This is not only physically exhausting but also poses a serious challenge to the mental state of the

A. Cunha et al. (Eds.): MobiHealth 2022, LNICST 484, pp. 61–68, 2023.
https://doi.org/10.1007/978-3-031-32029-3_6

patient. A person who was previously healthy is suddenly in permanent need of support to manage activities of daily living. The slow process of regaining the ability to perform the basic movements necessary to carry out trivial tasks that once were ordinary can become very frustrating for the patient.

Conventional physical therapy aims to restore motor functions as well as coordination through movement exercises done by the patient with the help of a therapist. While this process can significantly improve the medical state of the patient, it requires the constant attendance of a therapist or a doctor. As a result, physical therapy is a very staff-intensive and expensive process. This leads to challenges in the medical sector which is often understaffed and overburdened. Consequently, the patient often does not receive as many therapy sessions as would be necessary for his medical state or the interval of therapy sessions is larger than it should be. Therefore the therapy that is essential for the patient to recover his health and thereby regain his independent life back often has a slow progress rate and needs a lot of time. This can result in frustration and even depression and can lead to premature disengagement with the therapy.

An approach to solve that problem is the use of a force feedback capable haptic robot to support the physical therapy. Such a robot can be used by the patient to perform movement exercises independently of a therapist. By that, it is not intended to replace the therapist with the robot but to use the robot as an additional tool in the therapy. The therapist can give the patient exercises to train with the robot and then use the measured data to assess the rehabilitation progress. The gained independence results in an improved mental state of the patient and allows the therapist to focus on diagnosing the patient and developing a therapy plan while the patient can partially train the exercises on his own.

A further approach to improve the therapy process is to combine the haptic robot with a serious video game. Through this, the repetitive and arduous exercises are placed in an engaging and motivating environment. Furthermore, known mechanics from video games can be utilized by this. To beat a level or to set a new high-score in a video game can be a far more motivating goal than to successfully perform a therapeutic exercise. While the training of physical therapy may be seen as work, a serious video game has the potential to change this perception and make training an entertaining activity that people enjoy doing.

Seven different games for haptic desktop systems were found and analyzed to understand the current state of research and to identify the requirements and needs for the design process. Four of them [1,3,7,9] focused on the specific task of drawing and writing or for the hand to follow a trajectory. The other three systems [2,5,10] focused on more general hand movements in different game environments, like a virtual ice hockey system or a spaceship in a blood vessel.

After analyzing these systems, it was found that most systems do not provide sources for the trained movements. As a result, an analysis of requirements from physical therapy was conducted, which led to the selection of specific motions which were already used in conventional therapy and thereby have a proven benefit for the rehabilitation process. It was also found that most analyzed games are not more than a virtual simulation of the used movements. To allow for the biggest possible engagement of the patient, it was decided that the developed serious video game, while having the main focus on the trained movements, also should contain some amount of decision making.

2   Game Design

2.1   Used System

The touch X is a stationary haptic desktop device that can input precise positional and rotational information into a computer. Moreover, the touch X also can be used as an output device to apply forces or guide and restrict movements. The game was created in the Unity game engine.

2.2   Game-Play

Since the movement itself is already a challenge for the patient, the game mechanics should not be simple and easy to understand. To achieve this, the concept of a microworld [8] was deployed. The resulting game should be real enough so the situation and objective can be understood immediately but simple enough to understand the rules and the goal of the game. Subsequently, the game is a simplified version of a real-life scenario.

The chosen game scenario is a vastly simplified driving simulation. [Fig. 1.] It is a situation that everybody can identify and understand immediately. The objective of preventing a crash and staying on the road is natural in this situation and requires no further explanation, even for persons who have never driven a car before.

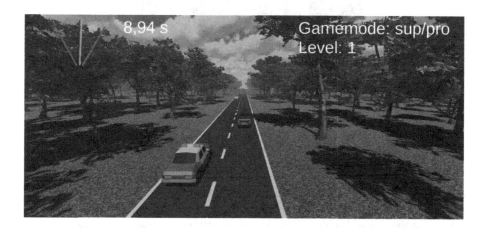

Fig. 1. Screenshot of the game-play

The central game object is a police car that is driving on a multi-lane highway. The car is constantly moving forward and thereby travels through the in-game environment. There are also other cars driving on the highway at a slower speed which have to be bypassed to prevent an accident. Therein lies the central gameplay challenge, which is to change the lane the car is driving in to always be on the free lane. This lane change is induced by the patient through the successful performance of a medical exercise. An exercise counts as successfully executed if the patient rotates his hand from the middle, neutral position to a predetermined angle threshold. A level is finished if the patient avoids all collisions until a timer runs out.

2.3   UI

To avoid frustration over an unclear game mechanic, it is essential to give clear feedback to the patient while the game is played. To achieve that, a graphical interface [Fig. 2.] was created to permanently provide information on the current position of the patient's hand in relation to the neutral position and the angle thresholds to the left and right. This is implemented through four coloured lines in the top left corner of the screen. The blue line in the upright position represents the neutral position. To the left and the right, two red lines represent the angle difference the patient has to overcome to successfully complete the exercise. While these lines are always stationary, the green line moves according to the patient's inputs. This line turns yellow if a movement exercise was started but is not finished yet.

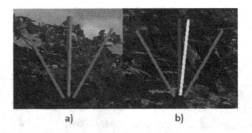

Fig. 2. Graphical interface a) Next exercise can be performed b) Patient has to return to neutral position

2.4   Adjustable Parameters

To allow the biggest possible usability throughout the therapy process, a number of game parameters can be freely adjusted for each level individually. Through that, the difficulty of the game and the difficulty of the movement exercise can grow with the progress the patient makes to keep the game interesting and challenging (Table 1).

Table 1. Available game parameters

Parameter	Explanation
Lanes	Number of lanes the highway has min.2 max.4
Movement angle left in degree	Threshold to complete the movement exercise in the left direction
Movement angle right in degree	Threshold to complete the movement exercise in the right direction
Movement angle neutral in degree	Threshold around the 0° position that counts as neutral position
Speed in $\frac{m}{s}$	Speed of the car the patient is controlling
Distance between obstacles in m	Minimal distance between cars, busses or trucks that block the lanes
Time in s	Time the level has to be played to complete it

Furthermore, the strength and mode of the force feedback can be freely adjusted. Three feedback modes are available. In the passive game mode, the hand of the patient is moved through the robot, which enables the system to employ passive training. In the active game mode, no force feedback is applied, and the touch X robot is used as an input device only. The active resistance game mode applies a force against the movement direction of the patient's hand to train strength and endurance. For all game modes, the amount of force is individually adjustable for each level.

2.5   Input and Output

For the integration of the developed system into the therapy process, it is necessary that the setup and use of the system can be done with only basic computer skills. To allow for an easy way to alter the adjustable parameters, two different input methods are provided. A fast and simple setup can be made in the menu of the game to allow for spontaneous use of the system. This menu also allows the patient to directly recreate the last used settings. For more complex inputs, an input document [Fig. 3.] exist, that is based on a standard spreadsheet document. Through that, a level structure can be created were each parameter can be set for each level individually. As a result, it is possible to always adjust the difficulty of the game and the trained movements to the specific needs and capabilities of the patient.

Furthermore, an output document exists, where important data for each movement, like direction, travelled distance and speed, is automatically tracked to allow the patient to receive feedback on his improvement and enable the

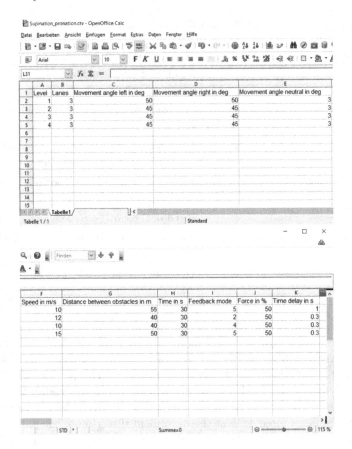

Fig. 3. Input document

therapist to assess the therapy progress. To make this easily usable, the output document also uses the format of a standard spreadsheet document.

2.6   Forearm Support Stand

Additionally to the serious video game, a mechanical stand [Fig. 4.] for the forearm of the patient was developed and constructed. This stand serves multiple purposes. Firstly it gives the patient physically support while playing, which is important since the strength of the upper extremity is severely limited after a stroke. Secondly, it allows for a better contact between the hand of the patient and the robot by providing a bigger surface to grasp the robot in order to play the game. Thirdly it has the role of restricting the possible movements, so no other motions than the desired medical exercise are possible. This is especially important for passive training, where the hand of the patient is moved by the robot while the patient himself can have very limited control of the hand. It is necessary to restrict the movement since the touch X cannot directly apply torque. Since the trained movements are, for the most part, rotatory motions, attachment points for the robot are integrated into the forearm support stand, which creates a stable axis of rotation for each movement exercise.

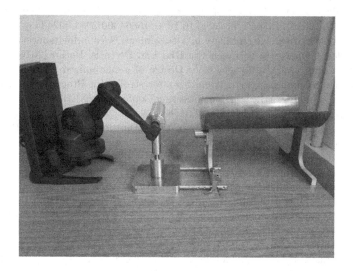

Fig. 4. System in the configuration for the ulnar and radial deviation game-mode

3   Conclusion and Future Work

In this work, a serious video game was developed that allows the patient to independently train medical exercises with the use of a haptic robot. The game features a simplified driving simulation in which the patient controls a car on a highway through the performance of medical exercises. The difficulty of the game and the exercises can be freely adjusted to allow for the biggest usability throughout the therapy process. The data for all movements are logged to be used by the therapist to evaluate the progress of the therapy. All inputs and outputs happen through standard spreadsheet documents or in the game itself to allow for an easy use of the system. Additionally, a mechanical support stand was constructed to support the patient while playing and restrict the possible movements.

To further verify the system and to receive feedback from therapists and patients, a patient trial is currently prepared.

References

1. Auguste-Rampersad, D., Medford, G., Kanneh, A.: Haptics and post stroke rehabilitation of the hand: immersive gaming using haptics to motivate patients to continue repetitive exercises needed for rehabilitation after stroke. In: 2018 IEEE Symposium on Computer Applications Industrial Electronics (ISCAIE), pp. 422–427 (2018). https://doi.org/10.1109/ISCAIE.2018.8405510

2. Broeren, J., Sunnerhagen, K.S., Rydmark, M.: Haptic virtual rehabilitation in stroke: transferring research into clinical practice. Phys. Ther. Rev. **14**, 322–335 (2009). https://doi.org/10.1179/108331909X12488667117212

3. Covarrubias, M., Bordegoni, M., Cugini, U.: Haptic trajectories for assisting patients during rehabilitation of upper extremities. Comput. Aided Des. Appl. **12**, 218–225 (2015). https://doi.org/10.1080/16864360.2014.962434

4. Robert Koch-Institut. Gesundheit in Deutschland. Gesundheitsberichterstattung des Bundes. Gemeinsam getragen von RKI und Destatis. Berlin (2015)

5. Lafond, I., Qiu, Q., Adamovich, S.V.: Design of a customized virtual reality simulation for retraining upper extremities after stroke. In: Proceedings of the 2010 IEEE 36th Annual Northeast Bioengineering Conference (NEBEC), pp. 1–2 (2010). https://doi.org/10.1109/NEBC.2010.5458130

6. Lisabeth, L.D., et al.: Acute stroke symptoms. Stroke **40**(6), 2031–2036 (2009). https://www.ahajournals.org/doi/abs/10.1161/STROKEAHA.109.546812, https://doi.org/10.1161/STROKEAHA.109.546812

7. Pareek, S., Chembrammel, P., Kesavadas, T.: Development and evaluation of haptics-based rehabilitation system. In: 2018 International Symposium on Medical Robotics (ISMR), pp. 1–6 (2018). https://doi.org/10.1109/ISMR.2018.8333298

8. Rieber, L.P.: Seriously considering play: Designing interactive learning environments based on the blending of microworlds, simulations, and games. Educ. Technol. Res. Devel. **44**, 43–58 (1996)

9. Wang, X., Li, J.: Feasibility of a tele-rehabilitation system with corrective-force. In: 2011 International Conference on Virtual Reality and Visualization, pp. 259–262 (2011). https://doi.org/10.1109/ICVRV.2011.14

10. Yang, X., et al.: Hand tele-rehabilitation in haptic virtual environment. In: 2007 IEEE International Conference on Robotics and Biomimetics (ROBIO), pp. 154—149 (2007). https://doi.org/10.1109/ROBIO.2007.4522150

Design and Optimization of a Mechanism, Suitable for Finger Rehabilitation

Alireza Abbasimoshaei$^{(\boxtimes)}$ ⓘ, Tim Siefke ⓘ, and Thorsten A. Kern ⓘ

Institute for Mechatronics in Mechanical Engineering, Hamburg University of Technology, Hamburg, Germany

{al.abbasimoshaei,tim.siefke,t.a.kern}@tuhh.de

Abstract. Due to demographic change and the aging of the population, diseases such as strokes are expected to increase over the years. In this situation, the medical sector is reaching its capacity limits, making any solution that takes over time-intensive treatments that can be standardised relevant for the future. In this paper, a mechanism for finger rehabilitation therapy is presented. After identifying the requirements, a detailed investigation of the current situation of hand rehabilitation devices is presented. A working prototype for fingers is designed and built to show the capabilities of the mechanism. It can be operated independently and is adaptable to different hand sizes. The prototype consists of a linear microdrive connected to the finger mechanism via Bowden cables. Additive manufacturing (AM) was mainly used as the production method. The prototype was successfully tested on four people with hands of different sizes. It allowed an actuation of 85 to 110° for all joints. Different settings of the Bowden cable allow the actuation of different sections of the finger. Different settings of the mechanism, actuator, control analysis and optimization are presented.

Keywords: Finger rehabilitation · Bowden cables · Control system

1 Introduction

The human hand is one of the most versatile limbs nature has ever created, and it plays a significant role in the evolution of the species. Strokes are one of the most common diseases affecting the neurological functions needed to control the human hand. More than 200,000 patients suffer from it every year, in Germany alone [1]. Studies show that immediate therapy involving repetitive movements of the paralyzed limb helps to regain normal function more quickly [2]. Depending on the focus of the work, different approaches can be used to classify hand rehabilitation devices. According to Yue et al. [3], devices are classified into three categories: Mechanical linkage, cable-controlled and pneumatic/hydraulic mechanisms. Mechanical linkage systems use a direct connection between an energy source such as a motor or actuator and the end effector, which is connected to the fingertip or joint. Cable-driven mechanisms for rehabilitation devices can be subdivided based on the use of cables or Bowden cables [3]. As the name suggests,

© ICST Institute for Computer Sciences, Social Informatics and Telecommunications Engineering 2023
Published by Springer Nature Switzerland AG 2023. All Rights Reserved
A. Cunha et al. (Eds.): MobiHealth 2022, LNICST 484, pp. 69–77, 2023.
https://doi.org/10.1007/978-3-031-32029-3_7

the Bowden cable relies on the pulling of the cables to generate torque for the joints. The movement of the Bowden cable is not as precise as that of the cable pull, as it is not under constant tension. For devices with a high number of degrees of freedom (DOF), Bowden cable mechanisms are used because they have a lower demand for actuators and cables. Hydraulic or pneumatic mechanisms with pneumatic power transmission are not common in rehabilitation or research applications. A disadvantage of the hydraulic approach is that handling a fluid in a medical environment can cause hygiene problems. At best it is water, at worst oil, but this always increases maintenance. Also, vibrotactile is a very useful idea for rehabilitation, but the use of different tactile systems makes the system expensive and difficult to control. So the main aim of this system is to propose a simple system that can be used alongside other vibrotactile systems [4].

2 Design of Mechanism

Some basic details of the motor functions and structures of the human hand are described here, which are needed to establish the requirements for the design process of the mechanism. Then a diagram of the functionality of the rehabilitation device, the requirements and the design steps and the derived units are explained.

2.1 Anatomy of the Hand

The fingers of the human hand have three joints: the MCP, PIP and DIP. They are all hinge joints that allow one degree of freedom. The thumb is an exception, as the MCP is positioned at the wrist and thus represents two DOF saddle joints (Fig. 1).

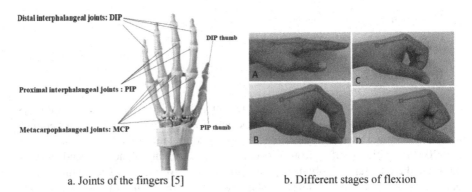

a. Joints of the fingers [5]   b. Different stages of flexion

Fig. 1. Schematic of finger and its flexion

Research has shown that studies that focused on a single movement of all three finger joints resulted in a very complicated and large device [6, 7]. This would clash with the requirement for a simple and cost-effective design. Therefore, this study focuses on the two proximal joints of the finger (MCP and PIP joints). Table 1 shows the different flexion angles of the individual joints according to Fig 1b.

Table 1. Joint angles in different stages of flexion

	MCP	PIP	DIP	SUM
A	0	0	0	0
B	50	40	20	110
C	45	55	40	140
D	65	95	55	215

2.2 Requirements

The first step in developing a mechanism for rehabilitating fingers is to define the requirements on which the following steps will then be based. Figure 2 shows the general structure of the desired device. All requirements in terms of weight, size, portability, operating
time, harmlessness and efficiency should be evaluated. This system should weigh less
than 1.5 kg and the flexion/extension angle should be between 100° and 140°.

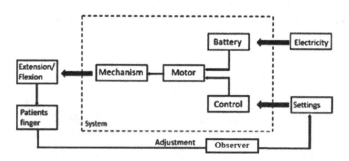

Fig. 2. Block diagram of the rehabilitation device functionality

2.3 Iterative Design

2.3.1 Approach

Based on a literature review and after weighing the advantages and disadvantages of the
approaches mentioned in the introduction, the decision was made in favour of cable-
controlled mechanisms. They can harness the potential of additive manufacturing (AM)
for efficient design at a low cost, while the solid and durable steel cable provides the
power transmission. This was preferred because the surface quality and durability of the
AM parts could not be guaranteed. The Bowden cable can perform movements in both
directions and requires only one drive, one fixation point and one guide for flexion and
extension of the finger. This advantage over cable mechanisms leads to the decision to
use the Bowden cable. Since this work develops a mechanism that can be used for all
kinds of devices, a versatile applicability should be ensured.

2.3.2 Design

In this step, two different design approaches were considered and tested, the problems of the first design were analyzed and a new approach for the second design was developed. The problem of unnatural movement of the fingers was solved by moving the mechanism to the back of the finger and passing the attachments through the side space only. The two cables on each side of the finger and their guides were combined in a bridge on the top of the finger (Fig. 3). On the back of the hand, the baseboard (Fig. 3a–4) is mounted, to which the first segment (Fig. 3a–1) of the mechanism is attached. This segment is identical to the most distal segment (Fig. 3a–3). The adjustable length for different finger sizes is solved by dividing the middle part of the mechanism (Fig. 3a–2), which lies on the first finger segment (phalanx proximal). Section A in Fig. 3a shows this in the top view of the mechanism.

Looking at a prototype for different fingers shows the principles that can be adapted to form a complete hand rehabilitation device. The mechanism is designed to be modular to fit all fingers, but the connections and details to build the whole device are not addressed. Nevertheless, a possible solution for the different mechanical situations on the thumb was considered. Cheng et al. used an extension of their base plate to reach the thumb [8]. This idea was taken up and extended. To make the system suitable for different uses, a rotation axis was added to the extension plate to allow different thumb positions for maximum applicability.

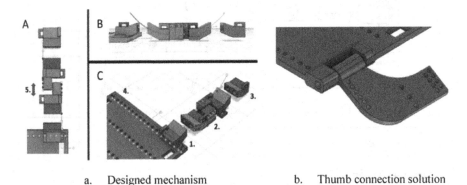

a.   Designed mechanism   b.   Thumb connection solution

Fig. 3. Designed mechanism and Thumb

The Bowden cable mechanism has already been identified as a practical way to transmit the force of the actuator and transfer the torque to the joint. Cheng et al. [8] used a 0.265 mm cable for the pulley mechanism in their development. Initially, a twisted steel cable with a diameter of 0.8 mm was chosen for the system, but it turned out that this size was too thin to transmit the force. A small resistance on the mechanism resulted in a bend before the first segment. After increasing the diameter to 1.5 mm, which could not be bent to a required radius, the perfect size of 1 mm was found. The tab at the end of the cable is connected to a pin or screw on the linear actuator and moves through the holes in the segments of the mechanism. Additive manufacturing is used as the crucial production technology. Better known as 3D printing, additive manufacturing enables new possibilities in engineering and design. As the name of the process suggests, an object is made by joining materials together.

2.4 Drive Units

To operate the stiff Bowden cable, it was decided to use a linear actuator. This allows a precise movement and defines the actuation of the cable. The Bowden cable does not bend around an axis of rotation, thus preventing frictional forces and deformation. After a complete research and a market comparison, the Actuonix L12/16 micro linear actuators (see Fig. 4) proved to be the best choice to meet the requirements.

In this system, the LAC board automatically reduces the input voltage from 12 V to 3.3 V at the P+/P− terminal for the potentiometer. The control is done by a voltage adjusted with a potentiometer. A potentiometer with 10 kilo-ohm (kΩ) and a rotation angle of the rotary switch of 270° was chosen. Measurements were taken to determine the actual speed at the different angles of rotation of the switch, and the average of four measurements was taken to reduce the error due to manual data collection. It is noticeable that the actuator is slightly faster on the way back than on the way out. This should be taken into account when setting the speed manually and not via the software. Table 2 shows the stroke times for different speeds.

Table 2. Stroke times for different speeds

Speed	100%		75%		50%		25%	
Time (s): Forward/Backward	6.0	5.6	6.7	6.3	7.5	7.1	13.4	12.6
mm/s	6.7	7.1	6	6.3	5.3	5.6	3	3.2

A 12 volt (V) lithium battery with 11 ampere hours (Ah) was chosen to supply the required energy. The actuator's data sheet gives a quiescent current of 650 milliamps (mA) at 12 V voltage. The device was tested on the left hands of four different people. Care was taken to include different hand sizes in the sample. In all cases, the prototype was attached to the hand and was able to actuate the finger in the desired manner. When the device was mounted, the connection between the mechanism and the actuator made the mechanical transmission of the force difficult. This led to a high risk of this part getting jammed. After you have attached the device to your finger and switched it on, you can control the stroke of the actuator with the rotary switch on the control box. When the settings are adjusted, you can control the speed, the accuracy and the end positions of the stroke with the small screws on the board LAC. When the settings have been changed, the board LAC must be switched on before the adjustments take effect.

You can see the extension and flexion in the two cable set-ups in Fig. 5a–B. The mechanism is able to flex the finger joints by 85° to 110°. The second set-up locks the MCP and only actuates the two distal joints of the finger (PIP and DIP). This allows a combined angle of 80° to 100° for these joints. Possible factors for the variation of the determined angle are Installation position and precision, finger size, actuator, influence

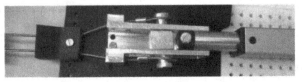

a.   Assembled connector

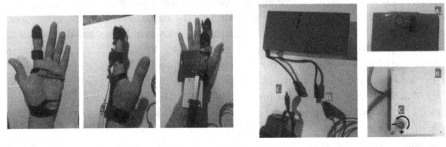

b.   Mounting of the device   c.   Electric components

Fig. 4. Designed and assembled mechanism

of the cable connection by the test person, hand orientation. Figure 5b shows the device for the whole hand.

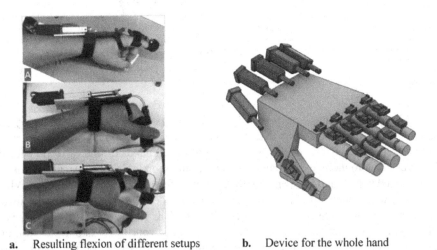

a.   Resulting flexion of different setups   **b.**   Device for the whole hand

Fig. 5. The designed mechanism, its flexibility, and 3-D geometry

2.5 Closed-Loop Controlling System

To ensure safe rehabilitation, such a positioning system needs adequate speed control. For this purpose, three control approaches were analyzed with Simulink, presented in the following section and ordered according to their complexity. In this study, three different variants of the Simulink models were analyzed in detail. The three variants are ordered according to their complexity. The first is a simple model of a unidirectional system. The second variant allows changing the direction and the type of movement. The third variant is the final, complete simulation that includes noise and disturbances. For each DoF of the system, there is a characteristic threshold angle. This angle represents the physiologically maximum permissible angle necessary to ensure patient safety [9]. This robot can be configured to allow flexion and extension of a finger. The third variant of the system is the final and most complete robot model. However, the second variant only represents an ideal situation in which the system block operates without interference or noise. To simulate a more realistic situation, noise and interference are necessary additions. To test and analyze the behaviour of the system with these external influences, one must consider the third variant of the model (Fig. 6).

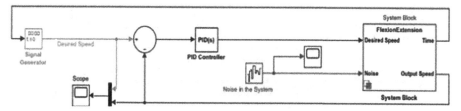

Fig. 6. The General Model of the 3rd Variant

The controller used is a PID controller. Three different tuning methods are implemented: manual tuning, MATLAB automatic tuning and Ziegler-Nichols tuning method, and after comparing the results, the manual tuning method is chosen. In manual tuning, the coefficients of the PID controller are changed manually depending on the main output. The aim of manual tuning is to design the controller in such a way that the overshoot remains close to zero, i.e. below 1%, and the rise time and settling time are significantly reduced. Ideally, the rise and settling time should be kept below 0.05 s. The results for the middle finger are shown in Table 3. From these results and the diagram shown in Fig. 7, it can be concluded that the tuned response is suitable for the system and that the system is stable.

Table 3. Variant 2 and variant 3 PID Parameters and Response (Manual Tuning)

Variant 2		Variant 3	
Controller Parameters		Controller Parameters	
P	10	P	20

(continued)

Table 3. (*continued*)

Variant 2		Variant 3	
Controller Parameters		Controller Parameters	
I	450	I	1000
D	0.01	D	0.01
N	100	N	100
Rest time	0.000612 s	Rest time	0,000296 s
Settling time	0.00111 s	Settling time	0.000846 s
Overshoot	0	Overshoot	5.73%
Peak	0.99	Peak	1.06
Gain margin	-	Gain margin	-
Phase margin	74.8deg@ 2.61e^{+03} rad/s	Phase margin	63.3deg@ 4.62e^{+03} rad/s
Closed-loop stability	Stable	Closed-loop stability	Stable

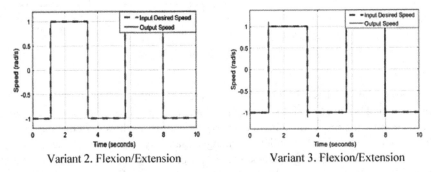

Variant 2. Flexion/Extension   Variant 3. Flexion/Extension

Fig. 7. Manually Tuned Response for variant 2 and variant 3

3   Conclusion

In this work, a mechanism was developed to allow external actuation of fingers. A prototype was made using additive manufacturing and connected to a structure that allows testing. It consists of a mechanism with two Bowden cables connected to a linear actuator Actuonix L16 with a stroke of 50 mm. This actuator is controlled by a circuit board that allows the adjustment of stroke length, speed and accuracy. A potentiometer was wired to the board to operate the actuator within the previously set end positions. The mechanism represents a way to implement hand rehabilitation into everyday life. It can actuate the paralyzed fingers and support the rehabilitation process. It can be operated in a mobile way and allows the patient to use it independently. The mechanism can support physiotherapists or provide quick and available rehabilitation when medical facilities reach their capacity limits. The mechanism is designed to fit all fingers. The variation of the middle segment by 6 mm to adjust its length allows for wide application. The segments can be assembled in different ways to suit the situation. For children or people with unusually short fingers, the mechanism may need to be adjusted to function precisely. A solution for the different mechanical situations on the thumb has also been introduced. It focuses on wide applicability in combination with the independent movement of each finger. Normally, rehabilitation devices with less functionality are in the range of 5,000 EUR. Taking into account typical margins, overheads and assembly costs, the purchased components of such a robotic system may not cost more than 1/5 of such a device, resulting in a maximum of 1,000 EUR. For the system presented, which provides a structure for all five fingers, the combined costs are well below this level, reaching 480 EUR in the bill of materials (BOM).

References

1. Wittchen, H.-U., et al.: Gesundheitsberichterstattung des Bundes Heft 21. Robert Koch-Institut, Berlin (2010)
2. Cumming, T.B., et al.: Very early mobilization after stroke fast-tracks return to walking. AHA J. Stroke **42**(1), 153–158 (2010)
3. Yue, Z., Zhang, X., Wang, J.: Hand rehabilitation robotics on poststroke motor recovery. Behav. Neurol. (2017). https://doi.org/10.1155/2017/3908135
4. Seim, C.E., Wolf, S.L., Starner, T.E.: Wearable vibrotactile stimulation for upper extremity rehabilitation in chronic stroke: clinical feasibility trial using the VTS Glove. J. Neuroeng. Rehabil. **18**(1), 1–11 (2021)
5. Khan, A., Giddins, G.: The outcome of conservative treatment of spiral metacarpal fractures and the role of the deep transverse metacarpal ligaments in stabilizing these injuries. J. Hand Surg. (Eur. Vol.) **40**(1), 59–62 (2015)
6. Chiri, A., et al.: HANDEXOS: towards an exoskeleton device for the rehabilitation of the hand. In: 2009 IEEE/RSJ International Conference on Intelligent Robots and Systems, pp. 1106–1111 (2009). https://doi.org/10.1109/IROS.2009.5354376
7. Wege, A., Zimmermann, A.: Electromyography sensor based control for a hand exoskeleton. In: 2007 IEEE International Conference on Robotics and Biomimetics (ROBIO), pp. 1470–1475 (2007). https://doi.org/10.1109/ROBIO.2007.4522381
8. Cheng, L., Chen, M., Li, Z.: Design and control of a wearable hand rehabilitation robot. IEEE Access **6**, 74039–74050 (2018). https://doi.org/10.1109/ACCESS.2018.2884451
9. Holzbaur, K.R.S., et al.: Upper limb muscle volumes in adult subjects. J. Biomech. **40**(4), 742–749 (2007). https://doi.org/10.1016/j.jbiomech.2006.11.011

Health Information Systems

Highlighting the Danger of Water Storage Zones in Baixo Tâmega Valley

Jorge Pinto[1], Sandra Pereira[1(✉)], Cristina Reis[2], Paula Braga[3], and Isabel Bentes[1]

[1] UTAD/CMADE, Vila Real, 5000-801 Vila Real, Portugal
{tiago,spereira,ibentes}@utad.pt
[2] UTAD/CONSTRUCT/INEGI, 5000-801 Vila Real, Portugal
crisreis@utad.pt
[3] UTAD/INEGI, 5000-801 Vila Real, Portugal
plsilva@utad.pt

Abstract. This paper intends to highlight the problem of water-related accidents using Baixo Tâmega Valley, in Portugal, as a study case. Water storage zones can be a threat. There is no yet specific Portuguese standard to guide these infrastructures. In rural areas, this kind of risk also exists. It is very likely to find rivers, brooks, river beaches, swimming pools, washing tanks, fountains, watering holes, and wells, among others, in this type of low-density population site. Unfortunately, every summer, there are always victims of drowning and other water-related kinds of accidents. In this region, during the summer of 2020, there was a significant boom in swimming pool construction due to the COVID-19 pandemic that made it impossible to go abroad. Therefore, some examples of the above-identified existing water storage zones will be presented, some figures concerning water-related accidents will be delivered, and some technical aspects that may avoid this type of accident will also be introduced. The obtained conclusions may be extended to other rural regions.

Keywords: Water storage zones · rural areas · safety · Baixo Tâmega Valley

1 Introduction

Baixo Tâmega Valley is located in the Douro Litoral county and near the border between this county and the Trás-os-Montes e Alto Douro county, Portugal. It is a hilly area. The Tâmega river dictates the landscape, and, in this part, it almost reaches the Douro river. It is a very green scenario because it is a rainy region. Therefore, there are a lot of pine trees and green wine vineyards. Agriculture has been one of the main activities.

Considering these remarks makes sense that it is very likely to find water reservoirs such as rivers, brooks, river beaches, swimming pools, washing tanks, fountains, watering holes, and wells, among other water storage zones.

On the other hand, tourism is also an emerging activity in this region. Principally due to the wine industry and the beauty of the landscape.

A. Cunha et al. (Eds.): MobiHealth 2022, LNICST 484, pp. 81–89, 2023.
https://doi.org/10.1007/978-3-031-32029-3_8

In this context, a boom of touristic accommodation has occurred and there has been a significant increase in building. Traditional dwellings have been reformulated to work as tourist accommodations.

In parallel, the COVID-19 pandemic has enormously changed daily life and resulted in considerable constraints in our way of living. Having holidayed in public places and abroad was banned, and people had to spend time at home or in private areas. These facts had unexpected results, such as selling off air conditioning and swimming pool accessories during the summer of 2020. There was a dramatic increase in interest in swimming pools and other water storage zones. Therefore, the risk of water accidents also increased.

Drowning has been a neglected health issue, largely absent from the global health and development discourse until the UN General Assembly (UNGA) adopted its first resolution on global drowning prevention in 2021 [1]. Some outlining issue characteristics are stated that interest for the present work: Over 2·5 million preventable deaths in the past decade; Drowning is largely unrecognised relative to its impact; Over 90% of drowning deaths occur in low-income and middle-income countries; Drowning takes place in rivers, lakes, domestic water storage, swimming pools, and coastal waters; Drowning affects children and adolescents in rural areas and presents as a social inequity issue; Drowning prevention could be a Sustainable Development Goal measure for child deaths, and could be framed as protecting investments in child development; Preventable and scalable, low-cost interventions exist.

There are several works published concerning this topic, such as Jonh Pearn et al., which analysed a consecutive series of 66 immersion accidents in swimming pool immersion accidents [2]. Joanna Chan et al. make some recommendations for swimming pools to avoid drowning [3], and Tracynda Davis encompasses new designs found in modern water parks and provides data for regulators to make better-informed judgements for the health and safety of pools [4]. Kyra Hamilton et al. explore the prediction of pool safety habits and intentions [5]. In addition, *Associação para a promoção das Segurança Infantil* (APSI) highlights the drowning tragedy worldwide [6]. American Academy of Pediatrics (AAP) also alerts to the need for measures to prevent drowning [7].

UNICEF states drowning, since 2001, when was the second cause of accidental death in children [8]. Many countries report drowning as the leading cause of childhood mortality, and drowning is among the ten leading causes of death globally for 5- to 14-year-olds [9]. Unfortunately, in Europe, about 5000 children (under 19 years old) drown stated to World Health Organization (WHO) [10]. In Portugal, this is also a tragedy. For instance, from 2002 to 2008, 144 children died by drowning reported by APSI [6] and European Child Safety Alliance (ECSA) [10].

Therefore, drowning is a priority, and there is much work to be done in this area.

Justin-Paul Scarr et al. identify three factors crucial to drowning prevention 1) methodological advancements in population-representative data and evidence for effective interventions; (2) reframing drowning prevention in health and sustainable development terms with an elevated focus on high burdens in low-income and middle-income contexts; and (3) political advocacy by a small coalition [11].

Thus, the main objective of this paper is precise to underling the danger related to water reservoir usage in the Baixo Tâmega region and as an example of the low population density territory of Portugal.

This paper is structured as follows. After this introduction, this region's existing traditional water reservoirs are identified. The next part reflects some technical aspects that may affect water accidents. Some mitigating measures to avoid water accidents are also considered. Finally, the main conclusions are delivered.

The danger of water storage zones in rural areas is highlighted, and some mitigating measures to reduce the risk of accidents are also presented.

2   Some Water Storage Zones in the Region

As stated above, this region is characterised by considerable rainfall. Therefore, it is expected to find different types of water storage zones. There are natural and artificial water storage zones.

In natural water storage zones, we can find rivers (Fig. 1.a) and brooks (Fig. 1.b).

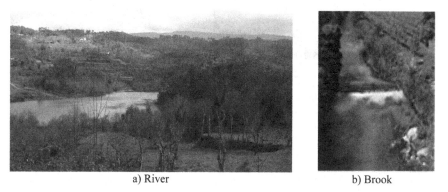

a) River   b) Brook

Fig. 1. Example of an existing river and a brook in the region of the Baixo Tâmega Valley.

In terms of artificial water storage zones, river beaches (Fig. 2.a), swimming pools (Fig. 2.b), washing tanks (Fig. 3.a), fountains (Fig. 3.b), watering holes (Fig. 4.a) and wells (Fig. 4.b) are some types that exist.

On the other hand, artificial water storage zones may be public or private. This fact is quite important because it defines the main entity responsible for the feature and influences the number of people who can access it.

In addition, the artificial water storage zones may have different purposes, such as agricultural (e.g. watering hole), domestic usage (e.g. washing tank and well), and leisure (e.g. river beach and swimming pool), among others.

It is worth adding that the wells in this region are still widely used in isolated houses, and rural areas, for domestic water supply and irrigation.

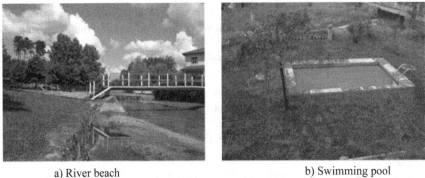

a) River beach   b) Swimming pool

Fig. 2. Example of an existing river beach and a swimming pool in the region of the Baixo Tâmega Valley.

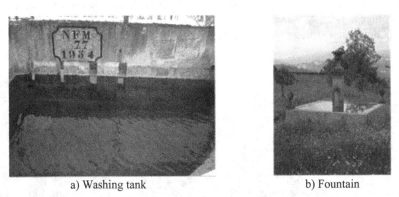

a) Washing tank   b) Fountain

Fig. 3. Example of an existing washing tank and a fountain in the region of the Baixo Tâmega Valley.

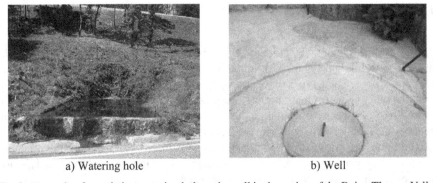

a) Watering hole   b) Well

Fig. 4. Example of an existing watering hole and a well in the region of the Baixo Tâmega Valley.

3 Some Technical Aspects that May Affect Water Accidents

UN General Assembly, in its first resolution on global drowning prevention, outlines some solutions that can be adopted in all countries: Appoint a national focal point for drowning prevention; Develop a national drowning prevention plan; Develop drowning prevention programming in line with WHO recommended interventions; Ensure the enactment and active enforcement of water safety laws across all relevant sectors; Include drowning within civil registration and vital statistics registers; Promote drowning prevention public awareness and behaviour change campaigns; Encourage the integration of drowning prevention within existing disaster risk reduction programmes; Support international cooperation by sharing lessons learned; Promote research and development of innovative drowning prevention tools and technology and Consider the introduction of water safety, swimming, and first-aid lessons as part of school curricula [1].

The above-identified water storage zones have a considerable amount of water and threaten people's safety.

The threat may increase if the purpose of the water storage zones is for leisure and if it is public because more activity may occur as more people use it.

Several kinds of accident consequences can occur in water storage zones, such as drowning, fracture of a human limb, contracting a disease by water contamination, stopping congestion, and falls.

Water flow, depth, accessibility, unpredictability, quality of water, the temperature of water and level of water surface are some technical aspects that can significantly influence the risk of an accident. Given their variability and extension, controlling the technical characteristics mentioned above in natural water storage zones is tough. In this case, displaying information concerning safety measures in critical points may be an excellent mitigating action to prevent accidents and also confining (when possible) access to hazardous areas.

On the other hand, in artificial water storage zones, it seems easier to control these technical aspects. For instance, on river beaches, the water flow and water depth can be controlled by building dams or floodgates. In the other type of water storage zones, such as swimming pools, the water depth can be controlled by considering floors with different levels. However, we must be aware that even very shallow water storage zones are enough to potentiate an accident if we think of an infant.

Accessibility is another important technical aspect that may avoid accidents. Automatic control of the access to the water reservoir by building a fence and having an intelligent control device, increasing the distance, using a rough pavement or using different levels may impede an infant's entrance to the water storage zones, as stated by the Consumer Product Safety Commission (CPSC) [12].

Avoiding unusual geometries and shapes of the reservoir and avoiding unexpected objects or devices below the water level may also reduce danger.

On the other hand, ensuring good water quality is also fundamental to reducing the risk of contracting a disease or accident. Therefore, the water should be tested often. The water treatment process also has to be considered to avoid threats because there may be certain health risks. The quality of the water can also be obtained using an intelligent control/action system.

The temperature of the water can also potentiate accidents. For instance, freezing water can cause a shock and result in a heart attack or digestion stops. The water surface level of the reservoir may also affect the risk of an accident.

The same pavement level and water surrounding the water storage zones may be hazardous. A high level of water surface may be difficult to reach. A deep level may potentiate falling.

These situations can be oblivious to using intelligent systems to control and actuate in dangerous situations, so there is much scientific work to be done in these areas.

4 Some Mitigating Measures

Traditionally, care has been taken to prevent water accidents.

Good evidence supports building and maintaining four-sided fenced polls to prevent drowning. Enclosing the pool (isolation fence) is better than surrounding the property and the pool together because it further reduces the risk of exposure. Recent European research confirms that fences should be at least 1,1m hight, without footholds, to be most effective. Ornamental bar fences are attractive, provide visibility and are harder to climb than chain-like fences, which young children can easily scale [10].

Metal and stone safety barriers were used. Figure 5 shows two examples in which the safety barrier was the technical measure adopted to avoid accidents in water storage zones. At the same time, the swimming pool, Fig. 5.b, was also considered a gate and flower bed borders to work as obstacles from the main house to the water reservoir.

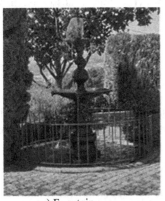 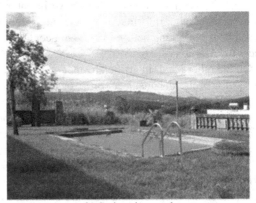

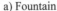

a) Fountain   b) Swimming pool

Fig. 5. Safety barrier, gate and flower bed border.

Creating a barrier between children and water by covering them with heavy grills reduces the risk of drowning. In Portugal, a national law was enacted in 2002 requiring newly constructed wells access points to be a minimum of 80 cm from the ground and have secure covers [10].

On the other hand, the distance between the main house and the water storage zone is another essential technical aspect that can save lives. In the case of Fig. 6, it was possible to have a distance of 9.0 m. There are also obstacles between the path, such as stone artefacts (detail A) and a flower bed border of 1.6 m width. Furthermore, a stone pavement of 2.6 m in width is made of rough granite stones (detail B, Fig. 6). There is also a difference of 1.0 m between the level of the pavement and the swimming pool. All these measures may hinder an infant's access to the swimming pool without them noticing it.

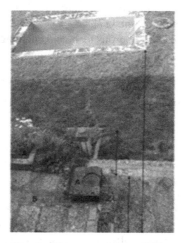

Fig. 6. Distance and accessibility.

At the same time, raising the water level from the soil level may also be an excellent procedure to reduce risk.

Having a proper stair also helps improve the safety of a water storage zone (Fig. 5.b).

When the water level is underground, it seems adequate to use a proper covering that meets all the standards for this type of use.

As the previous works cited show, shifting the response from drowning detection to drowning prevention is imperative.

Closed-Circuit Television (CCTV) cameras cannot prevent swimming pool drownings without image-correction capability, but Artificial Intelligence (AI) technology can transform standard CCTV cameras into intelligent cameras. They effectively see through the water and allow the system to track swimmers doing everything from diving to splashing around. Surface water disturbances, such as waves, ripples and glare, no longer pose a problem. Standard CCTV cameras can be converted into intelligent cameras that utilise AI image-correction software to see everything happening in the swimming pool. Machine learning algorithms recognise the predictable behaviours present when a swimmer is drowning. So combining algorithms and AI image correction can create a one-of-a-kind technology to prevent swimming pool drownings [13, 14].

Cepeda-Pacheco et al. developed a novel 5G and beyond child drowning prevention system based on deep learning that detects and classifies distractions of inattentive parents or caregivers and alerts them to focus on active child supervision in swimming pools [15].

A real-time system that will track swimmers in a pool using machine learning techniques and prevents drowning accidents is proposed by Abdel Alshbatat et al. The system consists of a Raspberry Pi with the Raspbian operating system, a Pixy camera, an Arduino Nano board, stepper motors, an alarm system, and motor drivers. The proposed approach is based on the colour-based algorithm to position and rescue drowning swimmers. The device then sends an alarm to the lifeguards [16].

Nasrin Salehi et al. developed software that can detect a drowning person in indoor swimming pools and sends an alarm to the lifeguard rescues if the previously seen person is missing for a specific amount of time [17].

Alvin Kam et al. investigated numerous technical challenges in developing a novel real-time video surveillance system capable of detecting potential drowning incidents in a swimming pool. In future work, they suggested expanding the sophistication of the existing descriptor set to facilitate more accurate event modelling [18]. This work provides several interesting insights into human detection and tracking within a dynamic environment and the recognition of highly complex events through the incorporation of domain expert knowledge.

5 Main Conclusions

Different existing water storage zone types in the Baixo Tâmega Valley were identified, such as rivers, brooks, river beaches, swimming pools, washing tanks, fountains, watering holes, watering tanks and wells. Most of them are built traditionally.

Several kinds of consequences of accidents related to water reservoirs were identified, and also some technical aspects that may affect this type of accident were indicated.

Some traditional mitigating measures to prevent water accidents were also presented. Safety barriers and gates are the main ones.

Policymakers should pass legislation or building codes to mandate four-sided isolation pool fencing for new and existing residential and non-residential pools.

Most hazards can be oblivious to using intelligent systems to control and actuate in dangerous situations, so there is much scientific work to be done in these areas.

Acknowledgements. This work was supported by the FCT (Portuguese Foundation for Science and Technology) through the project UIDB/04082/2020 (CMADE).

References

1. Assembly, U.G.: Global drowning prevention - Resolution adopted by the General Assembly on 28 April 2021, vol. 75, no. 273 (2021)
2. Pearn, J.H., Nixon, J.: Swimming pool immersion accidents: an analysis from the brisbane drowning study. Med. J. Aust. 3(4), 307–309 (1997). https://doi.org/10.1136/IP.3.4.307
3. Chan, J.S.E., Ng, M.X.R., Ng, Y.Y.: Drowning in swimming pools: clinical features and safety recommendations based on a study of descriptive records by emergency medical services attending to 995 calls. Singap. Med. J. **59**(1), 44 (2018). https://doi.org/10.11622/SMEDJ. 2017021

4. Davis, T.: Water quality of modern water parks. J. Environ. Health **71**(9), 14–19 (2009). https://www.jstor.org/stable/26327917. Accessed 17 Nov 2022

5. Hamilton, K., Peden, A.E., Smith, S., Hagger, M.S.: Predicting pool safety habits and intentions of Australian parents and carers for their young children. J. Safety Res. **71**, 285–294 (2019). https://doi.org/10.1016/j.jsr.2019.09.006

6. Afogamentos de Crianças - Relatório 2002/2010-Afogamentos em Crianças e Jovens em Portugal (2002). www.apsi.org.pt. Accessed 17 Nov 2022

7. Denny, S.A., et al.: Prevention of drowning. Pediatrics **143**(5) (2019). https://doi.org/10.1542/peds.2019-0850

8. Brenner, R.A.: Childhood drowning is a global concern. BMJ **324**(7345), 1049–1050 (2002). https://doi.org/10.1136/bmj.324.7345.1049

9. Meddings, D.R., Scarr, J.P., Larson, K., Vaughan, J., Krug, E.G.: Drowning prevention: turning the tide on a leading killer. Lancet Public Heal. **6**(9), e692–e695 (2021). https://doi.org/10.1016/S2468-2667(21)00165-1

10. Sethi, D., Towner, E., Vincenten, J., Segui-Gomez, M., Racioppi, F.: European report on child injury prevention. World Heal. Organ. (2008). https://apps.who.int/iris/handle/10665/326500. Accessed 17 Nov 2022

11. Scarr, J.P., Buse, K., Norton, R., Meddings, D.R., Jagnoor, J.: Tracing the emergence of drowning prevention on the global health and development agenda: a policy analysis. Lancet Glob. Heal. **10**(7), e1058–e1066 (2022). https://doi.org/10.1016/S2214-109X(22)00074-2

12. U.S Consumer Product Safety Commission, "Safety Barrier Guidelines for Home Pools," no. 362, p. Pub. No. 362

13. Prevention Over Detection: How Machine Learning Saves Lives - Lynxight. https://lynxight.com/blog/prevention-over-detection-how-machine-learning-saves-lives/. Accessed 17 Nov 2022

14. Artificial intelligence system aimed at preventing drownings ǀ AP News. https://apnews.com/article/corals-drownings-artificial-intelligence-easton-426055e1248e454cbb07407425a04b7b. Accessed 17 Nov 2022

15. Cepeda-Pacheco, J.C., Domingo, M.C.: Deep learning and 5G and beyond for child drowning prevention in swimming pools. Sensors **22**(19), 7684 (2022). https://doi.org/10.3390/s22197684

16. Alshbatat, A.I.N., Alhameli, S., Almazrouei, S., Alhameli, S., Almarar, W.: Automated vision-based surveillance system to detect drowning incidents in swimming pools. In: 2020 Advances in Science and Engineering Technology International Conferences (ASET) (2020). https://doi.org/10.1109/ASET48392.2020.9118248

17. Salehi, N., Keyvanara, M., Monadjemmi, S.A.: An automatic video-based drowning detection system for swimming pools using active contours. Int. J. Image, Graph. Signal Process. **8**(8), 1–8 (2016). https://doi.org/10.5815/IJIGSP.2016.08.01

18. Kam, A.H., Lu, W., Yau, W.-Y.: A video-based drowning detection system. In: Heyden, A., Sparr, G., Nielsen, M., Johansen, P. (eds.) ECCV 2002. LNCS, vol. 2353, pp. 297–311. Springer, Heidelberg (2002). https://doi.org/10.1007/3-540-47979-1_20

Measures to Improve Health Performing of an Accommodation Building. A Study Case

Isabel Bentes[1], Sandra Pereira[1(✉)], Teixeira Carla[2], and Jorge Pinto[1]

[1] UTAD/CMADE, Vila Real, 5000-801 Vila Real, Portugal
`{ibentes,spereira,tiago}@utad.pt`
[2] Módulo Curioso, Gabinete de Arquitetura, 5100-065 Lamego, Portugal
`geral@arquitetacarlateixeira.pt`

Abstract. Tourism has been a promising activity in Portugal. There has been an increasing interest in the interior part of this country as a destination. At the same time, there is still a lack of accommodation buildings to follow this trend. Therefore, rehabilitating traditional buildings has been a wise option to deal with this problem. During the rehabilitation process, several challenges emerge because each building has its specification. Thus, this research focuses on the relevance of ventilation to guarantee an adequate healthy environmental habitat. A study case of an accommodation building in Lamego city, Portugal, is used to give more practicality to this topic. At the same time, a ventilation solution is presented as a measure of assuring proper adequate inner air and some future works about automatic control/predictions are delivered. The presented results may give guidance for future rehabilitation processes or may have to solve existing problems concerning this issue.

Keywords: Inner air · Ventilation · Rehabilitation · automatic control

1 Introduction

Traditional dwellings can be rehabilitated for tourism accommodation purposes [1]. Several technical aspects, such as health and comfort in living, are still more critical in this context.

Some technical aspects that must be considered are the views, natural light, space, ventilation, thermal behaviour, acoustic, humidity, and smell.

Considering that traditional dwellings are likely to be placed in the city centres, these concerns tend to increase.

The main goal of this research is to emphasize a natural ventilation system proposed in a rehabilitation process of a traditional Portuguese dwelling in the North of the country that will be used as a tourist accommodation and to present the automatic control system used to manage the temperature, ventilation, and lightning.

The proposed ventilation solution ensured the air quality in the tourism accommodation building. The adopted solution was validated and can be applied in other future

A. Cunha et al. (Eds.): MobiHealth 2022, LNICST 484, pp. 90–99, 2023.
https://doi.org/10.1007/978-3-031-32029-3_9

works of rehabilitation projects - the air quality achieved in the studied building guaranty the health requirement standards of this type of building.

Therefore, this document is structured as follows. After this introduction, a brief description of traditional natural ventilation solutions is done. The introduction of the building used as a study case is presented afterwards, followed by the explanation of the ventilation solution applied in the study case. At this stage, the necessity of the required ventilation system is identified. The description of the adopted technical solution is delivered, and the evaluation of its efficiency is estimated. Finally, the main conclusion is also presented.

2 Traditional Natural Ventilation Solutions

In terms of ventilation, it can be natural or forced. Natural can be considered more sustainable. In contrast, a forced ventilation system may be more high-tech, requiring mechanical devices and energy consumption [2]. On the other hand, forced ventilation may be the only solution considering the specificities of traditional buildings. For instance, the existence of underground floors, the lack of windows or doors, the density of construction, the morphology of the landscape and the insulation can contribute to different ventilation system requirements (natural or forced).

A proper ventilation system allows good air quality in a building and contributes to accommodation comfort. It avoids inconvenient smells and health-related problems such as allergies and breathing difficulties.

At the same time, a proper ventilation system may avoid accidental scenarios such as high carbon monoxide levels that can cause death [3].

Systems like control and prediction are needed to detect other hazards like radon or gases that can be dangerous to health [4–6]. The comfort level of the accommodation is also a concern, and having some control over temperature, humidity, smell, and noise can also help [7–12].

Among traditional Portuguese dwellings, several building technical aspects guarantee natural ventilation. For instance, conventional timber frame windows and doors usually have poor isolation, Fig. 1a. The typical kitchen chimneys allow air circulation from inner and exterior spaces, Fig. 1b. The traditional fireplaces may achieve the same feature, Fig. 2a. Meanwhile, the typical timber pavements and roofs (Fig. 2b) are poorly isolated, allowing natural ventilation through different rooms. Thus, traditional dwellings may guarantee natural ventilation, even if inefficient.

On the other hand, new construction may behave differently, considering that they are much more isolated. Pavements tend to be reinforced and made of concrete, windows and doors are more sealed, and walls and roofs are more insulated. Therefore, there is a need to build proper ventilation systems using pipe networks and grills. Level differentiation off entrance and exit of air is recommended. For instance, bathrooms, closets or storerooms may require this type of system because they tend to be unprovided by a window.

When this type of natural ventilation is insufficient thus, it may be reinforced by forced ventilation which relies on a mechanical extractor.

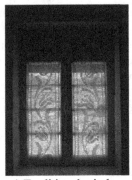
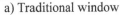
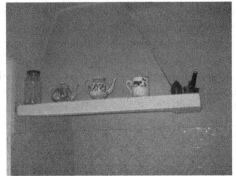

| a) Traditional window | b) Traditional kitchen chimney |

Fig. 1. Traditional natural ventilation solutions. Windows and kitchen chimneys.

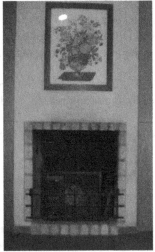
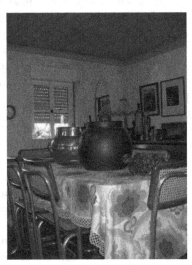

| a) Fireplace chimneys | b) Timber roofs |

Fig. 2. Traditional natural ventilation solutions. Fireplace chimneys and roofs.

3 Study Case

The traditional Portuguese dwelling used as a study case during this research work is shown in Fig. 3. It is a two-floor building located in the Lamego city centre, particularly in the historical part of this city near the castle.

Meanwhile, Lamego is located in the Douro Valley, rich in baroque architecture and religious buildings. It is an international tourist attraction.

As a typical dwelling of the North part of Portugal, it was built with exterior granite masonry and *tabique* walls. The pavements and roof were built with timber. Windows and doors were made with timber frames. The cover of the roof was made of ceramic tiles.

On the other hand, the building presented a lousy level of conservation in which the main structural elements were almost destroyed. There was no point in rehabilitating or reinforcing most of the building. Only the external walls were maintained Fig. 4.

At the same time, the municipality regulations only allow the use of timber or steel as structural building materials for this type of rehabilitation process in this area. Therefore, steel frames, glulam pavements and roofs were used, Fig. 3b.

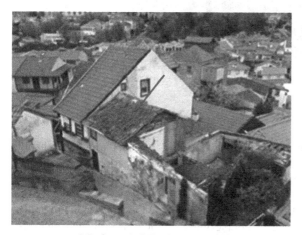
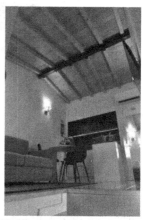

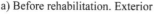

a) Before rehabilitation. Exterior

b) After rehabilitation. Interior of the top floor flat

Fig. 3. The study case building.

4 Ventilation Solution Applied in the Study Case

4.1 The Problem

At this stage, it is worth mentioning that this building was rehabilitated to be converted into a three-floor flat tourism accommodation (Fig. 3b and 5b).

This specific building is lacking in terms of space. It is placed between two other traditional buildings and shares the same lateral walls, Fig. 4. Therefore, only two exterior walls are allowed to have windows, Fig. 5b. Thus, natural light and natural ventilation can be potentiated by these two walls and the roof, where it will be possible to place windows and grills.

At the same time, approximately one and a half of the building is under the level road, Fig. 4 and 5b.

These building aspects created several difficulties concerning the air ventilation of the house and lighting.

Musty smell, humidity, stagnant air and dark spaces resulted from these building constraints and resulted in an unhealthy living dwelling. Thus, the original building could not meet the actual requirements of living comfort with quality.

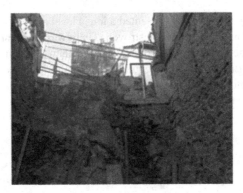

Fig. 4. Some highlights of the building constraints.

4.2 The Solution

Based on the above explanation, some building challenges existed during this rehabilitation process. Thus, the building solution proposed to solve the above-identified living
problems consisted of having an atrium on the left side of the building and next to the
façade facing South, Fig. 5a.

This atrium connects all the floors (from the basement to the first floor), Fig. 5b.

The roof of the atrium is made of double glass to allow natural light entrance,
Fig. 6a. This roof has surrounding grills in connection with the structure of the atrium.
This structure ensures air circulation from the inside to the exterior and vice-versa.

At each floor level (e.g. ground floor and first floor), each flat has a door and balcony
connecting the atrium, Fig. 5b. On these floors, the atrium has windows placed in the
main façade of the building, Fig. 5b and 6a.

It is relevant to add that each balcony is built with a steel grid pavement to allow air
circulation and natural light passage between floors, Fig. 6b.

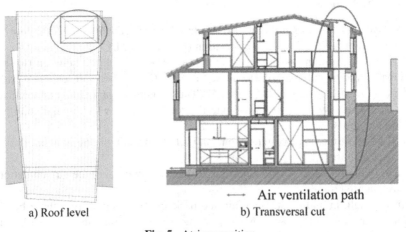

a) Roof level   ⟶ Air ventilation path
                                 b) Transversal cut

Fig. 5. Atrium position.

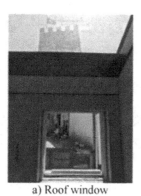
a) Roof window

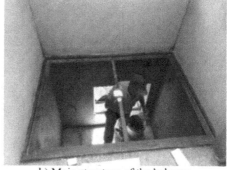
b) Main structure of the balcony

Fig. 6. Building details of the atrium.

At the basement pavement, a 200 mm diameter pipe network of PVC was considered to allow the air circulation between the interior of the atrium and the North face façade at this level, Fig. 7. There is approximately a 9 m height path to take into account. Therefore, the air circulation path of the atrium is graphically presented in Fig. 5b.

This air circulation path can have two directions throughout the year, depending on the temperature. Suppose the temperature at the top of the atrium is higher than the bottom (which is likely to occur during the warm temperature period of the year): in that case, the air tends to circulate from the bottom to the top of the atrium. On the other hand, the air will likely circulate from top to bottom. This last scenario may occur during autumn and winter. In addition, if the temperature reaches a high value at the top of the atrium (e.g. summer time), it can generate conditions that stop the natural circulation of the air. The above-identified problems may emerge in this case, particularly an unacceptable musty smell. It was noticed that this problem affects all three floors.

So the proposed natural air ventilation system had to be reinforced with a forced air ventilation system (another pipe network and an electrical extractor are the components of this additional forced air ventilation system). This reinforcement was also placed on the basement pavement floor and nearby the back window of this floor, Fig. 7b.

4.3 Remote Control Options

In this rehabilitation process, other technical aspects were also concerned with using the rehabilitated building during its lifetime, which required additional care. It is not an intelligent house, but it uses technology to reduce energy costs, increase comfort and facilitate management like touristic accommodations. For instance, to have more efficient energy-rehabilitated buildings, the air conditioning system of each flat is remote-controlled. It is possible to switch (on or off) the air conditioning devices using an online platform, Fig. 8. It is also possible to know the temperature of each flat remotely. The light system is also remote controlled as well as the ventilation. In this way, it is possible, without going to the place, to turn on the air conditioning before guests arrive, to have a cosy atmosphere. It is also possible to turn off all or part of the electrical system, namely the sanitary hot water heating systems when guests leave the apartments.

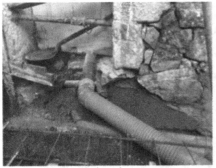 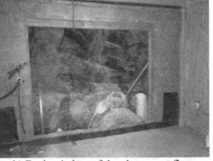

a) Ventilation pipe system   b) Back window of the abasement floor

Fig. 7. Additional building details of the atrium.

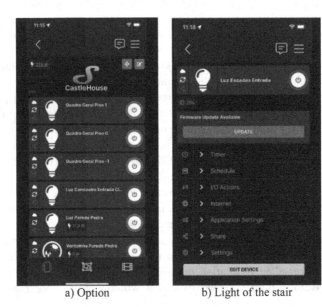

a) Option   b) Light of the stair

Fig. 8. Remote control platform

In addition, the blackout curtains are also remote-controlled. The respective device is shown in Fig. 9.

With this technical solution, it was possible to obtain a more technologically rehabilitated building and take a step toward innovative construction and an intelligent building approach.

4.4 The Degree of Satisfaction

To evaluate the efficiency of the built air ventilation, we are using the results of the typical inquiry of the booking companies concerning this specific tourism accommodation,

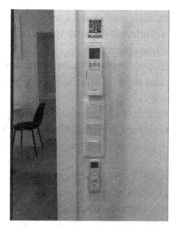

Fig. 9. Blackout curtain control devices

Fig. 10. The topic of the comfort of this inquiry indirectly indicates this ventilation solution may be efficient.

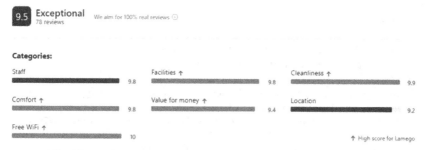

Fig. 10. Evaluation of the quality and comfort of the accommodation.

Based on the guest's degree of satisfaction, we may conclude that the ventilation system is working correctly [4]. Thus, health conditions have been guaranteed.

5 Main Conclusions

There has been an increasing demand for tourism accommodation, and rehabilitating traditional dwellings for tourism can help solve this problem.

However, the rehabilitation of traditional dwellings for accommodation purposes may present additional technical aspects to consider. Health issues are fundamental to avoid in this context. Also, good quality of the inner air is one of the aspects that is fundamental to guarantee.

A natural ventilation system may be a good option because it may be more environmentally friendly. When not enough, reinforcement with a forced ventilation system may be the required building option.

The remote-control options such as thermal control, ventilation control and access to accommodations have shown interest because they are energetically more efficient, less time-consuming and more convenient.

With this paper, the authors also intend to alert to the importance of using systems of control and prediction that can detect hazards, like the presence of dangerous gases that can bring health problems.

In this paper, a natural ventilation system solution was presented and described. It also introduced the required reinforcement of these systems. The success of the adopted technical solutions is shown by the satisfaction degree of the guests, which is quite positive.

The proposed solution may be applied in future rehabilitation processes.

As future works it is intended to undertake, a campaign of measurements over time of variables like outside/indoor temperatures, humidity and presence of CO/CO_2 gases. Another possibility is implementing a system of control and prediction that can provide quality health and comfort to the users.

Acknowledgements. This work was supported by the FCT (Portuguese Foundation for Science and Technology) through the project UIDB/04082/2020 (CMADE).

References

1. Teixeira, C., Moutinho, A., Bentes, I.: Reconstruction of "the castle house" in Lamego. In: Proceedings of the 8th International Conference on Safety and Ductility of Structures. ICOSADOS 2018. 23–25 May 2018. LLU, Latvia (2018)
2. Cardoso, P.J.S., et al.: Monitoring, Predicting, and optimizing energy consumptions: a goal toward global sustainability. In: Chapter 5 in Smart Systems Design, Applications and Challenges, pp. 80–107. IGI Global (2020). https://doi.org/10.4018/978-1-7998-2112-0.ch005
3. Pinto, J., Vasconcelos, V., Monteiro, R., Tapa, S., Bentes, I.: Um contributo na temática dos riscos tecnológicos em ambiente urbano. In: CONREA 2021 - O Congresso da Reabilitação. Livro de atas. UA Editora. 1ª edição - junho de 2021, pp. 127–133 (2021). ISBN 978-972-789-699-8. https://doi.org/10.48528/gy68-v843
4. Casado-Vara, R., et al.: Demand control ventilation strategy by tracing the radon concentration in smart buildings. In: Herrero, Á., Cambra, C., Urda, D., Sedano, J., Quintián, H., Corchado, E. (eds.) SOCO 2020. AISC, vol. 1268, pp. 374–382. Springer, Cham (2021). https://doi.org/10.1007/978-3-030-57802-2_36
5. Fromreide, M., Henne, I.; Smart control of HVAC based on measurements of indoor radon concentration. In: TOS Forum 2022, p. 441 (2022). https://doi.org/10.1255/tosf.172
6. Valcarce, D., Alvarellos, A., Rabuñal, J.R., Dorado, J., Gestal, M.: machine learning-based radon monitoring system. Chemosensors **10**, 239 (2022). https://doi.org/10.3390/chemosensors10070239
7. Bazzi, A., et al.: IoT-based remote health monitoring system employing smart sensors for asthma patients during COVID-19 pandemic, p. 6870358 (2022). https://doi.org/10.1155/2022/6870358. 1530-8669, Wireless Communications and Mobile Computing, Hindawi
8. Wu, Y., et al.: Effects of temperature and humidity on the daily new cases and new deaths of COVID-19 in 166 countries. In: Science of The Total Environment, vol. 729, p. 139051 (2020). https://doi.org/10.1016/j.scitotenv.2020.139051. ISSN 0048-9697

9. Kwon, N., Park, M., Lee, H.-S., Ahn, J., Shin, M.: Construction noise management using active noise control techniques. J. Constr. Eng. Manage. **142**(7) (2016). https://doi.org/10.1061/(ASCE)CO.1943-7862.0001121

10. Schieweck, A., et al.: Smart homes and the control of indoor air quality. Renew. Sustain. Energy Rev. **94**, 705–718 (2018). https://doi.org/10.1016/j.rser.2018.05.057. ISSN 1364-0321

11. Gao, G., Li, J., Wen, Y.: DeepComfort: energy-efficient thermal comfort control in buildings via reinforcement learning. IEEE Internet Things J. **7**(9), 8472–8484 (2020). https://doi.org/10.1109/JIOT.2020.2992117

12. Ramos, C.M., Andraz, G., Cardoso, I.: The role of ICT in involving the tourist and in sustainability of tourism destinations. In: Ratten, V. (eds.) Technological Progress, Inequality and Entrepreneurship, on Entrepreneurship, Structural Change and Industrial Dynamics, pp. 29–45. Springer, Cham (2020). https://doi.org/10.1007/978-3-030-26245-7_3. ISBN 978-3-030-26244-0

Medical and Healthcare Information Systems in Portugal: Short Literature Review

Bruna Rodrigues[1] , Rita Matos[1] , Silvana Guedes[1] , Ivan Miguel Pires[2] ,
and António Jorge Gouveia[1(✉)]

[1] School of Science and Technology of the University of Trás-os-Montes and Alto Douro, Vila Real, Portugal
{al66672,al66434,al64156}@utad.eu, jgouveia@utad.pt
[2] Instituto de Telecomunicações, Universidade da Beira Interior, Covilhã, Portugal
ivan.pires@lx.it.pt

Abstract. As the world comes to embrace technology, it becomes apparent that there is a progressive need to use information systems in all fields, especially in the medical one. While doctors and human resources will always be needed, technology can bring an enormous advantage. When using information systems an improvement can be seen while managing a hospital, diagnosing, and treating patients and even in reducing infection rates among hospital patients. There is a whole world for this new technology. Only, medical staff are not the keenest on this system, believing they would be replaced. Having this in mind it is important to have a balance between men and machine. This article aims to present a preliminary literature review that allows us to understand what medical and healthcare information systems are and how they are used.

Keywords: Medical · Healthcare · Information Systems

1 Introduction

Information systems is viewed has an integrated set of several components, including collecting, storing, and processing data [1]. However, they give information and knowledge as well. The development of this systems has been linked to changing needs in the healthcare industry. Governments all around the world are finding the need of a less doctor-centered healthcare, this can be implemented by information systems.

Information systems have the ability to manage healthcare costs, improve the care as well as decision support, this is helping doctors make an informed decision about a diagnosis, diminishing human error [2], not forgetting the ability to lower costs [3]. These are all big advantages for healthcare systems around the world seeing they are increasingly over pressured with the increase of patient's flow, and the aging population [2].

As a recent field with only about 60 years [4] under its belt, medical professionals are still on the fence about trusting the evolving information systems, while informatic

A. Cunha et al. (Eds.): MobiHealth 2022, LNICST 484, pp. 100–108, 2023.
https://doi.org/10.1007/978-3-031-32029-3_10

systems have been accepted to reduce paperwork and administrative work [4]. Help for diagnosis and patient care as not been accepted as well due to the fact medical professional believe they would be replaced. This is a common misconception seeing IT would serve as an aid for providing better care for patients while reducing the pressure exerted on doctors to not make any mistakes [2].

It is important to understand the beginnings of this field as well as the challenges it faces now, and where this could lead us. This article then aims to analyze the current information systems trends and future perspective in the medical field.

2 Background of Health Information Systems

Medicine and healthcare have changed a lot in the last 60 years, with major improvements in the last 20 [3]. Major companies have gotten into the development of software and hardware for health care [5], especially the emerging field of medical information systems. However, to understand the now it is important to understand the background of health information systems.

In the end of the 1950's [6] the first signs of this field appeared when talks about using computers to automate some of the medical personnel work started to appear. But it took 5 more years for one of the firsts software's for medical information systems to be developed in California [7]. But at this time not a lot of companies helped hospitals get computers. Then in 1967 the International medical informatics association (IMIA) was created, and the first meeting happened in the following year [8]. During this decade, the medical staff was used primarily for managing inventory and billings, all in a single database [9]. However, research into simulating and modeling biological processes had started as well as the first attempts to find decision support [10] and diagnosis tools.

As stated by Collen [11], during the 70's, departments relating to medical informatics popped up around the world. One of the first being the one Amsterdam followed by the former Soviet Union, besides that, professors from several countries published a paper discussing the term medical informatics. About this time, it was estimated that 10% of computers in the US had some form of informatic systems [12]. Getting to 1980 the first ever degree of this field was created in the Stanford University. It was also in the 1980's that European funding started to appear for research in this area [13]. During that decade, most paper records started to get digitalized and computer records were created. This was a big step to make medical informatics known worldwide, creating conferences, furthering the research, and making the rules for this field.

Reaching the 90's this fields has consolidated its positions as a separate discipline where most medical related degrees included classes on this matter [13]. Telemedicine research starts, medical imaging keeps improving and electronic health records keep improving to include data protection and confidentiality, with the European Data Protection Act in 1998 [14], turning into the norm the use electronic health records [5].

When getting closer to the present, new study areas related to information systems appeared as bioinformatics, hospital management, among others. New and improved technology appears, imaging, modeling of tissue, diagnosis tools. However, it is here we start to see problems emerge where the resistance against such technologies is faced by medical professionals [1], who mistakenly believe jobs would be lost, and older generations of patients who are not very trusting of things they do not understand.

Looking back at the past it can clearly be seen a big improvement over the years, with huge steps being taken in order to improve this area, with more and more research appearing. However, we must not forget that the level of medical information systems depends on the country as well as the socioeconomic context, as we see far more progress in first world countries [15].

3   Present

Nowadays, health information systems (HIS) have undergone a great development since its creation. This development allows us, not only to better manage healthcare data, but also to improve cost control, increase the timeliness and accuracy of patient care and administration information, among other things [1].

Currently, HIS has three main focuses, as we will see in the following subchapters.

3.1   How to Manage, Store and Transmit Health Data

One of the most developed areas of information systems in the medical field is managing the data. Data is constantly being produced in healthcare, ranging from prescriptions, exams and even billing. That being said, data collection allows healthcare workers to have an easier access and management of patient data by storing it electronically [16]. Which would create a faster and more convenient way of gathering patient records without wasting time in manually looking for them.

Transmitting health records could also assist in an easier connection between medical staff and patients, by allowing a faster spread of a patient's important information [2]. Electronic records would also assist in providing correct data between several medical organizations, improving the patient's chances for a better treatment [2].

Nonetheless, there are still issues regarding the electronic storage of data, most of which involving laws and patient safety. By using electronic records, medical data is more likely to get hacked and stolen than by keeping the records in paper [2]. Patients' rights and confidentiality are also a reason of concern, when medical records are kept electronically and shared in different healthcare organizations, since not all people agree in sharing all their information with different associations.

SClínico is a Portuguese clinical information system, created by SNS (Serviço Nacional de Saúde – National Health Service). The system allows medical personal to register patient data electronically in a shared database [17, 18].

PDS (Healthcare Data Platform - Plataforma de Dados da Saúde) allows medical workers from the SNS to have access to their patients' information database. With its use, it's possible to reduce the number of unnecessary duplicated exams and help professionals obtain the most important information regarding their patients [18, 19].

3.2   How to Help with Decision Support

Decision support is a big focal point in the development of HIS, as it would allow a wide range of improvements, such as patients' safety and cost control. These enhancements could be reached with the use of drug safety software, that would alert inappropriate dosing or recommend cheaper medicine options [2]. Another benefit would be the incorporation of decision support systems, which would provide a quick diagnosis with the use of the patient record [16].

Even though HIS brings amazing benefits to the medical field, the systems still have their pitfalls. For example, the workflow of the healthcare staff would need to be adapted to the system, resulting in wasting time training the medical team. The integration of a poor safety or managing software could also turn into a problem, causing inappropriate alerts, which would exhaust the personnel, who might begin to distrust and ignore the systems due to its lack of accuracy [2].

An example of the HIS's help in decision support is the online screening of the SNS. The National Health Service created an online page that allows patients to evaluate their symptoms and receive information and advice regarding their health [20]. Still, the results of the online check-up aren't one hundred percent trustworthy, as the evaluation mustn't replace one done by a professional worker.

3.3 How to Assist in Long Distance Patient Care

With the development of the internet, more and more forms of communication between doctors and patients have appeared. With the use of internet and its resources, the healthcare system can create a connection network that links several medical workers, to easily discuss patient care options and schedule appointments [2, 16].

Bearing in mind the transmission of patient information, the future HIS could also allow a quicker spread of the patient's symptoms and vital signs, making it possible for the doctor to communicate with the patient in-real time [2, 16].

Hospital da Luz has its own app (MY LUZ), with which the patients can manage health entries, control payments, check exams results and have online appointments with their doctors [21].

4 Current Difficulties

Despite HIS great evolution over the years, it hasn't efficiently been incorporated into healthcare systems yet. Many investors wonder what could be the cause for HIS's lack of integration in hospitals and why do the technologies keep failing when they show such amazing potential.

In spite of all its advantages and verified results, HIS still isn't used on a larger scale. The main reasons for the lack of use may be:

4.1 HIS Doesn't Have Much Support

The absence of HIS use can be co-related to its lack of support. That can be explained since hospitals don't want to waste time and money by exchanging their usual system and work ethics [1].

This difficulty could be potentially solved with the help of the government, by encouraging hospitals to keep their information in a digital database, as it would improve the transmission of the correct information no matter where the patient is taken care of.

4.2 Information Confidentiality

Medical information is highly sensitive, requiring an enormous level of security and confidentiality. With HIS, data as a higher risk of security breaches, medical data leaking or patients' data being exploited, when compared to paper records. The apparent risk of patient privacy being breached is a cause for concern, making them less inclined to share information [1].

4.3 Medical Staff is Afraid to Lose Their Jobs

In tune with the previous point, the lack of use of HIS can be linked with the fact that medical professionals feel that healthcare systems may take away their jobs, especially systems with a focus on decision support. When combining the lack of integration of HIS with professionals' fear of losing their jobs, healthcare systems gain a poor reputation that delays their implementation [1].

4.4 Patients Don't Trust It

Associated with the previous point, patients have trust issues regarding HIS, influenced by the opinion of the medical personal. The opinion of the professionals, then combined with the risk of their medical information leaking, makes the general public apprehensive to share sensitive personal information [1].

4.5 Lack of Communications Between Platforms

Nowadays there is a large number of information systems concerning healthcare, each single one with a wide variety of functions, uses and databases. While the extensive information gathered with the different platforms appears to be beneficial, the lack of connection between databases affects the availability to access records at any place [2, 18].

4.6 Expensive to Invest

While the incorporation of HIS can be extremely beneficial to healthcare, but the cost to implement it on a large scale is quite exorbitant. A wide application of HIS still requires an understanding of how it will work and where it will be applied, that can cause businesses not to invest in HIS implementation [2].

5 Future - Opportunities and Challenges

The constant development of medicine and all the technologies associated with it has led to a significant revolution in healthcare. Medical care has an evolutionary tendency to be increasingly preventive and patient-centered, this is possible through the improvement of the quality and availability of health information technologies, making it possible to have more intelligent, adaptable, and cost-effective medical services [22].

Health information technologies are still poorly suited tools due to a multifaceted environment, in which it is difficult to satisfy all the needs inherent to the patient, professionals and organizations. There is a need for technological change that can take all these factors into account and achieve interoperability between different systems [16].

Some examples of future opportunities and challenges in health information systems are:

The study, development and application of systems that allow health information exchange (HIE) between all hospitals through Electronic Medical Records (EMR) [16, 23]. HIMSS is a non-profit organization that helps companies work towards an electronic healthcare environment, consisting of the Electronic Medical Records Adoption Model (EMRAM) that incorporates methodology and algorithms to automatically score hospitals worldwide regarding their Electronic Medical Records (EMR) capabilities [16]. This model has 8 levels (0–7) that measure the adoption and use of electronic records (EMR) functions. The "HIMSS" level 7, allows continuous electronic information exchanges, allowing a fully functional electronic record that shares patient data with local health units, being accessible to the user and health professionals [24]. It also has the characteristic of being a continuous learning health system (LHS) which allows the use of data to improve care, quality, and safety. At this level, paper graphics and clinical decision support systems are not used 90% of the time [24]. "HIMSS" level 7 has already been reached by a Portuguese hospital - Hospital Cascais Dr. José Almeida, sharing the vanguard with a restricted elite of 3 hospitals in Europe and 6% in the USA, with its expansion being a future perspective [16, 25].

The evolution of data sharing between providers and the patient himself through a cloud, which alerts hospitals to an evolution in terms of management, security, storage, analysis, and interpretation of the data obtained [26].

Cybersecurity is also an important factor since computer attacks against hospital systems containing personal data are increasingly recurrent, which causes some fear in end-users to provide their data and personal information to third parties [22].

Consider the patient as a user, that is, the patient has access to his data, being able to edit or even delete them, having greater control over his records. This innovation can bring some associated risks to hospitals since the patient can function as a communication facilitator by being an active participant, or as an interfering participant, that is, not communicating the necessary data making the relationship between the health professional and the user [16].

Aggregation of data in order to cross organizational boundaries, with a very high number of benefits, however, organizational challenges also increase, due to the growing number of health organizations involved.

The growing development of intelligent devices capable of responding to electronic signals, such as bracelets with wireless communication devices that can exchange information with hospital computers, such as specific patient data or monitoring vital signs in real-time, which becomes to have numerous advantages from the point of view of hospital resources, reducing diagnostic tests and other procedures, and clinically.

The use of robots that are integrated into an HIE system to dispense medication or perform hospital disinfection.

6 Conclusion

Currently, healthcare has the future perspective of providing increasingly predictive and patient-centered medical care, this will be possible due to the real-time monitoring of the patient's health, the use of developing technologies such as smart devices, computers more powerful, intelligent processing and storage of data, and the interconnection of the entire healthcare ecosystem [22].

The globalization of the computer technology business associated with health is one of the main trends, currently, anyone is a potential consumer of data, and the possibilities of the IT market are still limitless. The main producers of these technologies include the USA, Japan, France, Great Britain, Germany, and Singapore, among others [5].

The implementation of HIS is not a constant work, there are several factors that change over time to which HIS must adapt, there is a need for a long-term perspective, that is, HIS must be seen as a journey that must be fulfilled in order to reach the goal, a future in which the wealth of data allows safe, efficient and high-quality care [16]. The increasing use of HIS is inevitable, and its variety will proliferate in the coming years, as we migrate to ubiquitous computing environments, however, there are ethical and even receptive aspects on the part of health professionals that cannot be forgotten because they are sources of gaps for this type of systems [27].

The future is promising for HISs that can support the provision of integrated patient-centered health care, that produce environments that are richer in data and more integrated models of care and information exchange with other professionals.

Acknowledgements. This work is funded by FCT/MEC through national funds and, when applicable, co-funded by the FEDER-PT2020 partnership agreement under the project **UIDB/50008/2020**.

This article is based upon work from COST Action COST Action CA19136 - International Interdisciplinary Network on Smart Healthy Age-friendly Environments (NET4AGE-FRIENDLY), supported by COST (European Cooperation in Science and Technology). COST is a funding agency for research and innovation networks. Our Actions help connect research initiatives across Europe and enable scientists to grow their ideas by sharing them with their peers. It boosts their research, career, and innovation. More information in www.cost.eu.

References

1. Fichman, R.G., Kohli, R., Krishnan, R.: The role of information systems in healthcare: current research and future trends. Inf. Syst. Res. **22**(3), 419–428 (2011). INFORMS Institute for Operations Research and the Management Sciences. https://doi.org/10.1287/isre.1110.0382

2. Goldschmid, P.G.: IT and MIS: implications of health information technology and medical information systems. Commun. ACM **48**(10), 68–74 (2005). https://doi.org/10.1145/1089107.1089141

3. Bogaevskaya, O.Y., Yumashev, A.V., Zolkin, A.L., Smirnova, O.A., Chistyakov, M.S.: Application of progressive information technologies in medicine: computer diagnostics and 3D technologies. J. Phys.: Conf. Ser. **1889**(5) (2021). https://doi.org/10.1088/1742-6596/1889/5/052001

4. Staggers, N., Thompson, C.B., Snyder-Halpern, R.: Healthy Policy and Systems Historical Influences of Information Systems in Clinical Care History and Trends in Clinical Information Systems in the United States (2001)
5. Vaganova, E., Ishchuk, T., Zemtsov, A., Zhdanov, D.: Health information systems: background and trends of development worldwide and in Russia. In: HEALTHINF 2017 - 10th International Conference on Health Informatics, Proceedings; Part of 10th International Joint Conference on Biomedical Engineering Systems and Technologies, BIOSTEC 2017, vol. 5, pp. 424–428 (2017). https://doi.org/10.5220/0006244504240428
6. Kaplan, B.: Development and acceptance of medical information systems: an historical overview. J. Health Hum. Resour. Adm. 11(1), 9–29 (1988). http://www.jstor.org/stable/257 80343
7. Lin, A.L., Chen, W.C., Hong, J.C.: Electronic health record data mining for artificial intelligence healthcare, Chap. 8. In: Xing, L., Giger, M.L., Min, J.K. (eds.) Artificial Intelligence in Medicine, pp. 133–150. Academic Press (2021). https://doi.org/10.1016/B978-0-12-821 259-2.00008-9
8. International Association of Engineering Insurers, History The historical development of IMIA. https://www.imia.com/history/. Accessed 19 Mar 2022
9. Collen, M.F., Hammond, W.E.: Development of medical information systems (MISs). In: Collen, M.F., Ball, M.J. (eds.) The History of Medical Informatics in the United States. HI, pp. 123–206. Springer, London (2015). https://doi.org/10.1007/978-1-4471-6732-7_3
10. Wasylewicz, A.T.M., Scheepers-Hoeks, A.M.J.W.: Clinical decision support systems. In: Kubben, P., Dumontier, M., Dekker, A. (eds.) Fundamentals of Clinical Data Science, pp. 153–169. Springer, Cham (2019). https://doi.org/10.1007/978-3-319-99713-1_11
11. Collen, M.F.: Medical Informatics Origins of Medical Informatics (1986)
12. Ball, M.J.: An Overview of Total Medical Information Systems (1971)
13. Hasman, A., Mantas, J., Zarubina, T.: An abridged history of medical informatics education in Europe. Acta informatica medica: AIM: J. Soc. Med. Inform. Bosnia Herzegovina: casopis Drustva za medicinsku informatiku BiH 22(1), 25–36 (2014). https://doi.org/10.5455/aim. 2014.22.25-36
14. Lawlor, D.A., Stone, T.: Public health and data protection: an inevitable collision or potential for a meeting of minds? (2001). https://www.imia.com/history/. Accessed 19 Mar 2022
15. Koumamba, A.P., Bisvigou, U.J., Ngoungou, E.B., Diallo, G.: Health information systems in developing countries: case of African countries. BMC Med. Inform. Decis. Mak. 21(1), 232 (2021). https://doi.org/10.1186/s12911-021-01597-5
16. Cresswell, K.M., Sheikh, A.: Health information technology in hospitals. Future Hosp. J. 2(1), 50 (2015). https://doi.org/10.7861/futurehosp.2-1-50
17. SClínico—Cuidados de Saúde Hospitalares (CSH) – SPMS. https://www.spms.min-saude. pt/2020/07/sclinico-hospitalar/. Accessed 06 May 2022
18. Pinheiro, A.P.: Os sistemas de informação na prática do médico de família: onde está a interoperabilidade? Revista Portuguesa de Medicina Geral e Familiar 34(4), 250–254 (2018)
19. Plataforma de Dados de Saúde (PDS). http://www.rcc.gov.pt/Directorio/Temas/ServicosCida dao/Paginas/Plataforma-de-Dados-de-Sa%C3%BAde-(PDS).aspx. Accessed 06 May 2022
20. SNS24: Avaliar sintomas. https://www.sns24.gov.pt/avaliar-sintomas/. Accessed 18 Jan 2021
21. MY LUZ: área pessoal online—Hospital da Luz. https://www.hospitaldaluz.pt/pt/hospital-da-luz/para-clientes/my-luz. Accessed 06 May 2022
22. Ahmad, K.A., Khujamatov, H., Akhmedov, N., Bajuri, M.Y., Ahmad, M.N., Ahmadian, A.: Emerging trends and evolutions for smart city healthcare systems. Sustain. Cities Soc. 80, 103695 (2022). https://doi.org/10.1016/j.scs.2022.103695
23. Electronic Medical Record Adoption Model. https://www.himssanalytics.org/emram. Accessed 06 May 2022

24. Who we are. https://www.himss.org/who-we-are. Accessed 06 May 2022
25. HIMSS Analytics: Hospital de Cascais classificado no nível 7 pelo modelo EMRAM do HIMSS Analytics. https://www.hospitaldecascais.pt/pt/comunicacao/noticias/Paginas/not icia-insights-himss-europe-dezembro-2017-.aspx. Accessed 06 May 2022
26. Staggers, N., Thompson, C.B., Snyder-Halpern, R.: History and trends in clinical information systems in the United States. J. Nurs. Schol. **33**(1), 75–81 (2001). https://doi.org/10.1111/j.1547-5069.2001.00075.x
27. Hackl, W.O., Hoerbst, A.: Trends in clinical information systems research in 2019. Yearb. Med. Inform. **29**(1), 121–128 (2020). https://doi.org/10.1055/s-0040-1702018

Page Inspector - Web Page Analyser

Francisco Filipe⬤ and António Jorge Gouveia(✉)⬤

School of Science and Technology, University of Trás-os-Montes and Alto Douro, Vila Real,
Portugal
jgouveia@utad.pt

Abstract. Web Accessibility refers to apps, websites, and digital tools designed to be accessible by all users, including those with disabilities. The web is a source of public information, education, employment, government, commerce, health, entertainment, and many others, and every person, regardless of ability, has the right to access it. Imagine missing out on thousands of new customers because your competitor has an easier-to-use, WCAG-compliant website [1]. The design and development consist of an open-source web platform, *PageInspector*, which allows anyone to analyze a website. It was built using JavaServer and Apache Tomcat. The platform provides a set of reports, spelling, accessibility, cookies, technologies, images, subdomains, Google Lighthouse and hyperlinks. In addition to these reports, it allows the user to view their website in real time, desktop and mobile versions, as well as the source-code. All reports are available through a dedicated API, so you also can integrate with your platforms.

Keywords: web · accessibility · sustainability · compliant · systematic literature review · websites · web page design · Web content accessibility guidelines (WCAG)

1 Introduction

Have you checked to see if your institution is creating websites and apps that follow the Web Content Accessibility Guidelines (WCAG)? If not, millions of people won't be able to use them. Since September 2018, all British Higher Education institutions have been legally required to upgrade their websites, online courses, and network resources to comply with the current Web Accessibility standards [1]. According to [2], digital services must meet at least Level AA of the Web Content Accessibility Guidelines (WCAG 2.1) to meet government accessibility requirements. Considering that higher education institutions often have thousands of pages of information to consider, this is a massively daunting task. The design and development consist of an open-source web platform, *PageInspector*, which allows anyone to analyze a website. It was built using JavaServer and Apache Tomcat. The platform provides a set of reports, spelling, accessibility, cookies, technologies, images, subdomains, Google Lighthouse and hyperlinks. In addition to these reports, it allows the user to view their website in real time, desktop and mobile versions, as well as the source-code. All reports are available through a dedicated API, so you can integrate them with your platforms.

A. Cunha et al. (Eds.): MobiHealth 2022, LNICST 484, pp. 109–117, 2023.
https://doi.org/10.1007/978-3-031-32029-3_11

The main objective behind the PageInspector is to allow anyone to analyse their webpages for free. This platform provides a set of detailed reports to help anyone to make their websites more accessible and more appealing to search engines. The platform provides a set of reports, spelling, accessibility, cookies, technologies, images, subdomains, Google Lighthouse and hyperlinks. In addition to these reports, it allows the user to view their website in real time, desktop and mobile versions, as well as the source-code. All reports are available through a dedicated API, so you can integrate them with your platforms. This paper is divided in four sections. Section 2 explains the though process behind the concept and development, Sect. 3 will address results and at last, Sect. 4 will address conclusions and future work.

2   Development

This section aims to present an exemplary modelling, through requirements gathering, use cases and activity diagram.

2.1   Requirements Gathering

Requirements gathering is closely linked to the quality of the produced software [3]. This subsection is a list with the specification of everything that must be implemented. The requirements can be divided into two categories, functional and non-functional requirements. Functional are related to the services that the system should offer. Non-functional are related to specific system characteristics or restrictions.

Functional requirements:

1. The *PageInspector* system should allow viewing of the intended website in real time;
2. The *PageInspector* system should allow selecting the view mode ("desktop" or "mobile");
3. The *PageInspector* system should allow consulting the website's source code;
4. The *PageInspector* system should allow for a spelling analysis;
5. The *PageInspector* system should allow for an accessibility analysis;
6. The *PageInspector* system should allow for a cookies analysis;
7. The *PageInspector* system should allow for a technologies analysis;
8. The *PageInspector* system should allow an images analysis;
9. The *PageInspector* system should allow a subdomains analysis;
10. The *PageInspector* system should allow for a Google Lighthouse analysis;
11. The *PageInspector* system should allow a hyperlinks analysis;
12. The *PageInspector* system should allow viewing of spelling errors in the page context;
13. The *PageInspector* system should allow for the identification of the more common spelling errors;
14. The *PageInspector* system should allow for the identification of the less common spelling errors;
15. The *PageInspector* system should allow viewing the number of occurrences of each misspelling.

16. The *PageInspector* system must allow CRUD (Create, Read, Update and Delete) operations of the user's dictionary;
17. The *PageInspector* system should allow viewing in the context of the page the accessibility errors;
18. The *PageInspector* system should allow viewing the accessibility error in the context of the source code;
19. The *PageInspector* system should allow informing the guideline of the error of accessibility;
20. The *PageInspector* system should allow informing the name and domain associated with a cookie;
21. The *PageInspector* system should allow informing which category of technologies is most used.

Non-functional requirements:

1. The *PageInspector* system must provide access to reports through from an API;
2. The *PageInspector* system must give the possibility to use cache when generating a report;
3. The *PageInspector* system must use an SSL certificate to ensure client-server security.

2.2 Use Cases

One of the ways of identifying and documenting the requirements previously enumerated is the use-case modelling. So, actors and use cases were identified [4]. To try and identify the actors that interact with the system, the authors tried to answer the following questions:

• Who uses the system? What roles does it play in the interaction?
• What other systems interact with the system?
• Who provides information to the system?
• Are there external events that affect the system?
• Who provides the data? Who uses the information?

Since the application developed is a fully autonomous and maintenance-free web page inspection tool, the only actor identified was the *User*.

Several use case diagrams have been developed to support all requirements. For space reasons, they are not presented in this paper.

2.3 Activity Diagram

The activity diagram presented in Fig. 1, refers to the base functioning of the platform, *PageInspector*. Activity diagrams allow you to model the flow of actions that are part of a larger activity. They are commonly used to specify use cases and class operations. It is very important that the diagram contains the minimum information necessary to communicate the message.

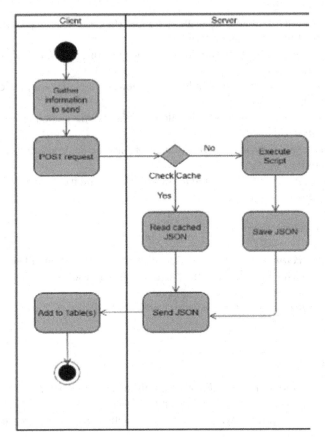

Fig. 1. Activity diagram

As a web page analysis platform, the following diagram represents the process to generate any report. The process starts by identifying the necessary information present on the website, for example, for the spelling report, the information will be the URL, the language, and the content. Then send that information to the server through a POST request. The requested report is checked to see if the requested report is cached, this check is made by the URL. If there is, then a JSON response is returned [5]. Otherwise, the dedicated script for each type of report is executed, the JSON is saved for future cache and finally the JSON is returned to the client. Finally, in the client, the JSON information is added to the desired table.

3   Results

This section aims to present the platform, as the API that supports it. Finally, an explanation of the platform's security.

3.1 Homepage

The platform's homepage allows the user to view the desktop version of the page to be analysed. The page can be loaded by entering the URL in the top bar, as well as selecting the page language and WCAG accessibility level. In the sidebar are the different views, "desktop", "mobile" and "code". In the desktop version, the page is loaded and displayed just as it would be on a desktop. The same goes for the mobile version. The view code allows the user to see the source code of the page. By default, the page is loaded in the desktop version. In the sidebar, the user can access the various reports. If the user wants to access the desired page directly, he can add the "URL" argument to the base URL. Users can also add the "lang" argument to indicate the language of the page to be analysed.

3.2 Spelling Report

The spelling report aims to make a spelling analysis of the page. Thus, allowing the user to view the spelling errors present on the page in order to correct them. The analysis is done through the open-source tool, LanguageTool [6, 7], developed in Java. This report, as we can see in Fig. 2, is available in the form of an API, receiving as arguments the URL, content and language of the page. The API returns a JSON response. If the user has not specified the language, then language detection is performed. If this argument cannot be found, a prediction is then made by the LanguageTool tool, finally, if both fail, the British English language is used by default. The user dictionary is managed through a cookie stored in the user's browser. In this way, it allows the user a more fluid and continuous experience.

```
let spellCheckJSON = await $.post("https://127.0.0.1/InspectorWS/LanguageTool", {
    content: spellTagsElem,
    langCode: langCode,
    url: siteUrl
}, function (result) {
    return result;
});
```

Fig. 2. API - Spelling Report

3.3 Accessibility Report

This report intends to present to the user the various accessibility errors of the page. This analysis allows you to verify whether the page complies with the Web Content Accessibility Guidelines (WCAG). This analysis is done through a library developed in NodeJS, HTML CodeSniffer [8]. This tool takes as arguments the URL of the page and the accessibility level, WCAG2A, WCAG2AA or WCAG2AAA [W3C 2022] – see Fig. 3. The API returns a JSON response. By default, the accessibility level is WCAG2AA.

```
let accessibilityJSON = await $.post("https://127.0.0.1/InspectorWS/Accessibility", {
    url: siteUrl, level: WCAGLevel
}, function (result) {
    return result;
});
```

Fig. 3. API - Accessibility Report

3.4 Cookies Report

The Cookies report seeks to show the user, as the name implies, which cookies are present on the analysed page. The analysis is done by a library developed by Google in NodeJS, Puppeteer [9]. This library allows controlling Chrome or Chromium through the DevTools protocol. The API takes the URL of the page as an argument and returns a JSON response, as we can see in Fig. 4.

```
let cookiesJSON = await $.post("https://127.0.0.1/InspectorWS/Cookies", {
    url: siteUrl,
}, function (result) {
    return result;
});
```

Fig. 4. API - Cookies Report

3.5 Technologies Report

This report, technologies report, aims to present the technologies used by the analysed page. This analysis is done by a library developed in NodeJS, Wappalyzer [10]. As we can see in Fig. 5, the API takes the URL of the page as an argument and returns a JSON response.

```
let wappalyzerJSON = await $.post("https://127.0.0.1/InspectorWS/Wappalyzer",
    url: siteUrl,
}, function (result) {
    return result;
});
```

Fig. 5. API – Technologies Report

3.6 Images Report

This report aims to present the images present on the analysed page to the user. The analysis is done by a library developed in Python, Pillow [11]. This library allows you to identify and analyse images present on a given page. The API takes the URL of the page as an argument and returns a JSON response – see Fig. 6.

```
let wappalyzerJSON = await $.post("https://127.0.0.1/InspectorWS/Wappalyzer",
    url: siteUrl,
}, function (result) {
    return result;
});
```

Fig. 6. API - Images Report

3.7 Subdomains Report

This report aims to present to the user the subdomains related to the domain of the analysed page. The analysis is done by a tool developed for Linux, Windows and MacOs. This CRT tool [12] allows you to analyse the certificate transparency logs (CRT) [13] of a domain. As is shown in Fig. 7, the API takes the URL of the page as an argument and returns a JSON response.

```
let domainsJSON = await $.post("https://127.0.0.1/InspectorWS/DomainDiscovery",
    url: siteUrl,
}, function (result) {
    return result;
});
```

Fig. 7. API - Subdomains Report

3.8 Google Lighthouse Report

This report aims to present to the user the report made by Google Lighthouse [14] of the analysed page. The analysis is done by a library developed in NodeJS, Lighthouse. It has performance audits, accessibility, progressive web applications, SEO. Lighthouse receives a URL, and it performs a series of audits on the page and then generates a report on the page's performance. As is shown in Fig. 8, the API takes as an argument the URL and the device to be used as a test (desktop or mobile) and returns a JSON response.

3.9 Hyperlinks Report

This report intends to present the hyperlinks present on the analysed page to the user. The analysis is done by a library developed in NodeJS, url-status-code [15]. This library allows you to identify and analyse the hyperlinks present on a given page. As we can see in Fig. 9, the API takes the URL of the page as an argument and returns a JSON response.

```
let lighthouseJson = await $.post("https://127.0.0.1/InspectorWS/Lighthouse",
    url: siteUrl, device: device
}, function (result) {
    return result;
});
```

Fig. 8. API - Google Lighthouse Report

```
let linkJSON = await $.post("https://127.0.0.1/InspectorWS/Links",
    url: siteUrl,
}, function (result) {
    return result;
});
```

Fig. 9. API - Hyperlinks Report

3.10 Security

The user does not need to have authentication or authorization to enjoy all the features of the platform. However, there are several other areas of computer security that have been considered throughout the development of the platform. To access the hosting service, two-factor authentication is required, that is, a username/password combination as well as a six-digit verification code, sent to the mobile phone or to a mobile application. Server access via SSH (Secure Shell Protocol) is also ensured. Each user has their individual access account, and a username/password combination is required as well as a private key. The version of Linux, Ubuntu Server, is the most current and to combat computer attacks updates are being made regularly.

To avoid data loss in the event of a catastrophic failure, a backup policy was adopted. This policy is known as 3-2-1:

- 3 backups;
- In 2 types of storage;
- With at least 1 at a distant physical location.

Therefore, every night 3 full copies of the server are made, a local copy, another on an external device and another on a cloud service.

4 Conclusions and Future Work

In addition to the development of the web platform described above, this project also had as its general objective the active participation in projects of a company at an international level. In order to acquire experience in the field of Information Systems and Computer Engineering, understand how the professional environment of a company works and its framework in the world of work. After several months of work, these objectives were successfully met.

4.1 Future Work

Throughout the development of this project, there were several challenges. The first was the decision of which technologies to use. It was decided to use Java Server as the platform support framework. This framework, in addition to being able to respond to all requirements, is also used in several platforms developed by Little Forest, thus contributing to the decision of its use. However, this framework is too complex for the type of platform developed. Thus, it is planned, in future versions, to use a lighter web framework, for example, Python Flask, and be able to meet the same requirements.

References

1. Filipe, F., Pires, I., Gouveia, A.J.: Why web accessibility is important for your institution. In: Paper Presented at the CENTERIS - International Conference on ENTERprise Information Systems, Lisboa, Portugal (2022)
2. Making your service accessible: an introduction. https://www.gov.uk/service-manual/hel ping-people-to-use-your-service/making-your-service-accessible-an-introduction. Accessed 31 Mar 2022
3. Ramesh, M.R.R., Reddy, C.S.: Metrics for software requirements specification quality quantification. Comput. Electr. Eng. **96**, 107445 (2021)
4. Barros-Justo, J.L., Benitti, F.B.V., Tiwari, S.: The impact of use cases in real-world software development projects: a systematic mapping study. Comput. Stand. Interf. **66**, 103362 (2019)
5. Crockford, D.: JSON. https://www.json.org/json-en.html. Accessed 19 Nov 2021
6. LanguageTool: LanguageTool - Online Grammar, Style & Spell Checker. https://languaget ool.org/. Accessed 23 Apr 2021
7. LanguageTool: LanguageTool: Style and Grammar Checker. https://github.com/languaget ool-org/languagetool. Accessed 25 Nov 2021
8. Squiz: HTML_CodeSniffer. https://squizlabs.github.io/HTML_CodeSniffer/. Accessed 26 Dec 2021
9. Google "Puppeteer.": https://github.com/puppeteer/puppeteer. Accessed 01 Jan 2022
10. Wappalyzer: Find out what websites are built with - Wappalyzer. https://www.wappalyzer. com/. Accessed 02 Jan 2022
11. Lundh, F.: Pillow. https://pillow.readthedocs.io/en/stable/. Accessed 05 Jan 2022
12. Cumulus: crt. https://github.com/cemulus/crt. Accessed 18 Feb 2022
13. Google "Certificate Transparency: Certificate Transparency.": https://certificate.transparency. dev/. Accessed 18 Feb 2022
14. Google "Lighthouse.": https://github.com/GoogleChrome/lighthouse. Accessed 18 Feb 2022
15. Zrrrzzt "url-status-code.": https://github.com/zrrrzzt/url-status-code. Accessed 18 Feb 2022
16. digicert "WHAT IS na SSL CERTIFICATE": https://www.digicert.com/what-is-an-ssl-certif icate. Accessed 24 Feb 2022

Medical, Communications
and Networking

Design of a Novel Reconfigurable Wearable Antenna Based on Textile Materials and Snap-on Buttons

Sofia Bakogianni[✉], Aris Tsolis, and Antonis Alexandridis

Institute of Informatics and Telecommunications, National Centre for Scientific Research 'Demokritos', Athens, Greece
sof.bakogianni@iit.demokritos.gr

Abstract. A novel wearable reconfigurable patch antenna is presented for wireless body-area applications at 2.4 GHz industrial, scientific, and medical (ISM) band. Textile and clothing materials are solely employed within the wearable antenna design process and reconfiguration mechanism. Specifically, by engaging or disengaging four pairs of metallic snap-on buttons, the textile antenna can exhibit an omnidirectional radiation pattern with linear polarization or a broadside radiation pattern with circular polarization enabling both on- and off-body wireless communication, respectively. A multi-layer tissue phantom is applied to emulate a realistic wearing environment. The resonance and radiation performance characteristics of the proposed antenna are examined in both radiation states. A parametric analysis regarding key design parameters is conducted. The specific absorption rate (SAR) is, also, assessed in terms of safety.

Keywords: Body-area networks · Reconfigurable antenna · Snap-on buttons · Textiles · Wearable antenna

1 Introduction

Wireless body-area networks (WBANs) are an emerging interdisciplinary technological field applied to improve personal and professional life routine in applications such as healthcare and entertainment, consumer electronics, military, and rescue services. Within the framework of WBAN systems, on-body and off-body wireless communication channels are established by integrating wearable antennas. The on-body links enable the wireless propagation of vital signals along human body; maximum antenna radiation is necessary along body surface [1]. In contrast, the off-body links allow communication between wearable antennas and external devices far away from the human body; maximum radiation is required in broadside direction normal to body surface [1]. The functionality of WBAN systems can be improved by applying antennas that achieve switching radiation properties. In practical, a radiation pattern reconfigurable antenna can support in a single wireless unit both the collection of vital physiological signals

A. Cunha et al. (Eds.): MobiHealth 2022, LNICST 484, pp. 121–129, 2023.
https://doi.org/10.1007/978-3-031-32029-3_12

from body-mounted sensor nodes and the data transmission in external base stations for remote healthcare monitoring, for instance [2].

Electronic switches integrated into the antenna structure are typically used to achieve the necessary reconfiguration. In [3], a conformal wearable antenna that electronically switches its radiation properties between broadside and monopole-like mode at 5.2 GHz has been proposed. Four PIN diodes were incorporated into the antenna to promote pattern reconfiguration. In [4], a textile antenna has been presented based on a metamaterial structure. Six switchable stubs enable antenna omnidirectional or broadside radiation at 2.4 GHz. In [5], a beam-steering patch antenna has been proposed for wrist-wearable applications at 6 GHz. Different beam directions are achieved by altering the state of two switches. Clothing accessories can, also, be used as passive switches. In [6], commercial metallic snap-on buttons have been applied as detachable shoring vias to split the radiation pattern of a textile patch antenna into two main beams at 3.6 GHz. In [7], two reconfigurable textile antennas that employ a conductive Velcro tape and zip fastener have been presented for operation at 2.4 GHz. Antenna polarization can be changed from linear to circular at will, by altering the state of the applied clothing components.

In this paper, a reconfigurable wearable antenna is designed for wireless on/off-body applications at 2.4 GHz industrial, scientific, and medical (ISM) band. The research challenge lies in the entirely use of textile and clothing materials within the antenna design process. A single-layer microstrip-fed patch antenna printed on textile fabric is adopted as the radiating element aiming at design simplicity and low-profile. The radiation-pattern and polarization reconfiguration mechanism are induced by incorporating four pairs of metallic snap-on buttons that serve as detachable shorting vias into the antenna structure. Circular polarization is achieved through antenna structure perturbation. The novelty of the proposed study lies in the design of a textile antenna that achieves both radiation pattern and polarization reconfiguration at fixed frequency of operation. Research works found in the literature present antenna designs with single radiation reconfiguration capabilities.

This paper is organized as follows. Section 2 presents the design of the proposed textile reconfigurable antenna and the equivalent tissue-simulating model. In Sect. 3, the simulation results including antenna resonance and radiation performance under both radiation configurations are featured. A parametric design analysis is conducted. Specific absorption rate (SAR) is, also, assessed. Conclusions follow in Sect. 4.

2 Antenna Design

The geometry of the proposed fully-textile reconfigurable patch antenna is shown in Fig. 1. A 0.97 mm thick felt material (relative permittivity ε_r of 1.64 and loss tangent $tan\delta$ of 0.033) is used as the antenna substrate. A square patch is printed onto the textile substrate with a full ground plane. The patch surface and the ground plane are made of conductive fabric (Nora-Dell, Shieldex) with a conductivity σ of 1.54×10^6 S/m and a thickness of 0.13 mm.

Four pairs of commercial metallic snap-on buttons are symmetrically located into the diagonal directions of the antenna structure, as depicted in Fig. 1 (S1, S2, S3, and S4 positions), to promote radiation-pattern and polarization reconfigurability at 2.4 GHz band. The snap-on buttons have been proved a robust mechanical and radio frequency connection for wearable systems since they can provide detachability with suitable RF performance up to 5 GHz [8]. In the proposed design concept, four male buttons are soldered into the patch surface and can serve as shorting vias when they are engaged to their female counterparts attached onto the ground plane layer. When the male parts are engaged to the female ones, the textile antenna operates in a monopole-like state exhibiting omnidirectional radiation for on-body wireless links. When the buttons are disengaged, the antenna operates as a conventional half-wave mode microstrip antenna presenting broadside radiation for off-body communication. Furthermore, to promote polarization reconfiguration the patch layer is corner-truncated and is loaded with a pair of diagonal stubs to efficiently produce a pair of degenerated modes. Hence, circular polarization (CP) is generated in the off-body radiation state. On the other hand, linear polarization is adopted within the on-body radiation mode.

Antenna feeding is realized through a stepping microstrip line instead of a coaxial cable to enhance wearer's comfort. The origin of the coordinate system is placed into the ground plane center. Ansys HFSS and CST MWS electromagnetic software packages are used for the antenna design process and the extraction of numerical results. The antenna design parameter values are recorded in Table 1.

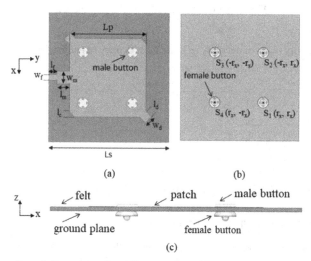

Fig. 1 Configuration of the proposed textile reconfigurable antenna: (a) top view showing the four male buttons on the patch surface, (b) bottom view showing the four female buttons on the ground plane layer, and (c) side view showing all antenna elements (not in same scale).

Considering antenna integration onto human body, a three-layered tissue model that consists of skin (thickness 1.3 mm), fat (thickness 10.5 mm) and muscle (thickness 20 mm) is employed as shown in Fig. 2 [2]. The dielectric constants of the applied tissues are evaluated at 2.44 GHz and are listed in Table 2 [9]. To emulate realistic wearing conditions, the antenna is placed at 3 mm distance from the tissue model. Felt material ($\varepsilon_r = 1.2$, $tan\delta = 0.001$) is used to fill the space.

Table 1. Antenna geometrical parameter values [in mm].

Name	Value	Name	Value
Ls	74	l_f	5.0
Lp	45	w_f	3.3
l_d	2.5	l_m	7.3
w_d	5.2	w_m	7.5
l_c	3.0	r_x	14.5

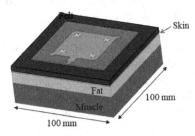

Fig. 2 Numerical three-layered tissue model.

Table 2. Permittivity (ε_r), conductivity (σ), and mass density (ρ) of the tissues used in this study.

Tissue	ε_r	σ (S/m)	ρ (kg/m^3)
Skin	38.01	1.46	1100
Fat	5.28	0.10	920
Muscle	52.74	1.73	1040

3 Reconfigurable Textile Antenna Performance

3.1 On-Body Antenna Operation State

Figure 3 (black line) illustrates the simulated reflection coefficient |S11| frequency response of the designed reconfigurable patch antenna when the snap-on buttons are engaged serving as shorting vias. The antenna presents a resonance frequency at 2.44 GHz and the obtained 10-dB impedance bandwidth is 87 MHz covering the ISM frequency band. A parametric analysis regarding snap-on buttons' position (r_x) within the antenna structure is, also, superimposed in Fig. 3. Based on the numerical results, a frequency shift of about 60 MHz is observed when the buttons are moved by 1 mm ($r_x = 15.5$ mm) towards the antenna's corners with respect to their initial location ($r_x = 14.5$ mm). This implies that proper buttons' positioning is significant to ensure the desired antenna operation at specific frequency.

Furthermore, the simulated normalized radiation patterns of the antenna in xz- and xy-planes are presented in Fig. 4(a) and (b), respectively. An omnidirectional radiation pattern with vertical polarization, normal to the patch surface, is achieved which fulfils the requirements for on-body communication. The calculated peak gain in the azimuth plane is −6.4 dBi. The maximum gain is calculated to be −1.5 dBi at 2.44 GHz.

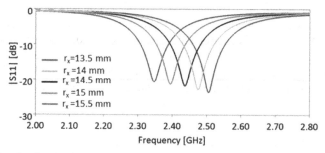

Fig. 3 Simulated reflection coefficient characteristics of the proposed reconfigurable antenna design for different snap-on buttons position (r_x) under monopole-like mode.

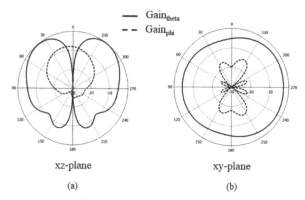

Fig. 4 Simulated normalized radiation patterns of the proposed reconfigurable antenna design at 2.44 GHz under monopole-like mode in: (a) xz-plane, and (b) xy-plane, respectively.

3.2 Off-Body Antenna Operation State

When the snap-on buttons are disengaged, the proposed textile antenna operates as a typical microstrip patch and its simulated reflection coefficient |S11| frequency response is illustrated in Fig. 5(a) (black line). The antenna presents a broadband resonance response around the 2.44 GHz frequency of interest. The 10-dB impedance bandwidth is 195 MHz fully covering the ISM frequency band. By implementing diagonal stub loading and corner truncation into the patch layer (see Fig. 1), the fundamental mode of the proposed antenna is split into modes f_{low} and f_{high}, as shown in Fig. 5(a). The two resonance modes produce the wide impedance bandwidth. In addition, the split modes satisfy the condition of equal amplitude and orthogonal phase to achieve circular polarization. The simulated axial ratio (AR) response of the proposed antenna is presented in Fig. 5(b) (black line). The 3-dB AR bandwidth is 43 MHz exhibiting satisfactory CP behavior.

A parametric analysis regarding the diagonal stubs' length (l_d) is, also, superimposed in Fig. 5(a) and (b). It is obvious that the variation of stubs' length impacts on the response of the mode f_{low}, while the higher mode seems to be nearly unaffected. Furthermore, Fig. 6(a) and (b) depicts the antenna |S11| and AR frequency response by altering the truncated corners' length (l_c). The design parameter l_c controls the upper mode f_{high}, while the lower frequency mode remains stable. It seems, also, that the diagonal stubs' length (l_d) exerts stronger influence on the AR response. It should be noted that in Figs. 5 and 6, black line represents the |S11| and AR when all antenna geometrical parameters are at their nominal values (see Table 1). Colored lines correspond to the numerical results when the value of one geometrical parameter of interest changes.

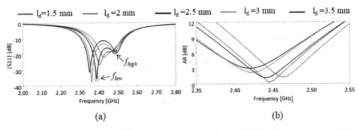

Fig. 5 (a) Simulated reflection coefficient characteristics and (b) AR response of the proposed reconfigurable antenna design varying diagonal stub's length (l_d) under broadside mode (rest of geometrical parameters are at their nominal values). (Color figure online)

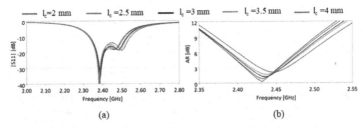

Fig. 6 (a) Simulated reflection coefficient characteristics and (b) AR response of the proposed reconfigurable antenna design varying truncated corner's length (l_c) under broadside mode (rest of geometrical parameters are at their nominal values). (Color figure online)

In Fig. 7, the simulated surface current distribution onto the patch layer is presented at 2.44 GHz, when the snap-on buttons are disengaged. As can be observed, the surface current rotates in the clockwise direction. This produces left-handed CP waves in the broadside radiation mode.

Furthermore, the simulated normalized radiation patterns of the textile antenna in xz- and yz-planes are presented in Fig. 8(a) and (b), respectively. A broadside radiation pattern with circular polarization is accomplished which is suitable for off-body channels. The peak gain is 1.1 dBi at 2.44 GHz. The cross-polarization level is below −20 dBi which allows good polarization purity.

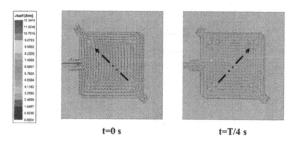

t=0 s   t=T/4 s

Fig. 7 Simulated surface current distribution at 2.44 GHz under broadside mode.

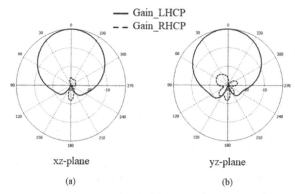

Fig. 8 Simulated normalized radiation patterns of the proposed reconfigurable antenna design at 2.44 GHz under broadside mode in: (a) xz-plane, and (b) yz-plane, respectively.

3.3 Antenna Radiation Safety Performance

Specific Absorption Rate (SAR) analysis is conducted to assess the electromagnetic power absorbed by the tissue model at 2.44 GHz. SAR calculation is realized in terms of radiofrequency radiation exposure safety and constitutes a sufficient electromagnetic dosimetry measure for wearable applications. When the proposed textile antenna is assumed to deliver 0.5 W, the simulated SAR distributions regarding the on- and off-body radiation modes are shown in Fig. 9(a) and (b), respectively. The maximum 1-g average values are 0.237 W/kg and 0.079 W/kg under both operation modes. This implies that the IEEE standards limiting 1-g and average SAR to a value of less than 1.6 W/kg are not violated [11].

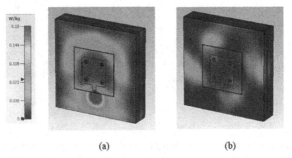

(a)   (b)

Fig. 9 Simulated SAR distributions averaged in 1 g of tissue for antenna input power = 0.5 W at 2.44 GHz under (a) monopole-like mode, and (b) broadside mode, respectively.

4 Conclusions

In this paper, a compact textile patch antenna with pattern and polarization reconfigurability has been proposed for WBAN applications at 2.4 GHz ISM band. When four snap-on buttons are engaged, a monopole-like radiation pattern with vertical polarization is achieved for on-body communication. Under disengaged buttons, the antenna radiates in a broadside direction with circular polarization which is suitable for off-body channels. Numerical results in terms of resonance, radiation, and safety performance indicate that the antenna is a suitable candidate for wearable healthcare applications. The textile antenna can be integrated into a patient's robe and dynamically select the optimum radiation mode to enable efficient remote health monitoring within hospital facilities or patient's house. In the on-body mode, a wearable control unit can wirelessly collect physiological parameters (e.g., heart rate and temperature) recorded by sensor nodes for data processing. The on-body unit can, then, transmit the data to an external base station via the off-body link for medical assessment.

In our future work, numerical evaluation of the antenna performance characteristics will be conducted by applying an anatomical human body model. The impact of the antenna structural deformation will be examined, as well. The study will be fulfilled with the fabrication and experimental measurement of the antenna design.

Acknowledgment. H.F.R.I. The research project was supported by the Hellenic Foundation for Research and Innovation (H.F.R.I.) under the "2nd Call for H.F.R.I. Research Projects to support Post-Doctoral Researchers", Project Number: 205, with title "Innovative Textile Structures for Mechanical Electromagnetic Reconfigurability of Wearable Antennas" (M-REWEAR).

References

1. Hall, P.S., et al.: Antennas and propagation for on-body communication systems. IEEE Antennas Propag. Mag. **49**(3), 41–58 (2007)

2. Zhu, X., Guo, Y., Wu, W.: Miniaturized dual-band and dual-polarized antenna for MBAN applications. IEEE Trans. Antennas Propag. **64**(7), 2805–2814 (2016)
3. Mohamadzade, B., et al.: A conformal, dynamic pattern-reconfigurable antenna using conductive textile-polymer composite. IEEE Trans. Antennas Propag. **69**(10), 6175–6184 (2021)
4. Yan, S., Vandenbosch, G.A.E.: Radiation pattern-reconfigurable wearable antenna based on metamaterial structure. IEEE Antennas Wirel. Propag. Lett. **15**, 1715–1718 (2016)
5. Ha, S., Jung, C.W.: Reconfigurable beam steering using a microstrip patch antenna with a U-slot for wearable fabric applications. IEEE Antennas Wirel. Propag. Lett. **10**, 1228–1231 (2011)
6. Chen, S.J., Ranasinghe, D.C., Fumeaux, C.: Snap-on buttons as detachable shorting vias for wearable textile antennas. In: Proceedings of International Conference on Electromagnetics in Advanced Applications (ICEAA), pp. 521–524 (2016)
7. Tsolis, A., Michalopoulou, A., Alexandridis, A.A.: Use of conductive zip and Velcro as a polarisation reconfiguration means of a textile patch antenna. IET Microw. Antennas Propag. **14**, 684–693 (2020)
8. Chen, S.J., Fumeaux, C., Ranasinghe, D.C., Kaufmann, T.: Paired snap-on buttons connections for balanced antennas in wearable systems. IEEE Antennas Wirel. Propag. Lett. **14**, 1498–1501 (2015)
9. Gabriel, S., Lau, R.W., Gabriel, C.: The dielectric properties of biological tissues: II. Measurements in the frequency range 10 Hz to 20 GHz. Phys. Med. Biol. **41**, 2251–2269 (1996)
10. Hall, P.S., Hao, Y.: Antennas and Propagation for Body-Centric Wireless Communications, 2nd edn. Artech House, Norwood (2012)
11. IEEE standard for safety levels with respect to human exposure to radiofrequency electromagnetic fields, 3 kHz to 300 GHz. IEEE Standard C95.1 (1999)

Signal/Data Processing and Computing
For Health Systems

Myocardial Infarction Prediction Using Deep Learning

Catarina Cruz[1], Argentina Leite[1,2] (ID), E. J. Solteiro Pires[1,2]([envelope]) (ID),
and L. Torres Pereira[1,2] (ID)

[1] Escola de Ciências e Tecnologia Universidade de Trás-os-Montes e Alto Douro,
Vila Real, Portugal
al70600@utad.eu, {tinucha,epires,tpereira}@utad.pt
[2] INESC TEC, Porto, Portugal

Abstract. Myocardial infarction, known as heart attack, is one of the leading causes of world death. It occurs when blood heart flow is interrupted by part of coronary artery occlusion, causing the ischemic episode to last longer, creating a change in the patient's ECG. In this work, a method was developed for predicting patients with MI through Frank 3-lead ECG extracted from Physionet's PTB ECG Diagnostic Database and using instantaneous frequency and spectral entropy to extract features. Two neural networks were applied: Long Short-Term Memory and Bi-Long Short-Term Memory, obtaining a better result with the first one, with an accuracy of 78%.

Keywords: Electrocardiogram · Myocardial infarction · Deep Learning · Long Short-Term Memory

1 Introduction

Coronary heart disease is one of the leading killer diseases in the world and the deadliest in the US [2]. In this disease type, myocardial infarction (MI) is characterized by a part of the heart not being supplied with blood due to an occlusion of a coronary artery. As a result, the heart muscle is permanently damaged if it is not intervened immediately, leading to the death of its tissue. Thus, early identification and diagnosis become crucial to avoid sequelae of MI, such as heart failure or arrhythmia. This is called silent disease, as patients only know they have a myocardial infarction when they suffer an attack. American Health Association published that 750,000 Americans have a heart attack once per year, and 210,000 have recurrent heart attacks. Reaching a value of 72% for silent heart attacks [1].

Myocardial ischemia is the initial step when patients develop MI, which results from an imbalance between oxygen supply and demand. Before a patient has MI, the ischemia has reversible effects, and the heart cells can recover. However, during myocardial infarction, the ischemia episode lasts longer, causing the heart muscle to die and the heart signal ECG change [3].

© ICST Institute for Computer Sciences, Social Informatics and Telecommunications Engineering 2023
Published by Springer Nature Switzerland AG 2023. All Rights Reserved
A. Cunha et al. (Eds.): MobiHealth 2022, LNICST 484, pp. 133–143, 2023.
https://doi.org/10.1007/978-3-031-32029-3_13

The acute myocardial infarction diagnosis usually uses an electrocardiogram (ECG) as an integral part of the patient's diagnosis with suspected MI. ECG abnormalities due to MI are detected in the PR segment, QRS complex, ST segment, or T wave signals [5]. The diagnosis of heart disease there is two devices used to perform the diagnosis of heart disease: the 12-lead ECG and the three-channel Frank. The standard ECG has some leads almost aligned or derived from the others and, consequently, contain redundant information, not presenting spatial information such as the cardiac vector orientation. Frank Orthogonal Leads uses fewer leads and capture more information compared to 12-lead Holter ECG, even spatial information [2].

In 2018 Mohammad Kachuee et al. [9] proposed a heartbeats classifier using deep convolutional neural networks. They used five different arrhythmia according to the AAMI EC57 standard, using the knowledge acquired for classifying myocardial infarction, obtaining a prediction with an average accuracy of 95.9%. Two years later, Makimoto et al. [10] also created an AI using a convolutional neural network (CNN) equipped with a 6-layer architecture to accurately recognize ECG images and patterns achieving an accuracy of 81.4%.

Ardan et al. [3], in a different approach to the convulsional neural networks used a fuzzy inference system and obtained the characteristics of the MI through the S and T peaks ending with a sensitivity in the detection system test of 73%.

Recently, Adyasha Rath et al. [13] applied three cycles of LSTM network with 256, 128, and 64 modules in each stage, employing 20% random drop-offs of weights between modules. With two types of training schemes and validation (80 and 20%) and (70 and 30%) dataset was obtained with the best performance of 86.98% in accuracy, 93.82% in precision, 88.02% in sensitivity, 71.60% in specificity, and 91.50% in F1-score, respectively. It should be noted that these results were obtained using the 12 conventional lead ECGs.

This study aims to predict possible MI patients from characteristics extracted from the 3 Frank lead ECGs using two approaches with different neural networks: one with long-term memory (LSTM) and another with Bi-Long Short-Term Memory (BiLSTM).

The remaining work is organized in the following sections: Sect. 2 describes the dataset, data augmentation, resource extraction, network, and methods used to classify the patients. Section 3 shows the results and discussion, and finally, Sect. 4 draws the main conclusions concerning the study.

2 Materials and Methods

2.1 Data

This work analyzes cardiovascular signals extracted from the PTB Diagnostic ECG Database of PhysioNet [6,8]. The dataset consists of ECG recordings from 290 patients, each containing 5 individual recordings. In each record, 15 signals were measured simultaneously: the conventional twelve leads and the three Frank lead ECGs, with each signal, digitized at 1000 samples per second. For this study, only the three Frank lead ECGs were used, as represented in Fig. 1.

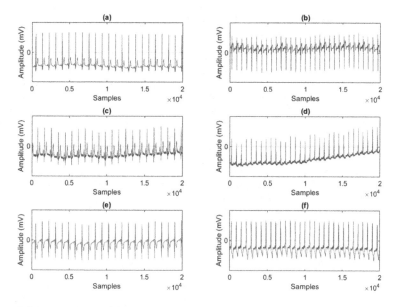

Fig. 1. ECG recordings. (a) Healthy Control with Frank Lead x, (b) MI with Frank Lead x, (c) Healthy Control with Frank Lead y, (d) MI with Frank Lead y, (e) Healthy Control with Frank Lead z, and (f) MI with Frank Lead z.

All 52 available control patients were used, and of the 148 patients with myocardial infarction, 52 were randomly selected to equate with the number of control, leaving the database with a total of 104 patients (52 with MI, 52 as healthy controls).

Each ECG record had an initial length of 115,200. As it was a long record and to increase the number of data, each ECG was divided into four identical parts, each record having a length of 28,800. Each part of the record was treated and added to the database as a new example patient, totaling 416 example patients, where 208 are healthy patients and 208 are patient with MI examples.

2.2   Feature Extraction

Extracting features from the data is critical to improving the classifier's performance. The characterization of ECG signals is achieved by time-frequency methods, such as spectrograms. Figure 2 illustrates this methodology for a healthy subject and a patient with MI.

Two-time parameters are used to extract sequences of features from the spectrograms: the instantaneous frequency and the spectral entropy.

The instantaneous frequency of a signal is a time sequence of features and is associated with the mean of the frequencies available in the signal as it

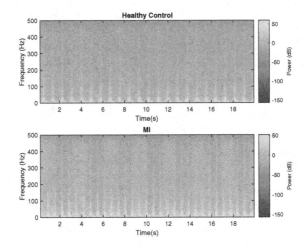

Fig. 2. Spectrum of a Healthy Control and a MI

changes over time. This approach estimates spectrogram using short-time Fourier transforms over time windows, where the time sequence of feature correspond to the centers of the time windows.

The spectral entropy of a signal is a parameter of its spectral power distribution. This parameter considers the normalized power distribution of the signal in the frequency domain as a probability distribution and calculates its entropy. As with instantaneous frequency, the function uses short time windows, and the time sequence of the feature corresponds to the center of the time windows [12]. These two-time sequences of features are represented in Fig. 3 and are then used as input for the LSTM and BiLSTM networks.

2.3   Neural Network

Long Short-Term Memory (LSTM) is a recurrent neural network that models how the human brain operates and discovers the underlying relationships in the sequential data provided with unknown duration time. It operates with a various RNNs that are capable of learning long-term dependencies, particularly in problems using sequence prediction. LSTM has feedback connections used to process the entire signal.

The primary role of the LSTM model is maintained by the memory cell known as the "cell state" which maintains its state over time.

Information can be added to or removed from the cell state. These gates could allow information to enter and leave the cell and contain a multiplication operation point and a sigmoid neural network layer that assists the mechanism (see Fig. 4).

On the other hand, Bi-Long Short-Term Memory (BiLSTM) is an LSTM model with two LSTMs layers [4], Fig. 5. The network is fed with two-time directions: a start-to-finish signal and an end-to-start signal, making the network flow

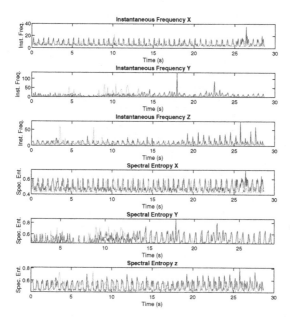

Fig. 3. Feature extracted from each Frank Lead: Healthy (blue) and Sick (red).

in both directions, contributing to the improvement of long-term dependency learning.

2.4   Classifier Performance

Five indicators are used to evaluate and analyze the effectiveness of the classifier's performance: accuracy (ACC) corresponds to the proportion of correct predictions to total predictions; sensitivity (SEN) is the proportion of true positives to the total positives present in the dataset; precision (PRE) is the ratio between true and total predicted positives; specificity (SPE) is the ratio between the true negatives and the total negatives; F1-Score (F1) combines the precision and sensitivity metric using their harmonic mean. The higher value, the more significant the balance between precision and sensitivity.

The following equations describe the performance classifiers used:

$$ACC = \frac{TP + TN}{TP + TN + FP + FN} \tag{1}$$

$$SEN = \frac{TP}{TP + FN} \tag{2}$$

$$PRE = \frac{TP}{TP + FP} \tag{3}$$

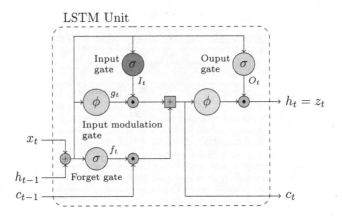

Fig. 4. LSTM unit [11].

$$SPE = \frac{TN}{TN + FP} \tag{4}$$

$$F1 = \frac{2.PRE.SEN}{PRE + SEN} \tag{5}$$

where TP is the true positives value, FP is the false positives value, TN is the value of the true negative, and FN is the value of the false negative.

The k-fold cross-validation method compares a large number of fitted models and avoids overfitting, evaluating the performance of neural networks. This method randomly splits the data into k portions. $k - 1$ portions are used for training and one for validation. This process is repeated k times. The general estimation error is the average test error of the iterations [7]. For this study, a k-fold with $k = 5$ was applied.

3   Results and Discussion

Each neural network was trained and tested two times with different training and test specification options. Two classes (healthy and sick) and six characteristics extracted from each patient were inserted into the neural networks, these being the instantaneous frequency and spectral entropy for each Frank lead ECG (v_x, v_y, v_z). The features for the two groups in the dataset are illustrated in Fig. 6. These features can characterize relatively well healthy and MI patients.

A 5-fold cross-validation was used, obtaining 80% of each group for training and 20% for testing. For all tests, a learning rate of $\alpha = 0.001$ was used, with two fully connected layers of size 20 and one of size 2 (two groups), followed by softmax and classification layers. The described model is illustrated in Fig. 7.

Initially, the LSTM neural network was used, with 100 Hidden Units and 80 MaxEpochs but varying the Mini Batch Size between 100 and 80. Table 1 and

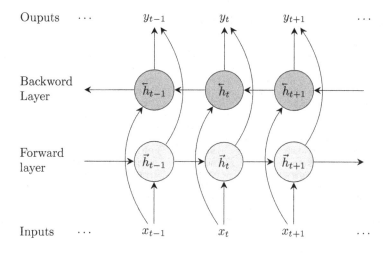

Fig. 5. Bi-LSTM layers [11].

Table 2 summarize the training and testing results, respectively. The best result was obtained when the Mini Batch Size was 80, obtaining test values of 78.13% for accuracy, 75.02% for sensitivity, 80.10% for precision, 81.27% for specificity, and 77.32% for F1-Score.

However, in BiLSTM, with the exact specifications used for the LSTM tests, there was a slight improvement in the training results, but the test results were lower when compared to the LSTM results. As with the LSTM, the best test results were achieved when the Mini Batch Size was 80, achieving 74.51% accuracy, 77.96% sensitivity, 74.96% accuracy, 71.24% specificity, and 75.37% of F1-Score. These results can be consulted in Tables 3 and 4 for training and testing, respectively.

Table 1. LSTM Train

NumHiddenUnits = 100, MaxEpochs = 80, MiniBatchSize = 100								
K=	TN	FN	TP	FP	ACC (%)	SEN (%)	PRE (%)	SPE (%)	F1 (%)
1	152	23	143	15	88.59	86.14	90.51	91.02	88.27
2	143	19	147	23	87.35	88.55	86.47	86.14	87.50
3	139	13	154	27	87.99	92.22	85.08	83.73	88.51
4	153	22	145	13	89.49	86.83	91.77	92.17	89.23
5	151	27	139	16	87.09	83.73	89.68	90.42	86.60
Mean ± std					88.10 ± 0.97	87.50 ± 3.15	88.70 ± 2.82	88.70 ± 3.59	88.02 ± 1.00
NumHiddenUnits = 100, MaxEpochs = 80, MiniBatchSize = 80								
K=	TN	FN	TP	FP	ACC(%)	SEN(%)	PRE(%)	SPE(%)	F1(%)
1	153	21	145	14	89.49	87.35	91.19	91.62	89.23
2	154	18	148	12	90.96	89.16	92.50	92.77	90.80
3	142	14	153	24	88.59	91.62	86.44	85.54	88.95
4	156	24	143	10	89.79	85.63	93.46	93.98	89.38
5	147	34	132	20	83.78	79.52	86.84	88.02	83.02
Mean ± std					88.52 ± 2.78	86.65 ± 4.56	90.09 ± 3.25	90.39 ± 3.50	88.28 ± 3.02

Table 2. LSTM Test

NumHiddenUnits = 100, MaxEpochs = 80, MiniBatchSize = 100								
K=	TN	FN	TP	FP	ACC (%)	SEN (%)	PRE (%)	SPE (%)	F1 (%)
1	32	13	29	9	73.49	69.05	76.32	78.05	72.50
2	32	6	36	10	80.95	85.71	78.26	76.19	81.82
3	30	9	32	12	74.70	78.05	72.73	71.43	75.29
4	29	7	34	13	75.90	82.93	72.34	69.05	77.27
5	35	16	26	6	73.49	61.90	81.25	85.37	70.27
Mean ± std					75.71 ± 3.10	75.53 ± 9.91	76.18 ± 3.77	76.02 ± 6.35	75.43 ± 4.46
NumHiddenUnits = 100, MaxEpochs = 80, MiniBatchSize = 80								
K=	TN	FN	TP	FP	ACC (%)	SEN (%)	PRE (%)	SPE (%)	F1 (%)
1	35	14	28	6	75.90	66.67	82.35	85.37	73.68
2	33	10	32	9	77.38	76.19	78.05	78.57	77.11
3	33	7	34	9	80.72	82.93	79.07	78.57	80.95
4	35	12	29	7	77.11	70.73	80.56	83.33	75.32
5	33	9	33	8	79.52	78.57	80.49	80.49	79.52
Mean ± std					78.13 ± 1.95	75.02 ± 6.42	80.10 ± 1.64	81.27 ± 3.01	77.32 ± 2.97

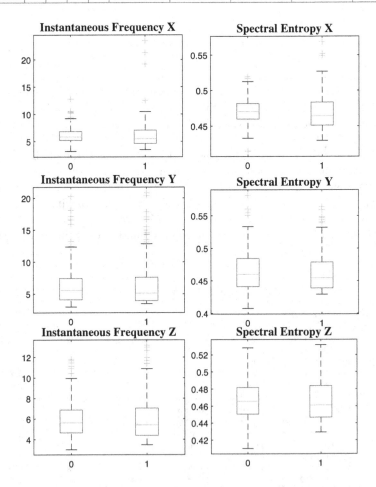

Fig. 6. Boxplot of the extracted features for two groups of patients: healthy (0) and sick (1).

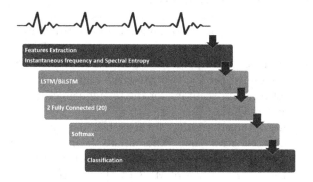

Fig. 7. Network structure

Table 3. BiLSTM Train

NumHiddenUnits = 100, MaxEpochs = 80, MiniBatchSize = 100								
K=	TN	FN	TP	FP	ACC (%)	SEN (%)	PRE (%)	SPE (%)	F1 (%)
1	146	5	161	21	92.19	96.99	88.46	87.43	92.53
2	164	20	146	2	93.37	87.95	98.65	98.80	92.99
3	155	4	163	11	95.50	97.60	93.68	93.37	95.60
4	155	21	146	11	90.39	87.43	92.99	93.37	90.12
5	165	21	145	2	93.09	87.35	98.64	98.80	92.65
Mean ± std					92.91 ± 1.86	91.46 ± 5.33	94.48 ± 4.29	94.35 ± 4.73	92.78 ± 1.95
NumHiddenUnits = 100, MaxEpochs = 80, MiniBatchSize = 80								
K=	TN	FN	TP	FP	ACC (%)	SEN (%)	PRE (%)	SPE (%)	F1 (%)
1	139	31	135	28	82.28	81.33	82.82	83.23	82.07
2	150	17	149	16	90.06	89.76	90.30	90.36	90.03
3	132	3	164	34	88.89	98.20	82.83	79.52	89.86
4	129	9	158	37	86.19	94.61	81.03	77.71	87.29
5	155	17	149	12	91.29	89.76	92.55	92.81	91.13
Mean ± std					87.74 ± 3.59	90.73 ± 6.35	85.91 ± 5.15	84.73 ± 6.63	88.08 ± 3.64

Table 4. BiLSTM Test

NumHiddenUnits = 100, MaxEpochs = 80, MiniBatchSize = 100								
K=	TN	FN	TP	FP	ACC (%)	SEN (%)	PRE (%)	SPE (%)	F1 (%)
1	33	11	31	8	77.11	73.81	79.49	80.49	76.54
2	36	17	25	6	72.62	59.52	80.65	85.71	68.49
3	32	21	20	10	62.65	48.78	66.67	76.19	56.34
4	30	10	31	12	73.49	75.61	72.09	71.43	73.81
5	32	15	27	9	71.08	64.29	75.00	78.05	69.23
Mean ± std					71.39 ± 5.36	64.40 ± 10.98	74.78 ± 5.69	78.37 ± 5.28	68.88 ± 7.76
NumHiddenUnits = 100, MaxEpochs = 80, MiniBatchSize = 80								
K=	TN	FN	TP	FP	ACC (%)	SEN (%)	PRE (%)	SPE (%)	F1 (%)
1	33	11	31	8	77.11	73.81	79.49	80.49	76.54
2	35	10	32	7	79.76	76.19	82.05	83.33	79.01
3	24	9	32	18	67.47	78.05	64.00	57.14	70.33
4	23	3	38	19	73.49	92.68	66.67	54.76	77.55
5	33	13	29	8	74.70	69.05	78.38	80.49	73.42
Mean ± std					74.51 ± 4.61	77.96 ± 8.90	74.12 ± 8.18	71.24 ± 14.03	75.37 ± 3.49

4   Conclusion and Future Work

In this work, a method was created for identifying myocardial infarction patients through the 3 Frank lead ECGsextracted from The PTB Diagnostic ECG Database from Physionet and applying two neural networks: LSTM and BiLSTM. The results obtained for the two networks were similar, with the LSTM obtaining a superior result in accuracy for the testing values of 78% for a testing value of 74% of the BiLSTM.

To improve the obtained results, future work may involve increasing or improving the characteristics that differentiate healthy patients from sick patients to optimize the classifier. Another approach for future work would be the separation of the different types of MI, with the criterion of separation being the location of the myocardial attack.

References

1. Acharya, U.R., Fujita, H., Oh, S.L., Hagiwara, Y., Tan, J.H., Adam, M.: Application of deep convolutional neural network for automated detection of myocardial infarction using ECG signals. Inf. Sci. **415**, 190–198 (2017)
2. Aranda, A., Bonizzi, P., Karel, J., Peeters, R.: Performance of dower's inverse transform and frank lead system for identification of myocardial infarction. In: 2015 37th Annual International Conference of the IEEE Engineering in Medicine and Biology Society (EMBC), pp. 4495–4498. IEEE (2015)
3. Ardan, A., Ma'arif, M., Aisyah, Z., Olivia, M., Titin, S.: Myocardial infarction detection system from PTB diagnostic ECG database using fuzzy inference system for ST waves. In: Journal of Physics: Conference Series, vol. 1204, p. 012071. IOP Publishing (2019)
4. Baldi, P., Brunak, S., Frasconi, P., Soda, G., Pollastri, G.: Exploiting the past and the future in protein secondary structure prediction. Bioinformatics **15**(11), 937–946 (1999)
5. Baloglu, U.B., Talo, M., Yildirim, O., San Tan, R., Acharya, U.R.: Classification of myocardial infarction with multi-lead ECG signals and deep CNN. Pattern Recogn. Lett. **122**, 23–30 (2019)
6. Bousseljot, R., Kreiseler, D., Schnabel, A.: Nutzung der ekg-signaldatenbank cardiodat der ptb über das internet (1995)
7. Ghojogh, B., Crowley, M.: The theory behind overfitting, cross validation, regularization, bagging, and boosting: tutorial. arXiv preprint arXiv:1905.12787 (2019)
8. Goldberger, A.L., et al.: PhysioBank, PhysioToolkit, and PhysioNet: components of a new research resource for complex physiologic signals. Circulation **101**(23), e215–e220 (2000)
9. Kachuee, M., Fazeli, S., Sarrafzadeh, M.: ECG heartbeat classification: a deep transferable representation. In: 2018 IEEE International Conference on Healthcare Informatics (ICHI), pp. 443–444. IEEE (2018)
10. Makimoto, H., et al.: Performance of a convolutional neural network derived from an ECG database in recognizing myocardial infarction. Sci. Rep. **10**(1), 1–9 (2020)
11. Monteiro, S., Leite, A., Solteiro Pires, E.J.: Deep learning on automatic fall detection. In: 2021 IEEE Latin American Conference on Computational Intelligence (LA-CCI), pp. 1–6 (2021). https://doi.org/10.1109/LA-CCI48322.2021.9769783

12. Pham, T.D.: Time-frequency time-space LSTM for robust classification of physiological signals. Sci. Rep. **11**(1), 1–11 (2021)
13. Rath, A., Mishra, D., Panda, G.: LSTM-based cardiovascular disease detection using ECG signal. In: Mallick, P.K., Bhoi, A.K., Marques, G., Hugo C. de Albuquerque, V. (eds.) Cognitive Informatics and Soft Computing. AISC, vol. 1317, pp. 133–142. Springer, Singapore (2021). https://doi.org/10.1007/978-981-16-1056-1_12

A Review on the Video Summarization and Glaucoma Detection

Tales Correia[1] , António Cunha[2,3] , and Paulo Coelho[1,4(✉)]

[1] School of Technology and Management, Polytechnic of Leiria, 2411-901 Leiria, Portugal
tales.correia@ipleiria.pt, paulo.coelho@ipleiria.pt
[2] Escola de Ciências e Tecnologias, University of Trás-os-Montes e Alto Douro, Quinta de Prados, 5001-801 Vila Real, Portugal
atcunha@utad.pt
[3] Institute for Systems and Computer Engineering, Technology and Science (INESC TEC), 4200-465 Porto, Portugal
[4] Institute for Systems Engineering and Computers at Coimbra (INESC Coimbra), DEEC, Pólo II, 3030-290 Coimbra, Portugal

Abstract. Glaucoma is a severe disease that arises from low intraocular pressure, it is asymptomatic in the initial stages and can lead to blindness, due to its degenerative characteristic. There isn't any available cure for it, and it is the second most common cause of blindness in the world. Regular visits to the ophthalmologist are the best way to prevent or contain it, with a precise diagnosis performed with professional equipment. From another perspective, for some individuals or populations, this task can be difficult to accomplish, due to several restrictions, such as low incoming resources, geographical adversities, and traveling restrictions (distance, lack of means of transportation, etc.). Also, logistically, due to its dimensions, relocating the professional equipment can be expensive, thus becoming inviable to bring them to remote areas. As an alternative, some low-cost products are available in the market that copes with this need, namely the D-Eye lens, which can be attached to a smartphone and enables the capture of fundus images, presenting as major drawback lower quality imaging when compared to professional equipment. Some techniques rely on video capture to perform summarization and build a full image with the desired features. In this context, the goal of this paper is to present a review of the methods that can perform video summarization and methods for glaucoma detection, combining both to indicate if individuals present glaucoma symptoms, as a pre-screening approach.

Keywords: Review · Glaucoma · Machine learning · Video summarization

© ICST Institute for Computer Sciences, Social Informatics and Telecommunications Engineering 2023
Published by Springer Nature Switzerland AG 2023. All Rights Reserved
A. Cunha et al. (Eds.): MobiHealth 2022, LNICST 484, pp. 144–156, 2023.
https://doi.org/10.1007/978-3-031-32029-3_14

1   Introduction

The human eyes take a key role in daily life, allowing humans to be able to see and perceive things all around their reach. Maintaining the eye in good health is extremely important, and the best way to keep track of its health is to have regular visits to the ophthalmologist. One of the most common eye checkups performed is the retinal fundus capture, which consists of the exposition of the back of the eye, where is located the macula and fovea, two of the principal areas where happens the actual formation of an image from the light incidence [1].

With the recent advances in studies in the fields of video summarization and machine learning, with a simple video recording taken from a smartphone using some gadgets with amplifying lens, is possible to convert it to a single image with the desired features to point out what could be an indication of glaucoma. This process doesn't intend to substitute the diagnosis process in a professional fundus machine, with specialist assistance, although it allows a quick summarization based on the captured video, to perform a pre-screening that may alert the individuals to seek professional assistance. Aiming to search for a method capable of performing retinal analysis based on low-quality imaging, thus, being capable of making pre-diagnosis with low-budget equipment, instead of professional medical equipment only found in clinics and hospitals. The idea is that with only a cell phone with a simple device, such as D-Eye attached, in hand, trained personnel can perform a retinal recording from patients that live in remote areas or have no facilitated access to other equipment. It is expected that it could help to orientate the most affected people to a further medical analysis, depending on the precision of the reading. Figure 1 shows a frame from a video captured of a patient eye using D-eye lens.

The advent of Video Summarization came from the need to gather important content from a significant amount of data, extracting the desired information from previously set keyframes that match the objective. With that in mind, selecting the keyframes and the features allied with the method to retrieve this information is crucial. Over the past years, many methods and techniques have been introduced and some of them will be shared later in this document, many of them being derived from machine learning, more specifically deep learning. Some examples of deep learning methods are Convolutional Neural Networks (CNNs), very useful for gesture recognition [2], speech recognition [3], and as will be presented in this document, video summarization [4–18]. Some of the reviewed works use advanced deep learning methods [19–21] and apply 3D-CNN methods, which are ideal when treating high volumetric data. It is also one of the objectives to include these methods of video summarization, applied to the lower-quality images.

Section 2 of this paper will be presented the criterion and methods that were used to select the reviewed works, and Sect. 3 will be presented the state of the art for both video summarization and glaucoma detection. Section 4 will present the conclusion and what can be done in terms of improvements in future works.

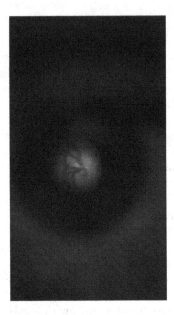

Fig. 1. Frame of retinal capture, using D-Eye lens.

2 Materials and Methods

2.1 Research Questions

This review was based on the following questions: (RQ1) Which methods can perform video summarization? (RQ2) Which methods can help identify glaucoma in a summarized image? (RQ3) From those methods which are realistic to be implemented specifically on low-quality acquired images? (RQ4) It is possible to adapt those methods in a multiple combination with other methods?

2.2 Inclusion Criteria

The study of the methods for both video summarization and glaucoma detection was performed with the following inclusion criteria: (1) studies that performed video summarization; (2) studies that performed glaucoma detection; (3) studies that apply deep-learning techniques; (4) studies with a relevant medical background; (5) studies that present their respective results/scores and datasets; (6) studies that were published between 2018 and 2022; (7) studies published in English.

2.3 Search Strategy

The reviewed studies with the selected inclusion criteria were searched in ScienceDirect and IEEE Xplore databases. The following research terms were used to research this review: "video summarization" AND "glaucoma detection". Every study was independently evaluated by the authors, determining their suitability with the agreement of all reviewers. There was a total of 44 reviewed studies and after more criterion selection, 18 studies were selected in the final analysis. The research was performed on 16 May 2022.

3   Results

As presented in Fig. 2, 42 studies were identified from the selected sources, without duplicated papers. Two additional records were added to the results, gathered from different queries to the databases. After analyzing each research article's metadata, namely the title, abstract, and keywords, 6 studies were excluded from the analysis because they were medically specific and did not directly relate to evaluating the video summarization or glaucoma detection. The full text of the remaining 38 articles was assessed considering the inclusion criteria, and consequently, 20 articles were excluded. Finally, the remaining 18 papers were examined and included in qualitative and quantitative syntheses. The criteria for organizing and presenting the articles description was based on the relevance of the study returned by the research platforms, followed by the year of publication, from the most recent to oldest.

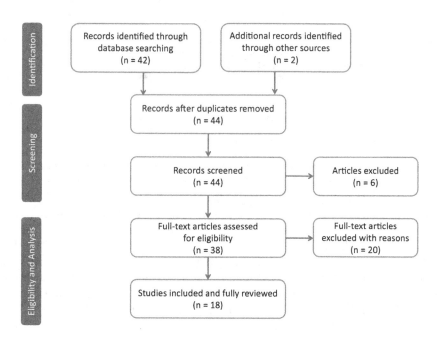

Fig. 2. Flow diagram of the selection of the papers.

3.1 Video Summarization

Some of the known techniques for video summarization rely on a set of tasks that the machine needs to perform to summarize relevant parts from video frames, taking into consideration the key features that have been selected to be present in the final set or image [22]. Figure 3 presents an example of the basic structure of how a video summarization algorithm performs. The input video is usually segmented frame by frame and based on what features the algorithm was trained to summarize, it will select the best shots or frames as output, depending on a chosen method or criteria.

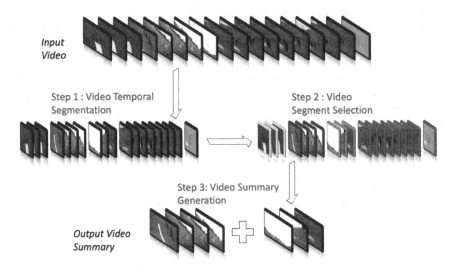

Fig. 3. Example of a video summarization algorithm structure - source [23].

The Long Short-Term Memory (LSTM) is a modern Recurrent Neural Network (RNN) useful to capture temporal dependencies between frames, but it has the issue of only being capable of handling short video segments, within a range from 30 to 80 frames. To overcome this, the method proposed by Lin et al. [4] employs a three-dimension Convolutional Neural Network (CNN) to extract features allied with a Deep Hierarchical LSTM Network with attention mechanism for Video Summarization (DHAVS) framework. This method was applied in SumMe [24], and TVSum [25] datasets and compared with recent results from other works with similar approaches. The F-Score obtained from DHAVS in SunMe was 45.2% and in the TVSum was around 60%.

In contrast to what was presented in [4], Zhao et al. [5] claims that RNN-based methods neglect global dependencies and multi-hop relationships between frames. To overcome that situation, a Hierarchical Multimodal Transformer (HMT) method is proposed for being capable of summarizing lengthy videos by hierarchically separating the layers of dependency between shots, thus reducing memory and computational consumption. The metrics were also like the previously mentioned work as well as the datasets, where this method achieved an F-Score of 44.1% on SunMe and 60.1% on TVSum.

An attention mechanism is proposed to work with a dual-path attentive network by Liang et al. [6] to overcome the systematical stiffness of the recurrent neural networks. It was stated that their method improves the processing time and reduces the computational power while is possible to train the model in parallel, thus being scalable in bigger datasets. The results for F-Score from training and testing in SumMe and TVSum, with 51.7% and 61.5% respectively, were higher than what was presented in [4] and [5].

Feng et al. [11] proposed a video summarization technique that uses two different feature extraction that converts frame-level features into shot-level features based on CNN which was named Video Summarization with netVLAD and CapsNet (VCVS). Their method improved computational and hardware work while using a feature fusion algorithm with capsule neural (CapsNet) networks to enhance the video features. The F-score presented is 49.5% on SumMe and 61.22% on TVSum.

Some video summarization methods [12–14], can only extract the content of static images of those videos. Huang et al. [15] comes with a method to do both video and motion summarization, relying on transitions effects detection (TED) for automatic shots segmentation, using CapsNet, and a self-attention method to summarize the results. The scores for this method were 46.6% on SumMe and 58% on TVSum.

A multiscale hierarchical attention approach is proposed by [16] for pattern recognition using intra-block and inter-block attention methods, exploring short and long-range temporal representations of a video. The implemented method was developed this way because the attention mechanism is easier to implement than RNN. The achieved results are scores of 51.1% on SumMe and 61.0% on TVSum.

Chai et al. [17] propose a graph-based structural analysis in a three-step method that can detect the differences in continuous frames and establish the correct summarization of the video. For the tests they used VSUMM and Youtube datasets [18], in which compared to similar analyzed works, they achieved an F-score of 67.5% and 56.7%, respectively.

Another interesting approach, presented by Hussain et al. [7] shows a survey on multi-view video summarization (MVS), claiming that this technique is not addressed regularly as other mainstream summarization methods. Consisting in gathering video records from simultaneous cameras within different angles, the paper reviews the recent and most significant works that englobe MVS.

A self-attention binary neural tree (SABTNet) method is proposed by Fu et al. [8] to perform video summarization, subdividing the video and then extracting it to shot-level features, altogether with a self-attention imbued. This work is the first to introduce such an approach, and similarly to the previously presented, the method was tested on SumMe and TVSum datasets, with F-scores of 50.7% and 61.0% respectively.

The work from Harakannanavar et al. [9] an approach based on ResNet-18, a CNN with eighteen layers, was used with kernel temporal segmentation (KTS) for the videos to create a temporally consistent summary. This method was benchmarked with the usual datasets SumMe and TVSum, obtaining 45.06% and 56.13% on F-scores respectively.

An interesting method is proposed in [10], a CNN with a Global Diverse Attention (SUM-GDA) mechanism, implying that the GDA provides relations within pair-frames and those pairs with all others in the video, stating that it overcomes the long-range issue from RNN models. They performed tests with supervised, unsupervised, and semi-supervised scenarios, with the usual datasets with the addition of VTW dataset [26]. The F-scores obtained from the tests were, as expected, higher in the supervised training, in which was obtained 52.8% on SumMe, 61% on TVSum, and 47.9% on VTW. Table 1 presents a resumed overview of the previously mentioned methods.

Table 1. Summary of the study analysis for video summarization.

Method	F-Score (%)		Remarkable Features
	SumMe	TVSum	
3D-CNN with DHAVS [4]	42.2	60	Employs LSTM to long videos.
HMT [5]	44.1	60.1	Reduces computational consumption by separating dependency between shots.
Dual-Path Attentive Network [6]	51.7	61.5	Improves computational consumption, improves process time and the model can be trained in parallel.
VCVS with CapsNet [11]	49.5	61.22	Improves computational and hardware work.
TED with CapsNet [15]	46.6	58	Summarization can be done in video and motion, not only in static images.
Multiscale Hierarchical Attention [16]	51.1	61	Captures of short and long-range dependencies also can perform motion detection.
SABTNet [8]	50.7	61	Shot-level segmentation and feature extraction.
ResNet-18 with KTS [9]	45.06	56.13	Temporal consistent summarization.
SUM-GDA [10]	52.8	61	Provides pair-frame relations within all video

It is relevant to imply that all those works are the most recent in terms of video summarization, making them a starting point as testing approaches to glaucoma detection. The following papers to be presented are more oriented to methods that have a direct impact on this matter.

3.2   Glaucoma Detection

A multimodal model to automatically detect glaucoma was proposed by [27] to combine deep neural networks focused on macular optical coherence tomography (OCT) and color fundus photography (CFP). Their dataset consisted of the UK Biobank dataset [28] with 1193 healthy and 1283 healthy and glaucomatous frames respectively. The OCT developed model was based on Densenet with MRSA initialization. For the CFP model, transfer learning with Inception Resnet V4 model, pre-trained on ImageNet data was used. Then it was introduced a gradient-boosted decision tree with XGBoost to create four separate baseline models (BM1 to BM4), enhancing specific features that they wanted to highlight. After testing the model, it was stated that mixing demographic and clinical features boosted the accuracy of diagnosis, obtaining around 97% of precision in correct results.

Trying to solve the issues of overfitting and big sets of data for training, Nayak et al. [29] proposed a method with a feature extraction called evolution-ary convolutional network (ECNet) to perform automated glaucoma detection. They also applied an evolutionary algorithm named real-coded genetic algorithm (RCGA), which maximizes the inter-class distance and minimizes the intra-class variability to optimize the weight of the layers. Then a set of classifiers is applied, such as K-nearest neighbor (KNN), extreme learning machine (ELM), backprop-agation neural network (BNN), and support vector machine (SVM), and kernel ELM (K-ELM), to enhance the model. They used a dataset, obtained from Kas-turba Medical College, Manipal, India using a Zeiss FF 450 fundus camera, containing 1426 retinal fundus images, 589 healthy, and 837 with glaucoma. As for the results, the classifier that made the best score was SVM with 97.2% of obtaining the correct diagnosis. Figure 4 illustrates the difference between a normal eye and glaucoma affected with a picture taken from the fundus of the retina, exposing the optic disc and cup. The difference in size between the optic cup and optic disc, also known as CDR (cup to disc ratio) is one of the most common clinical glaucoma diagnoses.

Li et al. [30] proposed an attention-based CNN for glaucoma detection (AG-CNN), using large-scale attention-based glaucoma (LAG) database [31], a large-scale fundus image that has 5824 images within positive and negative glaucoma, obtained from Beijing Tongren Hospital. When this work was proposed, there was no other work that incorporated human attention in medical recognition. These attention maps were obtained through a simulated eye-tracking experiment and incorporated into the LAG dataset. The method had an accuracy of 95.3%.

An artificial intelligence technique method presented by Venugopal et al. [32] relies on Phase Quantized Polar Transformed Cellular Automaton (PQPT-CA) for training on fundus images for glaucoma detection in early stages, using ACRIMA database, with 705 fundus images within glaucoma and normal ones. This approach was chosen because of the recent results in image processing, slightly changing the existing architecture of the automaton to fit the proposed method, they could use it to extract the features boosting the accuracy by around 24%, being 21% faster, and reducing the false-positive results in 54%.

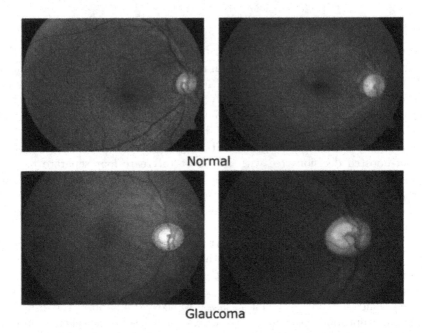

Fig. 4. Optic disc and optic cup comparison - source [29].

As for Zulfira et al. [33], they proposed a method that uses the classical parameter cup-to-disc ratio (CDR) allied with peripapillary atrophy (PPA) to enhance the precision of classification. They use an active contour snake (ACS) to segment the desired areas to calculate the CDR and Otsu's segmentation and threshold technique to acquire the PPA, and then the features are extracted with a grey-level co-occurrence matrix (GLCM). To classify glaucoma, dynamic ensemble selection (DES) is applied to make the final discrimination. The model was evaluated with three different databases where the ground truth was provided by ophthalmologists. Applying this method to RIM-ONE dataset [34] it was obtained an accuracy score of 96%.

Proposing the usage of 3D spectral-domain OCT, claiming that are potential information in these scans to help in glaucoma detection, Garcia et al. [35] brings a new perspective by presenting a method that uses the spatial dependencies of the features extracted from a B-scan of an OCT. Their database was composed of 176 healthy and 144 ill eyes. The method employed consisted of a slide-level feature extractor and a volume-based predictive model. They also used an LSTM network to combine the recurrent dependencies that will be further mixed into the latent space to provide a holistic feature vector that was generated by the proposed method of sequential-weighting module (SWM). The best results were achieved by using RAGNet-VGG16 architecture with an accuracy of 92%.

Gupta et al. [36] comes with a robust network to detect glaucoma in retinal fundus images based on CDR. They used two main modules, CLAHE [37] to improve the retinal images and the second module to find the CDR after the image segmentation based on EfficientNet and U-net. They performed the tests in DRISHTI-GS and RIM-ONE datasets. The result for this method using the Dice coefficient for similarity was 96%, and the pixel accuracy for optic disc and cup was 96.54% and 96.89% respectively.

Table 2 presents a resumed overview of the previously mentioned methods.

Table 2. Summary of the study analysis for glaucoma detection.

Method	Dataset/Number of images	Accuracy (%)
OCT & CFP & Systemic & Ocular Model [27]	UK Biobank/2476	97.0
RCGA with SVM [29]	Kasturba Medical College/1426	97.2
Full AG-CNN [30]	LAG/5824	95.1
DES-MI [33]	RIM-ONE/250	96.0
RAGNet-VGG16 with SWM [35]	Private Dataset/905	92.0
CLAHE with EfficientNet + U-Net [36]	RIM-ONE/766	99.6

4   Conclusions

It is noticeable that in the past years, new methods and algorithms have been implemented to bring solutions to recurring problems, and more than ever machine learning is taking a huge part in those approaches. As instigated before in (RQ2), when talking about specific objectives, like glaucoma detection, it is known that the algorithm must adapt to extract the correct and desired key features.

Answering (RQ1), some of the works showed that RNNs and LSTM are not the best methods to treat long video summarization due to limitations on data length, being more useful on short length videos, within 30–80 frames range, like speech recognition videos. CNNs have presented some of the best results within long-length video summarization, thus being useful in some areas like medical, face recognition, security, and summarization of large data in general. Most of the reviewed articles were dependent on CNN methods, due to their excellent performance, but it is important to note that being a powerful tool also means that it will need an equivalent computational power.

Overall, the key to achieving satisfactory results in video summarization depends on a good comprehension of the features needed to be summarized and choosing the method or combinations of methods that best suit the desired outcome, also selecting an ideal classifier can help achieve better results, that answers the (RQ4). In glaucoma detection, there is a great field of study that still can be developed.

From what (RQ3) brought, it is also important to state that in the reviewed papers, all of them used public or private databases from high-quality images or videos, and one of the main ideas of this work is the pursuit of the best method that can provide a reliable summary with low computational consumption, due to the usage of smartphones with lower-quality image acquisition.

Aiming for early detection with a fast and trustworthy algorithm is what this paper intends to propose for its next iteration. Instead of the conventional methods proposed in past works, a new algorithm capable of using a low-quality smartphone video of fundus recording and converting the resulting video to a single image with relevant features to finally bring a significant diagnostic, and of course, with a professional medical validation for those results.

Acknowledgements. This work is funded by FCT/MEC through national funds and, when applicable, co-funded by the FEDER-PT2020 partnership agreement under the project UIDB/00308/2020.

References

1. Cowan, C.S., et al.: Cell types of the human retina and its organoids at single-cell resolution. Cell **182**(6), 1623–1640 (2020)
2. Xu, L., Zhang, K., Yang, G., Chu, J.: Gesture recognition using dual-stream CNN based on fusion of sEMG energy kernel phase portrait and IMU amplitude image. Biomed. Sig. Process. Control **73**, 103364 (2022). https://doi.org/10.1016/j.bspc.2021.103364
3. Atila, O., Şengür, A.: Attention guided 3D CNN-LSTM model for accurate speech based emotion recognition. Appl. Acoust. **182**, 108260 (2021)
4. Lin, J., Zhong, S.H., Fares, A.: Deep hierarchical LSTM networks with attention for video summarization. Comput. Electr. Eng. **97**, 107618 (2022). https://doi.org/10.1016/j.compeleceng.2021.107618
5. Zhao, B., Gong, M., Li, X.: Hierarchical multimodal transformer to summarize videos. Neurocomputing **468**, 360–369 (2022). https://doi.org/10.1016/j.neucom.2021.10.039
6. Liang, G., Lv, Y., Li, S., Wang, X., Zhang, Y.: Video summarization with a dual-path attentive network. Neurocomputing **467**, 1–9 (2022). https://doi.org/10.1016/j.neucom.2021.09.015
7. Hussain, T., Muhammad, K., Ding, W., Lloret, J., Baik, S.W., de Albuquerque, V.H.C.: A comprehensive survey of multi-view video summarization. Pattern Recogn. **109**, 107567 (2021). https://doi.org/10.1016/j.patcog.2020.107567
8. Fu, H., Wang, H.: Self-attention binary neural tree for video summarization. Pattern Recogn. Lett. **143**, 19–26 (2021). https://doi.org/10.1016/j.patrec.2020.12.016
9. Harakannanavar, S.S., Sameer, S.R., Kumar, V., Behera, S.K., Amberkar, A.V., Puranikmath, V.I.: Robust video summarization algorithm using supervised machine learning. Global Transitions Proc. **3**(1), 131–135 (2022). https://doi.org/10.1016/j.gltp.2022.04.009
10. Li, P., Ye, Q., Zhang, L., Yuan, L., Xu, X., Shao, L.: Exploring global diverse attention via pairwise temporal relation for video summarization. Pattern Recogn. **111**, 107677 (2021). https://doi.org/10.1016/j.patcog.2020.107677
11. Feng, X., Zhu, Y., Yang, C.: Video summarization based on fusing features and shot segmentation. In: Proceedings of 2021 7th IEEE International Conference on Network Intelligence and Digital Content, IC-NIDC 2021, pp. 383–387 (2021)

12. Badre, S.R., Thepade, S.D.: Summarization with key frame extraction using thepade's sorted n-ary block truncation coding applied on haar wavelet of video frame. In: 2016 Conference on Advances in Signal Processing, CASP, pp. 332–336 (2016)

13. Fei, M., Jiang, W., Mao, W.: Memorable and rich video summarization. J. Vis. Commun. Image Represent. **42**, 207–217 (2017). https://doi.org/10.1016/j.jvcir.2016.12.001

14. Mehmood, I., Sajjad, M., Rho, S., Baik, S.W.: Divide-and-conquer based summarization framework for extracting affective video content. Neurocomputing **174**, 393–403 (2016). https://doi.org/10.1016/j.neucom.2015.05.126

15. Huang, C., Wang, H.: A novel key-frames selection framework for comprehensive video summarization. IEEE Trans. Circ. Syst. Video Technol. **30**(2), 577–589 (2020)

16. Zhu, W., Lu, J., Han, Y., Zhou, J.: Learning multiscale hierarchical attention for video summarization. Pattern Recogn. **122**, 108312 (2022). https://doi.org/10.1016/j.patcog.2021.108312

17. Chai, C., et al.: Graph-based structural difference analysis for video summarization. Inf. Sci. **577**, 483–509 (2021). https://doi.org/10.1016/j.ins.2021.07.012

18. De Avila, S.E.F., Lopes, A.P.B., Da Luz, A., De Albuquerque Araújo, A.: VSUMM: a mechanism designed to produce static video summaries and a novel evaluation method. Pattern Recogn. Lett. **32**(1), 56–68 (2011). https://doi.org/10.1016/j.patrec.2010.08.004

19. Huang, S., Li, X., Zhang, Z., Wu, F., Han, J.: User-ranking video summarization with multi-stage spatio-temporal representation. IEEE Trans. Image Process. **28**(6), 2654–2664 (2019)

20. Agyeman, R., Muhammad, R., Choi, G.S.: Soccer video summarization using deep learning. In: Proceedings - 2nd International Conference on Multimedia Information Processing and Retrieval, MIPR 2019, pp. 270–273 (2019)

21. Riahi, A., Elharrouss, O., Al-Maadeed, S.: EMD-3DCNN-based method for COVID-19 detection. Comput. Biol. Med. **142**, 105188 (2022). https://doi.org/10.1016/j.compbiomed.2021.105188

22. Apostolidis, E., Adamantidou, E., Metsai, A.I., Mezaris, V., Patras, I.: Video summarization using deep neural networks: a survey. Proc. IEEE **109**(11), 1838–1863 (2021)

23. Lei, Z., Zhang, C., Zhang, Q., Qiu, G.: FrameRank: a text processing approach to video summarization. In: Proceedings - IEEE International Conference on Multimedia and Expo, vol. 2019, pp. 368–373 (2019)

24. Gygli, M., Grabner, H., Riemenschneider, H., Van Gool, L.: Creating summaries from user videos. In: Fleet, D., Pajdla, T., Schiele, B., Tuytelaars, T. (eds.) ECCV 2014. LNCS, vol. 8695, pp. 505–520. Springer, Cham (2014). https://doi.org/10.1007/978-3-319-10584-0_33

25. Song, Y., Vallmitjana, J., Stent, A., Jaimes, A.: TVSum: summarizing web videos using titles. In: Proceedings of the IEEE Computer Society Conference on Computer Vision and Pattern Recognition, 07–12 June, pp. 5179–5187 (2015)

26. VTW Dataset. http://aliensunmin.github.io/project/%0Avideo-language/

27. Mehta, P., et al.: Automated detection of glaucoma with interpretable machine learning using clinical data and multimodal retinal images. Am. J. Ophthalmol. **231**, 154–169 (2021). https://doi.org/10.1016/j.ajo.2021.04.021

28. Sudlow, C., et al.: UK biobank: an open access resource for identifying the causes of a wide range of complex diseases of middle and old age. PLoS Med. **12**(3), 1–10 (2015)

29. Nayak, D.R., Das, D., Majhi, B., Bhandary, S.V., Acharya, U.R.: ECNet: an evolutionary convolutional network for automated glaucoma detection using fundus images. Biomed. Sig. Process. Control **67**, 102559 (2021). https://doi.org/10.1016/j.bspc.2021.102559

30. Li, L., Xu, M., Wang, X., Jiang, L., Liu, H.: Attention based glaucoma detection: a large-scale database and CNN model. In: Proceedings of the IEEE Computer Society Conference on Computer Vision and Pattern Recognition, pp. 10563–10572 (2019)

31. Li, L., et al.: A large-scale database and a CNN model for attention-based glaucoma detection. IEEE Trans. Med. Imaging **39**(2), 413–424 (2020). https://ieeexplore.ieee.org/document/8756196/

32. Venugopal, N., Mari, K., Manikandan, G., Sekar, K.R.: Phase quantized polar transformative with cellular automaton for early glaucoma detection. Ain Shams Eng. J. **12**(4), 4145–4155 (2021). https://doi.org/10.1016/j.asej.2021.04.018

33. Zulfira, F.Z., Suyanto, S., Septiarini, A.: Segmentation technique and dynamic ensemble selection to enhance glaucoma severity detection. Comput. Biol. Med. **139**, 104951 (2021). https://doi.org/10.1016/j.compbiomed.2021.104951

34. RIM-ONE (2020). https://www.ias-iss.org/ojs/IAS/article/view/2346

35. García, G., Colomer, A., Naranjo, V.: Glaucoma detection from raw SD-OCT volumes: a novel approach focused on spatial dependencies. Comput. Methods Programs Biomed. **200**, 105855 (2021)

36. Gupta, N., Garg, H., Agarwal, R.: A robust framework for glaucoma detection using CLAHE and EfficientNet. Vis. Comput. 1–14 (2021). https://doi.org/10.1007/s00371-021-02114-5

37. Pizer, S.M., et al.: Adaptive histogram equalization and its variations. Comput. Vis. Graph. Image Process. **39**(3), 355–368 (1987). https://linkinghub.elsevier.com/retrieve/pii/S0734189X8780186X

A Generalization Study of Automatic Pericardial Segmentation in Computed Tomography Images

Rúben Baeza[1,2(✉)] [iD], Carolina Santos[3], Fábio Nunes[3,4] [iD], Jennifer Mancio[4] [iD], Ricardo Fontes-Carvalho[3,4] [iD], Miguel Coimbra[2,5] [iD], Francesco Renna[2,5] [iD], and João Pedrosa[1,2] [iD]

[1] Faculdade de Engenharia da Universidade do Porto, Porto, Portugal
up202103374@up.pt
[2] Instituto de Engenharia de Sistemas e Computadores, Tecnologia e Ciência, Porto, Portugal
[3] Faculdade de Medicina da Universidade do Porto, Porto, Portugal
[4] Centro Hospitalar de Vila Nova de Gaia e Espinho, Vila Nova de Gaia, Portugal
[5] Faculdade de Ciências da Universidade do Porto, Porto, Portugal

Abstract. The pericardium is a thin membrane sac that covers the heart. As such, the segmentation of the pericardium in computed tomography (CT) can have several clinical applications, namely as a preprocessing step for extraction of different clinical parameters. However, manual segmentation of the pericardium can be challenging, time-consuming and subject to observer variability, which has motivated the development of automatic pericardial segmentation methods.

In this study, a method to automatically segment the pericardium in CT using a U-Net framework is proposed. Two datasets were used in this study: the publicly available Cardiac Fat dataset and a private dataset acquired at the hospital centre of Vila Nova de Gaia e Espinho (CHVNGE).

The Cardiac Fat database was used for training with two different input sizes - 512×512 and 256×256. A superior performance was obtained with the 256×256 image size, with a mean Dice similarity score (DCS) of 0.871 ± 0.01 and 0.807 ± 0.06 on the Cardiac Fat test set and the CHVNGE dataset, respectively.

Results show that reasonable performance can be achieved with a small number of patients for training and an off-the-shelf framework, with only a small decrease in performance in an external dataset. Nevertheless, additional data will increase the robustness of this approach for difficult cases and future approaches must focus on the integration of 3D information for a more accurate segmentation of the lower pericardium.

This work is financed by National Funds through the Portuguese funding agency, FCT - Fundação para a Ciência e a Tecnologia, within projects DSAIPA/AI/0083/2020 and LA/P/0063/2020.

A. Cunha et al. (Eds.): MobiHealth 2022, LNICST 484, pp. 157–167, 2023.
https://doi.org/10.1007/978-3-031-32029-3_15

Keywords: Pericardium Segmentation · Deep Learning · U-Net ·
Computed Tomography

1   Introduction

Coronary artery disease (CAD) is the most common type of heart disease and
the leading cause of death worldwide [10]. CAD happens when the coronary
arteries become hardened and narrowed causing the reduction of blood flow to
the heart muscle, leading to ischemia. This is due to the buildup of deposits of
calcium, fatty lipids, and inflammatory cells, called plaque, on the inner walls
of coronary arteries (atherosclerosis). As a result, the heart muscle is deprived
from the blood or oxygen it needs, which can lead to chest pain (angina) and
myocardial infarction.

Many risk factors increase the probability of CAD including cholesterol, diabetes, smoking, being overweight, or family history of heart disease. In these
cases, it is advisable to test for CAD [6]. Nowadays, quantifying calcium deposits
in the coronary arteries through calcium scans is the most common non-invasive
technique for screening CAD. A coronary calcium scan uses computerized tomography (CT) to detect calcium deposits in the coronary arteries of the heart. A
higher coronary calcium score suggests a higher chance of the presence of a
plaque and a higher risk of a future myocardial infarction [2].

However, CAD especially in people below 50 years of age, can be present without calcium (non-calcified plaque) and may not be detected by this technique
which leads some patients to be misdiagnosed. Early studies suggest that changes
in epicardial adipose tissue (EAT) may play an important role in the pathogenesis of CAD, emerging as a relevant factor for cardiovascular risk stratification
[14]. These structures can be visualized in non-contrast cardiac CT performed
for assessment of coronary calcium [9]. EAT assessment typically implies a prior
segmentation of the pericardium - a thin sac that covers the heart composed by
a double layered membrane. However, manual segmentation of the pericardium
is user-dependent, due to the difficulty of correctly identifying the area among
multiple observers and remains a tedious task, not suitable for clinical practice
[4], being essential to enhance the repeatability of the results and to reduce time.

In recent years, several research studies investigated the automatic segmentation of the pericardium and EAT on CT using machine and deep learning
algorithms. One of the first studies assessing a technique for the segmentation
of the fat surrounding the heart compartments was reported by Rodrigues et
al. [11]. They proposed a feature extraction method comprising an intersubjec-
tive registration based on the creation of an atlas and then, classification. This
method can obtain an ideal performance in the Dice similarity score (DSC) (97.9
%) for the segmentation of EAT. However, several issues must be considered in
the case of atlas-based techniques as the performance depends heavily on the
registration step [8]. Commandeur et al. [4] used a deep learning approach consisting of a multitask computational graph CNN network where the pericardium
was first segmented and then its inner region. This study reported a high correlation between deep learning quantification and manual segmentations of EAT

of two experienced tracers (r = 0.973 and r = 0.979; P < 0.001). Zhang et al. [15] proposed a method based on the U-Net framework, applying dual U-Nets with a morphological layer on cardiac CT scans. The first U-Net is used to detect the pericardium and the second to find and segment the epicardial fat from the pericardium. The proposed method achieves a mean DSC of 91.19%. Although many of these studies show promising results, the effectiveness of these tools has not yet been demonstrated in large populations. Furthermore, there are still challenges to be overcome namely in the integration of 3D and prior information (e.g. pericardial geometry).

The work presented in this report is a preliminary study towards the automatic segmentation of the pericardium in CT imaging. A state of the art architecture is trained for this purpose using publicly available data. Furthermore, a generalization analysis of the considered segmentation solution is performed using a private external dataset.

2 Methods

2.1 Datasets

In this work two datasets were employed: the publicly available Cardiac Fat dataset from Rio de Janeiro and a private dataset acquired from the hospital centre of Vila Nova de Gaia e Espinho (CHVNGE).

Cardiac Fat Dataset. The Cardiac Fat database [1] was acquired in Rio de Janeiro and released publicly by Rodrigues et al. [11]. The dataset includes 20 CT scans with 878 slices belonging to 20 patients as DICOM images (512 × 512 pixels). The CT scans were obtained with two different scanners (Phillips and Siemens) with a slice thickness of 3 mm. The average age of the patients is 55.4. The original ground truth was obtained via manual segmentation by a physician and a computer scientist who labeled the epicardial fat, pericardial fat (mediastinal), and finally, the pericardium layer. It is relevant to point out that CTs were manually centred and cropped to the pericardium and thresholded to the adipose tissue range of $[-200, -30]$ Hounsfield Unit (HU). Manual annotations of different structures are made available for these images. For this reason it is not possible to make a direct match of the labels with the original DICOM images. An example of a CT slices and the corresponding manual segmentations is shown in Fig. 1(a).

CHVNGE Dataset. The CHVNGE dataset is a subset of 20 patients randomly selected from the EPICHEART (The influence of EPICardial adipose tissue in HEART diseases) Study (ClinicalTrials.gov: NCT03280433), collected at the CHVNGE in Vila Nova de Gaia, Portugal. The EPICHEART study is a translational study designed to investigate the association between EAT and CAD, left atrial remodelling and postoperative atrial fibrillation, and frailty syndrome in patients with symptomatic severe aortic stenosis referred to aortic valve

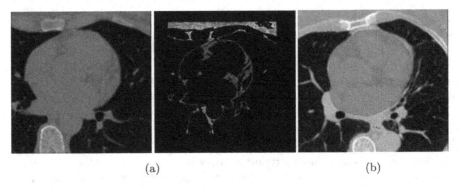

(a)   (b)

Fig. 1. Dataset overview. (a) Cardiac Fat dataset. Left: DICOM images; right: DICOM in fat HU range and manual segmentations of cardiac fat. Red indicates epicardial fat, green indicates mediastinal fat. (b) CHVNGE Dataset. DICOM images with pericardium in light red. (Color figure online)

replacement. This is a prospective cohort including 574 patients who underwent pre-operative assessment, intra-operative samples collections, and follow-up in hospital and at 6 months after surgery. All data was anonymized prior to analysis for the purposes of this study. The dataset includes 20 CT scans with 909 slices as DICOM images (512 × 512 pixels). All CT scans were acquired on a Siemens Somatom Sensation 64 with an ECG-triggered scanning protocol (tube voltage 120 kV, tube current 190 mA, gantry rotation 330 ms, collimation 24 × 1.2 mm, pitch 0.2) and a slice thickness of 3 mm. The pericardial segmentation was obtained via manual segmentation by one of the authors (CS). An example of a CT slice and manual pericardial segmentation is shown in Fig. 1(b).

2.2   Image Registration

Given the mismatch between the labels and original DICOMs due to the manual cropping and centering of CT slices for labelling, an image registration methodology was used to align the labels to the DICOM images. In this way, full DICOM images can be used to train a deep learning segmentation model without the need for centering and cropping on external datasets.

First, the DICOM images were converted to the same range as labeled images of $[-200, -30]$ HU to facilitate the recognition of key points between the two images. Image registration was then performed between pairs of DICOM and labeled CTs using the ORB (Oriented FAST and Rotated BRIEF) algorithm [13]. The process consists first of finding the key points using an algorithm called FAST, which mainly uses an intensity threshold between the central pixel and a circular ring around the center. Then, ORB uses BRIEF (Binary Robust Independent Elementary Features) descriptors to describe each keypoint. BRIEF is a bit string description constructed from a set of binary intensity tests between n pairs (x, y) of pixels which are located inside the patch (a key point is in the center of the patch). For further details, the reader is referred to the original publications of the ORB algorithm [13]. Next, a brute-force matcher was used to match the key points of the two images, selecting the best results while removing the noisy ones. The default parameters and the hamming distance were used for the ORB and the matcher, respectively. Finally, using the RANSAC algorithm it is possible to highlight the inliers (correct matches) and find the transformation matrix [7].

It should be noted that the images are misaligned in exactly the same way within each patient, therefore only one manually chosen transformation matrix is applied per patient. With this, there will be 20 transformation matrices corresponding to the 20 patients in the database.

2.3 Pericardial Segmentation

In this section, the strategy adopted to obtain the pericardial reference segmentations is initially presented. Finally, the models developed will be described, as well as the data preprocessing.

Pericardium Labelling. While the Cardiac Fat dataset has pericardial contours available, label inconsistencies were found in some images. Therefore, to train and test the segmentation model, only the EAT label was used to obtain an approximation of the pericardial mask using a Convex Hull [3]. This algorithm was applied to all binary masks of the EAT and an example is shown in Fig. 2.

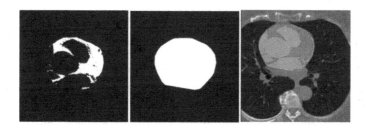

Fig. 2. Convex hull pericardium labelling example. Left: EAT mask; middle: generated pericardium label using convex hull; right: EAT (red) and Pericardial (yellow) labels registered and overlapped with DICOM images. (Color figure online)

Data Preprocessing. Before training the network, the CT slices were first clipped to [−1000, 1000] HU and then normalized to a range between 0 and 1. A total of 121 slices from the original dataset that did not include pericardium labels were also removed during training.

Model Architecture. Pericardial segmentation was then performed using a U-Net architecture [12], as show in Fig. 3. The U-Net is a popular framework for deep learning models, it often obtains excellent performance in image segmentation, especially in the area of medical image processing. This model was trained from scratch with a total number of 31,031,685 parameters. Two different input sizes were tested to evaluate the importance of contextual information and network receptive field: 512 × 512 (the original image size) and 256 × 256.

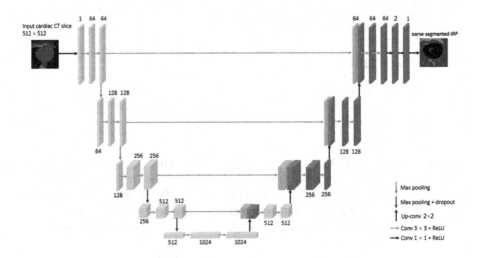

Fig. 3. U-Net architecture used for pericardial segmentation (adapted from [15]).

Training Setup. For the training, validation and testing of the model, the Cardiac Fat dataset was randomly divided as follows: 60% of the CT scans for training, 20% of the CT scans for validation, and the remaining 20% for testing. A patient-wise division was applied to avoid bias given that different CT slices of the same patient are highly correlated. The CHVNGE data was used for external testing of the automatic segmentation network and were thus not used for training.

The two models were trained with the binary cross-entropy loss function and using the adaptive moment estimation (Adam) optimizer. The binary cross-entropy is defined by the Eq. (1).

$$Loss = -\frac{1}{N} \sum_{i=1}^{N} y_i \log(p(y_i)) + (1 - y_i) \log(1 - p(y_i)) \qquad (1)$$

where y is the label and $p(y)$ is the predicted probability of the pixel being from the label for all N pixels.

A batch size of 2 and learning rate of 0.0001 was used for the first model. For the model trained with 256×256 images, a batch size of 12 and a learning rate of 0.001 was used. These hyper-parameters were selected based on empirical experiments, taking into account the memory constraints of the workstation used. An early stopping callback method was also used to stop training when the validation loss did not improve for 7 consecutive epochs. The two deep learning models were trained using Tensorflow and an NVIDIA GTX 1080 GPU.

Model Evaluation. Evaluation of the segmentation performance was done using the DSC [5], defined as:

$$DCS(A, B) = \frac{2 A \cap B|}{|A| + |B|}, \cdot \tag{2}$$

where A and B are the pericardial masks of the manual and automatic segmentations. The value of DCS ranges from 0, indicating no spatial overlap between the two segmentations, to 1, indicating complete overlap.

It should be noted that the model returns an array with the dimension of the image in which each pixel has a value from 0 to 1 that corresponds to the probability of it belonging to the pericardium. Thus, to create the predicted binary mask, this array was thresholded at 0.5.

3 Results and Discussion

3.1 Image Registration

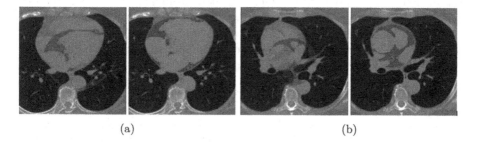

(a)   (b)

Fig. 4. Two examples ((a) and (b)) before (left) and after (right) image registration.

The result of the image registration for two patients is shown in Fig. 4. It can be seen that before the application of image registration for this patient, the labels were out of alignment with the DICOM image. After registration, a correct alignment of the mask with the DICOM image is verified as seen in Fig. 4. The registration results were evaluated qualitatively and a successful alignment was verified for all patients.

Table 1. DSC of the automatic segmentation for the Cardiac Fat dataset.

Size	Metric
	DCS (mean ± standard deviation)
256 × 256	0.871 ± 0.01
512 × 512	0.831 ± 0.02

3.2   Pericardial Segmentation

Cardiac Fat Dataset. The DCS mean values for the test images with 256 × 256 and 512 × 512 pixels are presented in Table 1. It can be seen that higher DSC was obtained for the 256 × 256 image size, with a DCS mean of 0.871 ± 0.01 for 256 × 256 images and 0.831 ± 0.02 for 512 × 512 images.

Two examples of automatic segmentations predicted by both models are presented in Fig. 5. It can be seen that the images predicted by the 256 × 256 model present slightly better results, being more similar to the corresponding label. In the case of the 512 × 512 images, there are some flaws in the classification of pixels and even inside the pericardium, some pixels are not attributed to it. The bottom row of Fig. 5 highlights the difficulty in segmenting the lower portion of the pericardium due to the presence of other organs in the CT slice.

The observed worse performance for the 512 × 512 images is likely due to the fact that the larger image size results in a decrease in the size of the receptive field thus giving less contextual information to the network, which can be important for segmentation. However, the use of different hyperparameters for the two models (batch size and learning rate) can also play a role. Even so, in both models a satisfactory DCS was obtained, taking into account that a standard U-Net architecture was used. Furthermore, the pericardium labels used for training, validation and testing on the Cardiac Fat dataset were obtained based on the convex hull of the EAT masks, which necessarily means that they will have missing sections, particularly on the lower and upper slices of the pericardium.

Table 2. DSC of the proposed automatic segmentation for the CHVNGE dataset.

Size	Metric
	DCS (mean ± standard deviation)
256 × 256	0.807 ± 0.06
512 × 512	0.769 ± 0.06

CHVNGE Dataset. The models trained on the Cardiac Fat dataset were then evaluated on the CHVNGE dataset to evaluate performance in an external dataset. The mean DCS for the 20 patients and the respective standard deviation are presented in the Table 2. It can be seen that, again, images with 256 × 256

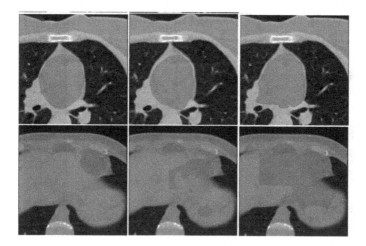

Fig. 5. Examples of pericardium segmentation for the Cardiac Fat dataset. Left: manual segmentation; middle: 256 × 256 automatic segmentation; right: 512 × 512 automatic segmentation).

showed better results with a DCS mean of 0.807 ± 0.06 for images with 512 × 512 pixels and 0.769 ± 0.06 for 512 × 512 images.

Two examples of automatic segmentations by both models are presented in Fig. 6. On the top row, it can again be seen that the results are better using 256 × 256 images and that the prediction is more similar to the corresponding label. However, examining the bottom row of the Fig. 6, it can be seen that the significant calcification of the aortic valve in this patient led to a failure of the segmentation network with a large portion of the center of the pericardium excluded from the segmentation. This example shows the need to train the model with a larger amount of data and especially with as much variability as possible with the aim of making the model more generalizable.

Still it is noteworthy that the results were only moderately worse compared to those obtained in the Cardiac Fat dataset (Table 1) with a difference of about 0.06 relative to the DCS metric. This decrease in performance was however expected since the model was trained for the Cardiac Fat dataset. In addition, the data from the hospital has more patients tested, increasing the variability and consequently the difficulty for the model to predict correctly.

3.3   Limitations and Future Work

In spite of the promising results obtained in this work, significant limitations remain as mentioned throughout the report.

First, the quantity and quality of the data and annotations that were used for training is clearly insufficient. While the 878 CT slices that compose the Cardiac Fat dataset are a significant number, it should be noted that these come from only 20 patients. As such, they are highly correlated and do not adequately

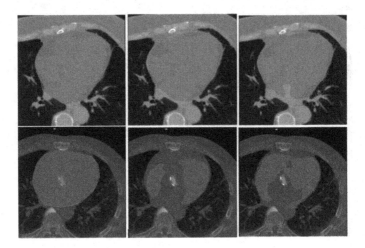

Fig. 6. Examples of pericardium segmentation for the CHVNGE dataset. Left: manual segmentation; middle: 256 × 256 automatic segmentation; right: 512 × 512 automatic segmentation).

represent the variability existing in the population. This was the observed on the CHVNGE dataset, with lower mean DSC and particularly for the example shown in Fig. 6. Furthermore, the labelling used for training is also not ideal as it was obtained from EAT labels and can be incomplete. As such it would be crucial to train the model with more patients and a more consistent pericardium labelling.

Second, in terms of segmentation performance, while the model can detect and locate the pericardium reasonably well throughout most axial slices, it can often fail, particularly for the lower pericardium and for slices where there is no pericardium (below or above). The use of 3D or 2.5D networks to provide further context during segmentation would thus be an extremely important strategy to improve performance in these slices which will be explored in future work.

4   Conclusions

In conclusion, a U-Net segmentation network for automatic pericardial segmentation was proposed, trained on the public Cardiac Fat dataset. A mean DCS of 0.831 ± 0.02 and 0.871 ± 0.01 was obtained on the public dataset using input sizes of 512 × 512 and 256 × 256, respectively. A private CHVNGE dataset was then tested and an expected worse performance with a DCS mean of 0.807 ± 0.06 for the 256 × 256 images and 0.769 ± 0.06 for 512 × 512 images. Overall, these results indicate that reasonable performance can be obtained with a small number of patients and only a small decrease in performance in an external dataset. Future work to improve performance and robustness must focus on increasing the quantity and variability of training and testing data and integrating contextual information to increase performance in the lower pericardium.

References

1. Cardiac fat database - computed tomography. http://visual.ic.uff.br/en/cardio/ctfat/index.php. Accessed 20 Feb 2022
2. Alexopoulos, N., McLean, D.S., Janik, M., Arepalli, C.D., Stillman, A.E., Raggi, P.: Epicardial adipose tissue and coronary artery plaque characteristics. Atherosclerosis **210**(1), 150–154 (2010)
3. Barber, C.B., Dobkin, D.P., Huhdanpaa, H.: The quickhull algorithm for convex hulls. ACM Trans. Mathem. Softw. (TOMS) **22**(4), 469–483 (1996)
4. Commandeur, F., et al.: Fully automated CT quantification of epicardial adipose tissue by deep learning: a multicenter study. Radiol. Artif. Intell. **1**(6), e190045 (2019)
5. Dice, L.R.: Measures of the amount of ecologic association between species. Ecology **26**(3), 297–302 (1945)
6. Hajar, R.: Risk factors for coronary artery disease: historical perspectives. Heart Views Official J. Gulf Heart Assoc. **18**(3), 109 (2017)
7. Li, X., Liu, Y., Wang, Y., Yan, D.: Computing homography with RANSAC algorithm: a novel method of registration. In: Electronic Imaging and Multimedia Technology IV, vol. 5637, pp. 109–112. SPIE (2005)
8. Militello, C., et al.: A semi-automatic approach for epicardial adipose tissue segmentation and quantification on cardiac CT scans. Comput. Biol. Med. **114**, 103424 (2019)
9. Morin, R.L., Gerber, T.C., McCollough, C.H.: Radiation dose in computed tomography of the heart. Circulation **107**(6), 917–922 (2003)
10. Okrainec, K., Banerjee, D.K., Eisenberg, M.J.: Coronary artery disease in the developing world. Am. Heart J. **148**(1), 7–15 (2004)
11. Rodrigues, É.O., Morais, F., Morais, N., Conci, L., Neto, L., Conci, A.: A novel approach for the automated segmentation and volume quantification of cardiac fats on computed tomography. Comput. Methods Programs Biomed. **123**, 109–128 (2016)
12. Ronneberger, O., Fischer, P., Brox, T.: U-net: convolutional networks for biomedical image segmentation. In: Navab, N., Hornegger, J., Wells, W.M., Frangi, A.F. (eds.) MICCAI 2015. LNCS, vol. 9351, pp. 234–241. Springer, Cham (2015). https://doi.org/10.1007/978-3-319-24574-4_28
13. Rublee, E., Rabaud, V., Konolige, K., Bradski, G.: ORB: an efficient alternative to SIFT or SURF. In: 2011 International Conference on Computer Vision, pp. 2564–2571. IEEE (2011)
14. Talman, A.H., Psaltis, P.J., Cameron, J.D., Meredith, I.T., Seneviratne, S.K., Wong, D.T.: Epicardial adipose tissue: far more than a fat depot. Cardiovas. Diagn. Ther. **4**(6), 416 (2014)
15. Zhang, Q., Zhou, J., Zhang, B., Jia, W., Wu, E.: Automatic epicardial fat segmentation and quantification of CT scans using dual U-Nets with a morphological processing layer. IEEE Access **8**, 128032–128041 (2020)

A Platform Architecture for m-Health Internet of Things Applications

Pedro Mestre[1,2,4]([✉]) [iD], Ertugrul Dogruluk[1] [iD], Carlos Ferreira[1] [iD],
Rui Cordeiro[1] [iD], João Valente[1] [iD], Sérgio Branco[1] [iD], Bruno Gaspar[3] [iD],
and Jorge Cabral[1,4] [iD]

[1] CEiiA Centro de Engenharia e Desenvolvimento de Produto,
4450-017 Matosinhos, Portugal
{pedro.mestre,ertugrul.dogruluk,carlos.ferreira,rui.cordeiro,
joao.valente,antonio.branco,jorge.cabral}@ceiia.com
[2] Universtity of Trás-os-Montes e Alto Douro, Vila Real, Portugal
[3] Mobile Centric Architecture and Solutions, NOS Technology, Lisbon, Portugal
bruno.gaspar@nos.pt
[4] ALGORITMI Research Centre/LASI, University of Minho,
4800-058 Guimarães, Portugal
https://www.ceiia.com,https://www.utad.pt,https://www.nos.pt,
https://algoritmi.uminho.pt

Abstract. In the last few years, several researchers have been focusing their research work on some specific applications of the Internet of Things, such as the Health Internet of Things (m-Health IoT). As in other IoT applications, integrating IoT devices and applications/platforms from different manufacturers/developers in Health-IoT can be challenging. Even though standards are available and used, there are many possible standards and different devices use different communication protocols and data formats. Also, the integration leads to the need to develop new ad hoc code that will fit only that particular integration. This paper presents a proposal for a platform that uses a modular architecture and enables the seamless integration of different components of an m-health IoT platform. Components can be dynamically added or removed from the platform, in run-time without impacting the already existing components and without the need of downtime of the platform to include the new components.

Keywords: m-Health · IoT · Dynamic Configuration · Seamless Integration · gRPC

1 Introduction

The Internet of Things (IoT) can be defined as an interaction between computing devices via the Internet. Based on their configuration, these devices are

A. Cunha et al. (Eds.): MobiHealth 2022, LNICST 484, pp. 168–179, 2023.
https://doi.org/10.1007/978-3-031-32029-3_16

responsible for sending and receiving data. IoT devices can cover several applications, such as automobiles, smart industries, smart cities, smart homes, and healthcare applications. Also, the IoT ecosystem has several entities such as consumers, smart devices, communication, security protocols, and platform to communicate, which are used to connect with the IoT services, e.g., healthcare applications [2,8].

Therefore, all IoT devices must be considered critical, especially those health-related. The IoT healthcare applications can provide services for hospitals, emergency transport vehicles such as ambulances, nursing, stakeholders, and allow the consumers to analyze or store the collected data.

In recent works, several authors have focused their research on health Internet of Things applications. For instance, authors of [12] studied and implemented remote health monitoring on wearable vital sensors to alert critical measurements to hospital monitors. This application is supported by cellular such as NB-IoT protocols to provide efficiency and reliability.

The work [9] studied non-contact Internet-of-Medical-Things (IoMT) systems that are implemented between cloud platforms and edge nodes for cardiopulmonary functions. IoMT application was applied to analyze the recovery performance of respiratory results for COVID-19 patients.

In [10], IoT e-health services architecture was studied to increase the data processing, availability, and low-cost management of fog and cloud computing. This work also discusses the research challenges of providing a good e-health application based on performance, availability, and accessibility to achieve the lowest maintenance cost and deployment.

The work [16] implemented an intelligent Heath-IoT platform to serve IoT devices such as wireless wearable sensors and medicine packages for healthcare applications. Das et al. [5] proposed an IoT-enabled health automated monitoring platform that is used to monitor emerging conditions of the patient. This platform provides various vital conditions and parameters such as an electrocardiogram (ECG), blood oxygen level, heartbeat, and body temperature for the patients.

In this area of Heath-IoT, as in other IoT areas, as we can see from the above implementations, there are many possible types of devices and applications. Consequently, several data formats, communication technologies, and protocols can be used by IoT devices and platforms. Integration of devices from these different manufacturers/developers with applications and platforms from diverse providers/developers is a challenge.

In fact, integration can be a very time-consuming task and not as seamless as it would be desirable. Either because of the different formats and protocols used and because the architectures might be different or new code must be written, not only for data conversion but also to code link between the components to be integrated.

This is a problem that also arises in health IoT services, where equipment from different manufacturers need to be integrated, for example, in hospital patient monitoring software or in software to track, in real-time, the location of emergency services (e.g., ambulances).

Even if the standards are used, there are standards for different types of applications, there are standards that are niche specific, and when researchers need to integrate applications from different areas, sooner or later, they end-up with an integration problem to solve. For instance, if the civil authorities and the hospitals need to know the location of ambulances in real time, we might be dealing with several and various standards that need to be integrated.

From a simplified point of view, a seamless way to integrate devices and applications is required. This integration must have a low impact on the already running platforms and require a minimal need for an integration platform. This paper presents a modular architecture (that can be implemented using micro-services) that allows the seamless integration of different components of an IoT platform (including those that are used in the case study in this paper, i.e., Health Services) that allows in run-time new components (e.g., adding a service or feature) to be added and establishment of links between components.

This work is organized as follows: Introduction, the current section, summarizes the related works within the motivation of this paper for the IoT health-care services and presents the motivations and objectives. Section 2 summarizes the literature on IoT healthcare transport services and IoT platforms. Section 3 introduces the main contribution of this work by presenting the IoT platform architecture. Section 4 presents the implementations and results related to the m-health IoT platform. Finally, Sect. 5 concludes this work.

2   Internet of m-Health Things

In recent years an increasing demand for wirelessly connected devices and IoT applications is evolving new communication technologies. Especially emerging health-related IoT applications use wireless sensor networks (WSN) to manage, sense, and monitor the application needs. For instance, several WSN are defined to increase IoT device battery lifetime, reliability, communication coverage, and efficient data rate. The latest LPWAN technologies can be identified as LoRaWAN, Sigfox, and the fifth generation (5G) family, including narrowband IoT (NB-IoT) and LTE-M. These technologies are selected depending on the m-health IoT application, or device [6,7].

Even though these technologies all use standard protocols (TCP/IP) for transmitting information, the upper layer protocols (Application Layer) can be different. Also, the way these devices use the network may impact the way protocols and platforms have to work. For example, NB-IoT and LTE-M have different latency values (around 300 ms with good network coverage for NB-IoT and 50–100 ms for LTE-M), which can impact how these devices are integrated with an application, for example, IoT healthcare.

The survey [14] studied the challenges with frameworks and IoT trends in IoT Forensics by highlighting IoT security practices. The work also stated that the IoT healthcare applications market size is placed as 3rd by following Smart Cities and Industrial IoT applications market sizes.

2.1   Mobile Health (m-Health)

In IoT architectures, mobile computing, emergency services, and medical IoT sensors technologies are defined as the Internet of m-Health Things in healthcare-related devices. To create reliable m-health applications, the latest low power-based design (LPWAN), such as narrowband NB-IoT with 4G and the latest 5G communication technologies, are engaging in several m-health related IoT applications. For instance, wearable sensors are used to monitor patient health conditions, trace emerging services (ambulance, firefighter, patient tracking, and more services) to serve the patient as soon as possible, and so on [2].

Smart monitoring devices in IoT infrastructures provide health services. For instance, in the m-health IoT approach, health-related information such as patient records, hospital billing, emerging transportation management, insurance records, etc. Because of these critical systems, keeping the integrity of confidentiality, data security, and data privacy are also stated as important, as described in [1].

2.2   Internet of m-Health Things Platform

Considerable m-health applications are proposed for various applications, e.g., iMedBox [16], wearable IoT application for safety and health use cases [15], low-powered based NB-IoT devices for various sensing technologies (humidity, temperature, etc.) [3,11], Cardiopulmonary monitoring [9], provide healthcare solution called eHealthCare defining the non-adherence to health medication for elderly individuals by using NB-IoT and artificial intelligence algorithms [13], and other m-health related IoT applications.

Managing distinctive IoT device brands, protocols, and database sets can be a challenge to communicating with other emerging m-health IoT applications. For instance, hospital records (billing, data, medical records, etc.) must be unified or simplified with other related IoT services (insurance company, accessible information for doctors, database structure, and more).

Figure 1 illustrates the Internet of m-health Things platform architecture with its main components. In this architecture, the m-health IoT platform is mainly responsible for the unification of the IoT services between the m-health IoT hardware (e.g., NB-IoT connected devices, such as patient monitoring, hospital records, etc.) and the m-health IoT applications (e.g., hospital billings, emerging messages, emerging transportation, health software, etc.).

To obtain such an m-health IoT platform, several entities are required. For instance, the API translation is responsible for translating different programming languages or database sets into one readable place. Also, other services such as bare-metal server configurations, data security, data management, Kubernetes pods, and databases are the entities used for robust communication, platform integrity, and load balancing of the platform services.

The next section presents a proposal for a platform to support m-health IoT applications.

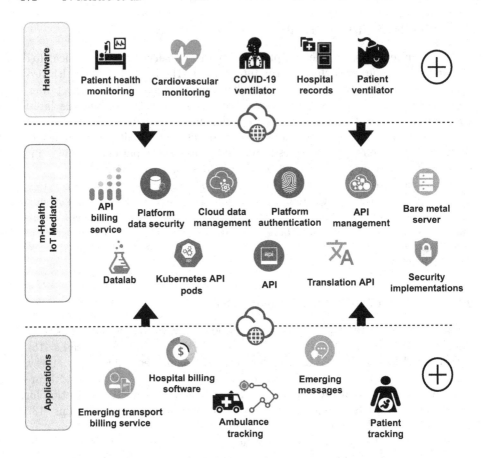

Fig. 1. Internet of m-health Things Platform Architecture

3 Internet of m-Health Things Platform (IoT-mP) Architecture

The rationale behind the platform architecture is the ability to link any data source(s) to any data sink(s), independently of the data formats and/or protocols that are used. It is an objective of the proposed platform to allow, dynamically, and at run-time, to link any data source to any data consumer, without "hard-coding" these links in the software application, or even to restart it. This means that we can have a set of devices that connect to the platform using CoAP (Constrained Application Protocol [4]), and another set that uses MQTT (Message Queuing Telemetry Transport). The data from these devices are simultaneously sent to a database (e.g., MongoDB) for storage, and some are sent to Artificial Intelligence (AI) algorithm for processing. Later, during the lifetime of the platform, the data can also be sent to another consumer without impacting its already existing components. Because of its modular architecture, the platform

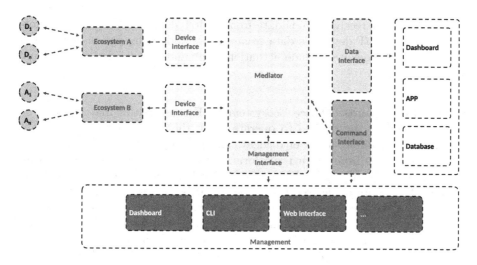

Fig. 2. Health IoT Platform structure

is ready to use any protocol, even those that are still not available at the time of its development and/or deployment.

As a case study, the platform was built having as a starting point a custom protocol (called Black-Wing), the same protocol as used in [11], and later, without the need to modify the architecture, MQTT and CoAP were also integrated into the platform, and tested successfully.

One can describe the developed platform either from the point of view of its functional components or through a set of interfaces that were developed to allow the flow of information, as it is shown in Fig. 2.

3.1   Platform Functional Architecture and Components

From the functional point of view, the architecture comprises five components, which provide the main functions of the architecture. To be noticed that a software component can implement more than one function. These five functions are:

- Mediator: the core of the platform;
- Device Ecosystems: that provide interface with the IoT devices;
- Data Consumers: which are the sinks of the data;
- Command Producers: that generate commands to be sent to the IoT devices.

Mediator. In the core of the platform, there is a component called the Mediator, which is responsible to know what paths data must follow. These data paths are set dynamically at run-time, allowing the data paths to change to accommodate any change needed, such as new data sources, new data sinks, new processing algorithms, etc.

The Mediator receives/sends data from/to IoT devices. Typically the information sent by IoT devices is data from sensors and configuration values, and data sent to the devices include actuation commands, configuration data, and firmware updates.

Device Ecosystems. Device Ecosystems (DE) are entities that provide the infrastructure for the devices to operate using their own protocols and data formats. For example, a set of devices can use MQTT to send its data and receive commands from the IoT platform. Besides providing the infrastructure for devices to communicate, DE is the bridge between the Mediator and the devices. When data is received from a device, it is the responsibility of the DE to send it to the Mediator. Also, when a command has to be sent to a device, the DE receives that command and forwards it to the device. The devices do not need to be aware of the existence of the Mediator, which allows the integration of already existing platforms and protocols. The Mediator does not need also to be aware about the communication details of the devices, making it device/platform/protocol agnostic. The DE might also include some data adaptation or translation functions to allow the data to arrive correctly to the consumers. However, it is not mandatory to have the data translation in this layer. In fact, any component of the platform can provide these services.

Data Consumers. After processing the messages arriving from the Device Ecosystems, the Mediator forwards data to their consumers. A consumer can be any application to which data has meaning (Dashboard, Database, APP, etc.). As previously stated, these consumers are defined in run-time, and therefore consumers can be added or removed without impacting other consumers. We can have multiple consumers that receive the same data.

Command Producers. Besides receiving data from devices, the mediator also handles instructions that are sent to the devices. These instructions can be actuation commands, configuration instructions, or even firmware updates, and are generated by entities called Command Producers (CP). When a CP needs to send a command to a device, it sends it to the Mediator, that will forward the request to the corresponding DE. When (if any) answer from the command is sent back to the Mediator, it will be forwarded to the origin Command Producer.

3.2   Interfaces

Although a sophisticated technology was used for communication between the components and functions of the platform, a set of "standard" technology and protocol-independent interfaces were specified. These interfaces allow communication between the platform components, as well as extend it and add new features to the platform or even use it in different target applications. This means that, for example, new algorithms that calculate which emergency team should go to a call can be easily added, without impacting the other elements of the platform, or that patient monitoring applications can be built on top of this platform.

As a case study, these interfaces were implemented using gRPC, but they can be implemented using any other technology. For this case, the interface that is used for management was also implemented using REST Web-services, to be compatible with web browsers.

There are four interfaces used to interconnect the functional components:

- Device Interface (DE-Interface);
- Data Interface (D-Interface);
- Command Interface (C-Interface);
- Management Interface (M-Interface).

Device Interface. Used for communications between the Device Ecosystems and the Mediator, defines all functions needed by the Device Ecosystem to forward data from devices to the Mediator, and to send back to the Mediator the response to the instructions received from the Command Producers.

Data Interface. Data from devices is sent to the Data Consumers using the Data Interface. Upon the arrival to the Mediator, the rules established by the administrator are matched against the ID of the device, if there is a match, data is sent to the Consumer.

Command Interface. In the opposite direction (in comparison to the Data Interface), requests for the devices are sent to the Mediator using the Command Interface. This is also the interface that is used by the Device Ecosystems to send the response to these requests to the Mediator.

Management Interface. It is the Management Interface that allows the administrator to setup the rules in the Mediator. The administrator, using, for example, a Command Line Interface (CLI), a Web Interface, or any other tools, can add/remove Device Ecosystems, Devices, Data Consumers, and Command Producers, as well as define a set of links between these components. How the data will flow inside the Mediator is set using this interface.

4   Implementation and Results

4.1   Implementation

The above-presented architecture can both be implemented in a monolithic or in a distributed way. While the first can be interesting in very specific situations, where a very low memory footprint is one of the main constraints (e.g., in a low-level embedded system), in most computing systems, a distributed approach using micro-services is better. Using a distributed approach allows us to achieve the desired run-time flexibility, and we can, if needed, use load-balancing strategies between the nodes of the platform.

Therefore the distributed approach, using a micro-services architecture, was chosen. In this architecture, each node is one of the functional components of the architecture. To provide the computational power, a Kubernetes cluster is being used. Kubernetes (K8S) provide us with features related to scaling and self-healing that are very useful in a system with a low tolerance for failure. Besides that, K8S provides a very flexible way to automate the deployment of the components and manage their life cycle.

To implement the Mediator, Java was the chosen programming language. Even though Java was chosen, any otter programming language with a stable support gRPC can be used. However to be noticed that performance was always the top requirement when implementing it, because it needs to route as fast as possible all the messages that are sent to it. Its current speed and memory footprint are suitable to run it in some of the mid-level computational platforms such as Raspberry Pi 4 and Orange Pi 0. The final performance and memory needs will depend on the number of rules, the number of associated nodes, the number of messages arriving at the Mediator and the available bandwidth.

4.2   Tests and Results

Preliminary tests with these platforms allow to conclude that the platform can be used from the bottom to the top in a distributed architecture for IoT systems. This makes this architecture also very useful for edge computing and data aggregation.

To test the proposed platform, it was implemented a test platform that consists of:

- A Device Ecosystem that receives data from devices using CoAP;
- A Device Ecosystem that receives data from devices using the protocols described in [11];
- One Mediator;
- One Data Consumer that receives data from the devices and sends it via web-socket to a Web Application;
- An example web application (Fig. 3) that shows the data.

For CoAP devices, a simulator was used, built in Java, which sends a set of pre-recorded coordinates, was used. For the other protocol, it was used a CPS Cyber-Physical System), a device that is under development, and an Android application. The data sent by the devices are the GPS coordinates.

While the simulator allowed to do performance and stress tests to the platform, the use of the CPS device and the Android Applications allowed for monitoring, in real-time, the location of the system.

Using an 11th Gen Intel(R) Core(TM) i7-1185G7 @ 3.00 GHz PC, with 16 GBytes of RAM, running Ubuntu Linux 22.04 and Java 11, without any load

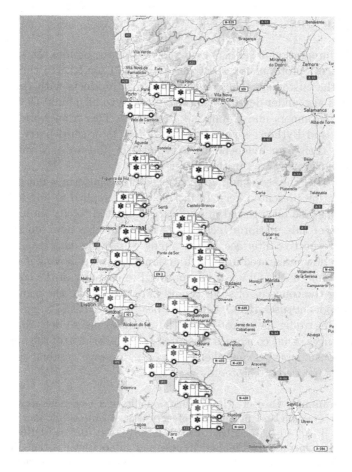

Fig. 3. Example of an output dashboard.

balancing strategy it was possible to achieve the following indicative values, when flooding the system with a message:

- Send messages between Device Ecosystem and Mediator (messages are validated and then dropped), around one million messages per minute;
- Send messages from a device (using CoAP) to a DE, the DE then sends the message to the Mediator that validates the message and then drops it, around 380K messages in a minute;
- The same as above, but the messages are sent to a Consumer that decodes the message and makes it available to the front-end (as the one presented in Fig. 3), around 285K messages per minute.

5   Conclusions

To make the integration of services even more seamless, besides the specification of the interfaces (protobuf for gRPC and OpenAPI for REST) that are made available to the customers that want to integrate products with the platform, currently, it is also under development a framework to help build Device Ecosystems, Data Consumers and Command Producers. This framework, developed both in Java and Python, is currently under test by a third party, which had already built their own independent IoT platform and are now integrating it with the platform presented in this paper.

Obviously that the scope and applications of the platform is not limited only to the application presented here. In fact, it can be applied to any IoT application, and it has also been tested in applications related to city mobility. Future developments of this platform include the inclusion of a new functional component, and respective interface, that is going to provide data translation (this component is now integrated in other functional blocks, removing it into a standalone functional block will allow an improved re-usability of the components).

Regarding the concerns of security and data protection, the communication between components uses gRPC, which can be done over HTTPS, providing data encryption. Regarding data protection, the platform per se does not store any data from devices. That concern is delegated to the providers of the applications, e.g., Data Consumers, because the Mediator is message content agnostic and therefore does not need to store any user data.

Acknowledgements. Project "(Link4S)ustainability - A new generation connectivity system for creation and integration of networks of objects for new sustainability paradigms [POCI-01-0247-FEDER-046122—LISBOA-01-0247-FEDER-046122]" is financed by the Operational Competitiveness and Internationalization Programmes COMPETE 2020 and LISBOA 2020, under the PORTUGAL 2020 Partnership Agreement, and through the European Structural and Investment Funds in the FEDER component.

References

1. Almotiri, S.H., Khan, M.A., Alghamdi, M.A.: Mobile health (m-Health) system in the context of IoT. In: Proceedings - 2016 4th International Conference on Future Internet of Things and Cloud Workshops, W-FiCloud 2016, pp. 39–42 (2016). https://doi.org/10.1109/W-FiCloud.2016.24

2. Bhuiyan, M.N., Rahman, M.M., Billah, M.M., Saha, D.: Internet of things (IoT): a review of its enabling technologies in healthcare applications, standards protocols, security, and market opportunities. IEEE Internet Things J. 8(13), 10474–10498 (2021). https://doi.org/10.1109/JIOT.2021.3062630

3. Borges, M., Paiva, S., Santos, A., Gaspar, B., Cabral, J.: Azure RTOS ThreadX design for low-End NB-IoT device. In: Proceedings - 2020 2nd International Conference on Societal Automation, SA 2020 (2020). https://doi.org/10.1109/SA51175.2021.9507191

4. Bormann, C., Lemay, S., Tschofenig, H., Hartke, K., Silverajan, B.: CoAP (constrained application protocol) over TCP, TLS, and WebSockets. Technical report (2018). https://doi.org/10.17487/RFC8323, https://www.rfc-editor.org/info/rfc8323

5. Das, A., Katha, S.D., Sadi, M.S., Ferdib-Al-Islam: an IoT enabled health monitoring kit using non-invasive health parameters. In: 2021 International Conference on Automation, Control and Mechatronics for Industry 4.0, ACMI 2021 (July), pp. 8–9 (2021). https://doi.org/10.1109/ACMI53878.2021.9528227

6. Kanj, M., Savaux, V., Le Guen, M.: A tutorial on NB-IoT physical layer design. IEEE Commun. Surv. Tutor. **22**(4), 2408–2446 (2020). https://doi.org/10.1109/COMST.2020.3022751

7. Khalifeh, A., Aldahdouh, K., Darabkh, K.A., Al-sit, W.: A survey of 5G emerging wireless technologies. In: 2019 International Conference on Wireless Communications Signal Processing and Networking (WiSPNET), pp. 561–566 (2019)

8. Lee, E., Seo, Y.D., Oh, S.R., Kim, Y.G.: A survey on standards for interoperability and security in the internet of things. IEEE Commun. Surv. Tutor. **23**(2), 1020–1047 (2021). https://doi.org/10.1109/COMST.2021.3067354

9. Liu, J., Miao, F., Yin, L., Pang, Z., Li, Y.: A noncontact ballistocardiography-based IoMT system for cardiopulmonary health monitoring of discharged COVID-19 patients. IEEE Internet Things J. **8**(21), 15807–15817 (2021)

10. Monteiro, K., Rocha, E., Silva, E., Santos, G.L., Santos, W., Endo, P.T.: Developing an e-health system based on IoT, fog and cloud computing. In: Proceedings - 11th IEEE/ACM International Conference on Utility and Cloud Computing Companion, UCC Companion 2018, pp. 17–18 (2019). https://doi.org/10.1109/UCC-Companion.2018.00024

11. Paiva, S., Branco, S., Cabral, J.: Design and power consumption analysis of a NB-IoT end device for monitoring applications. In: IECON Proceedings (Industrial Electronics Conference), vol. 2020-Octob, pp. 2175–2182 (2020). https://doi.org/10.1109/IECON43393.2020.9254374

12. Pathinarupothi, R.K., Durga, P., Rangan, E.S.: IoT-based smart edge for global health: remote monitoring with severity detection and alerts transmission. IEEE Internet Things J. **6**(2), 2449–2462 (2019). https://doi.org/10.1109/JIOT.2018.2870068, https://ieeexplore.ieee.org/document/8464257/

13. Pinto, A., Correia, A., Alves, R., Matos, P., Ascensão, J., Camelo, D.: eHealthCare - a medication monitoring approach for the elderly people. In: Gao, X., Jamalipour, A., Guo, L. (eds.) MobiHealth 2021. Lecture Notes of the Institute for Computer Sciences, Social Informatics and Telecommunications Engineering, vol. 440, pp. 221–234. Springer, Cham (2022). https://doi.org/10.1007/978-3-031-06368-8_15

14. Stoyanova, M., Nikoloudakis, Y., Panagiotakis, S., Pallis, E., Markakis, E.K.: A survey on the internet of things (IoT) forensics: challenges, approaches, and open issues. IEEE Commun. Surv. Tutor. **22**(2), 1191–1221 (2020). https://doi.org/10.1109/COMST.2019.2962586

15. Wu, F., Wu, T., Yuce, M.R.: Design and implementation of a wearable sensor network system for IoT-connected safety and health applications. In: IEEE 5th World Forum on Internet of Things, WF-IoT 2019 - Conference Proceedings, pp. 87–90 (2019). https://doi.org/10.1109/WF-IoT.2019.8767280

16. Yang, G., et al.: A health-IoT platform based on the integration of intelligent packaging, unobtrusive bio-sensor, and intelligent medicine box. IEEE Trans. Industr. Inf. **10**(4), 2180–2191 (2014). https://doi.org/10.1109/TII.2014.2307795

A Review on Deep Learning-Based Automatic Lipreading

Carlos Santos[1], António Cunha[2,3]🆔, and Paulo Coelho[1,4(✉)]🆔

[1] School of Technology and Management, Polytechnic of Leiria, 2411-901 Leiria,
Portugal
2180284@my.ipleiria.pt
[2] Escola de Ciências e Tecnologias, University of Trás-os-Montes e Alto Douro,
Quinta de Prados, 5001-801 Vila Real, Portugal
atcunha@utad.pt
[3] Institute for Systems and Computer Engineering, Technology and Science (INESC
TEC), 4200-465 Porto, Portugal
[4] Institute for Systems Engineering and Computers at Coimbra (INESC Coimbra),
DEEC, Pólo II, 3030-290 Coimbra, Portugal
paulo.coelho@ipleiria.pt

Abstract. Automatic Lip-Reading (ALR), also known as Visual Speech
Recognition (VSR), is the technological process to extract and recognize
speech content, based solely on the visual recognition of the speaker's
lip movements. Besides hearing-impaired people, regular hearing people
also resort to visual cues for word disambiguation, every time one is
in a noisy environment. Due to the increasingly interest in developing
ALR systems, a considerable number of research articles are being published. This article selects, analyses, and summarizes the main papers
from 2018 to early 2022, from traditional methods with handcrafted feature extraction algorithms to end-to-end deep learning based ALR which
fully take advantage of learning the best features, and of the evergrow-
ing publicly available databases. By providing a recent state-of-the-art
overview, identifying trends, and presenting a conclusion on what is to be
expected in future work, this article becomes an efficient way to update
on the most relevant ALR techniques.

Keywords: Automatic Lip-reading · Deep Learning · Audio-visual
Automatic Speech Recognition

1 Introduction

Human speech is one of the most important forms of communication, through
which we rapidly convey information, concepts, and ideas, therefore being a
key driver of Human Evolution. It also allows to enhance the performance of
teaching/learning and, as we are social beings, gossip, which makes up a large
portion of our human-to-human interactions.

© ICST Institute for Computer Sciences, Social Informatics and Telecommunications Engineering 2023
Published by Springer Nature Switzerland AG 2023. All Rights Reserved
A. Cunha et al. (Eds.): MobiHealth 2022, LNICST 484, pp. 180–195, 2023.
https://doi.org/10.1007/978-3-031-32029-3_17

Phoneticians call Phonemes the basic speech structures (or minimal units of speech), that enable to distinguish one word from another (e.g.: the phoneme /p/ is what distinguishes the word pat from bat) [1]. Visemes are a shortened version of the phrase visual phonemes and refer to any individual and contrastive visually perceived unit [2].

Lip reading or visual speech recognition is a procedure used to recognize and interpret the speech by analyzing the lip's movement. It is used to complete relayed information by people with hearing difficulties, either by being congenitally deaf or just by a significant decrease in speech-to-noise ratio, i.e., by augmenting the noise level and maintaining the speech level or by maintaining the noise level but diminishing the speech level [1]. Bauman's study [3] reported that hearing-impaired people understood 21% of speech, just using residual hearing, 64% if they combined residual hearing with either a hearing aid or with speechreading, and 90% if they used their residual hearing, hearing aids, and speechreading.

Video Speech Recognition, may be considered lip-reading based on artificial intelligence techniques, and also contributes to: speech synthesizing; multi-view mouth rendering; silent passwords; audio-less videos transcriber; speech recognition under noisy conditions; isolation of individual speakers; forensic study on surveillance videos; and face liveness detection.

Within approximately a single human generation, lip-reading evolved from a 4-grey layered template recognition model as the first Audio-Visual Automatic Speech Recognition (AV-ASR) [4], to recent, powerful, and more complex end-to-end deep neural network models [5–9], where linear considerations try to answer a non-linear question. ALR techniques vary in ways to find Regions of Interest (RoI) from frames, extract features, transform them, and to classifying in simple utterances up to full sentences, in real-time or for forensic analysis. In this time span, research on ALR has evolved from a limited number of researchers, to multinational, multicultural, ever-growing, and diversifying teams of researchers, producing an equally growing number of papers [10–14].

As a survey on the specific field of ALR, this document mainly aims and contributes to: (1) select a considerable number of recent relevant literature, as state-of-the-art; (2) summarize the selected literature; (3) identify patterns and tendencies; (4) establish a review that serves as a critical basis for the most recent methods, strategies and results that allow the development of works related to this area of knowledge.

Section 2 of this paper presents the criteria and methods used to select the reviewed works, Section 3 presents the state of the art in automatic lip-reading, along with a brief author's discussion, and Section 4 presents the conclusions and what can be done in terms of improvements in future works.

2   Materials and Methods

2.1   Research Questions

The systematic review that follows is based on a set of research questions: RQ1 - Which methods are more suitable for visual clues only automatic lip-reading?; RQ2 - Which methods are mainly used to support the analysis of lip-reading data? RQ3 - Which methods are specifically studied with the available datasets?; RQ4 - What challenges are still open for lip-reading solutions?

2.2   Inclusion Criteria

The research included only studies that fitted the following cumulative criteria: (1) ALR, VSR or AV-ASR related; (2) published from 2018 onwards; (3) traditional or end-to-end methods applied to ALR or VSR; (4) presented original research; (5) documents written in English; (6) publicly available; (7) for corpora in the English language; (8) for single view video corpora. Few exceptions were made, to include either historic articles, eminent authors, or articles referenced by previous or posterior readings that did not appear in the search results. The only exclusion criteria were applications and devices-oriented research, for being outside of the scope of this paper.

2.3   Search Strategy

The data used for this study were collected between 14 and 18 May 2022, using Science Direct and Scopus search engines, enabling easy access to abstract reading for exclusion purposes, classifying papers in subject areas, and showing a relevant bulk of papers. Google Scholar and IEEE were also firstly included, however, these comparably underperformed. The terms used in the research were "lip-reading" and "audiovisual automatic speech recognition". There was a total of 43 screened studies and after more meticulous selection, 23 studies were selected for the final analysis.

3   Results

Figure 1 summarizes as a flow diagram the steps for the gathering and analysis of the source papers for the review. Initially, were Identified 49 studies from the selected sources, and 8 of these papers were duplicated. Two additional records were added to the results, gathered from different queries to the databases. After analyzing each research article's metadata, namely the title, the keywords, and the abstract, 9 of such studies were eliminated from the analysis due to the lack of relation to computer-based lip-reading. The full text of the remaining 34 articles was evaluated considering the aforementioned inclusion criteria, and therefore, 13 articles were also dismissed. The remaining 21 papers were fully assessed.

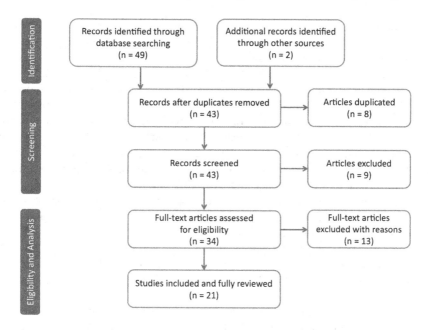

Fig. 1. Flow diagram depicting the selection of the papers.

Nowadays, with the deep learning techniques and the vast databases publicly available, some works are showing promising results. This section presents the current state of the art from the most recent studies and methods on ALR. As a criteria for the presentation of the studies, these were grouped in terms of focus of the methods, that is, these were grouped considering the characteristics that are intended to be obtained with each specific method (lip detection, features, homophemes, visemes), followed by which the specific objective (extraction of words, words and sentences, characters and sentences, speech).

Also, each of the following papers will have a description of their relevant characteristics, followed by a critical analysis/discussion from the authors.

Lopez et al. [15] aimed to study the upper bound of visual-only speech recognition in controlled conditions. Since the literature is not clear on who are the better lip-readers, the authors compared the lip-reading abilities of 15 normal-hearing and 9 hearing-impaired people. A database was constructed, and the speakers were instructed to facilitate lip-reading. Another study was to compare the performances of human and VSR systems, under optimal and directly comparable conditions. In the authors' tests, hearing-impaired participants just nearly outperformed normal-hearing participants. When comparing humans' performance to visual-only automatic systems, a 44% to 20% spoken message decoding decrease gap was observed. However, similar performances were obtained in terms of phonemes, suggesting that the difference between automatic and human speech-reading could be more influenced by the context than the ability to interpret mouth appearance.

Rethinking the RoI for ALR is the aim of Zhang et al. [16]. This paper questions the standard RoI for ALR papers, as human lip-readers do not just look at the lips, during a conversation. [15] states that facial expressions help to decode the spoken message, and context framing the speech (e.g.: a sad expression augments the probability of sad-related words/sentences). Using state-of-the-art VSR models at word level and sentence level, a thorough study is presented assessing the effects of extraoral information, including the upper part and the entire face, the cheeks, and the mouth. The author's proposed model [16] was trained on large-scale "in-the-wild" VSR datasets, depicting many real-world variables, such as variable lighting conditions, cluttering backgrounds, different human poses, expressions, accents, speaking manners, etc. According to the study, using crop augmentation (similar to drop pixels) with face-aligned inputs can produce stronger features, improving recognition by also making the model learn fewer evident extraoral cues from the data.

Using only the mouth entrances makes VSR an isolated problem, as the process will not consider other parts of the human face. Therefore, there has been no consensus on choosing RoIs, and intuition still plays a large role in RoI cropping.

Lu et al. [17] also propose a lip-segmentation method, but now in the framework of the maximum a posteriori Markov random field (MAP-MRF), a statistical segmentation method that considers the spatial relations between image pixels into account. The proposed method sets up a multi-layer hierarchical model, in which each pixel of each layer corresponds to the four nodes in a quad-tree structure (QTS). The probability of a branch node can be derived from the probability of the previous one, throughout the tree structure. Then a Markov random field derived from the model is obtained, so the unsupervised segmentation is formulated as a labeling optimization problem. The method also proposes a variable weight segmentation approach, to improve the robustness of over-segmentation.

Results show that the proposed method has better performance than the related methods, however, it runs between 3 and 4 s, therefore it is not suitable for real-time applications. Lip segmentation accuracy plays an important role in automatic lip-reading and can directly affect the recognition rate.

Lu and Liu [18] propose a localized active contour model-based method, using two initial contours in combined color space: a rhombus as the initial contour of a closed mouth; a combined semi-ellipse as the initial contours of both outer and inner lip boundaries for an open mouth. The method first applies illumination equalization to RGB images to reduce interference of uneven illumination, then adopts a combined color space, which involves the U component in the CIE-LUV color space and the sum components of the Discrete Hartley Transform (DHT). Finally, the shape of initial contours is determined, due to the positions of four key points in the combined color space.

The method improves segmentation results and gets more similar to the true lip boundary, compared with using a circle as the initial contour to segment grey images and images in combined color space.

Das et al. [2] show a refinement in automatic lip contour extraction, using pixel-based segmentation. This embodies an alternative to pixels classification of different color planes, a potential difficulty to lip contours detection in adverse conditions like variations in illumination and clothing. The mouth region is extracted, by k-means clustering binary classification based on Red/Green ratio thresholding. To avoid false detection, a big connected region around the center of the cropped image is considered to be the RoI. Next, the upper and lower lip areas are detected by k-means clustering algorithm binary classification, of Green plane and to weighted RGB plane respectively. The combined lip area is further processed to detect the centrally located big connected region. By finding the centrally located big connected region, rather than the biggest connected region in the whole binary classified image, variations in illumination and clothing effects are overcome and RoI is restricted around the mouth region. For smooth edges, piece-wise polynomial fitting is employed with a higher degree for the upper lip and a lower degree for the lower lip.

The proposed method works well, even for images with varying illumination and clothing effects. A future aim is to use this algorithm to obtain the best possible lip contour.

Visual Speech Recognition (VSR) is highly influenced by the selection of visual features, which can be categorized into static (geometrically based) and dynamic (motion-based). Radha et al. [19] propose a three-viseme model study, one as the control group and two considering both categories, one fused at the features level and the other fused at the model level. For dynamic-motion features extraction, Motion History Image (MHI) is calculated from all the visemes, from which Discrete Cosine Transform (DCT), Wavelet, and Zernike coefficients are extracted. For static-geometric features extraction, an Active Shape Model (ASM) is used. Fusion models are individually built by Gaussian Mixture Model Left-to-Right Hidden Markov Model (GMM L-R HMM).

The results show an improvement in performance due to the fusion, and the presence of complementary cues in the motion-based and geometric-based features, and that geometric cues provide better discrimination of visemes.

Weng and Kitani [20] experiment on word-level visual lipreading from video input with no audio, by replacing shallow 3DCNN + a deep 2DCNN with deep 3DCNN two-stream Inflated Convolution Networks (I3D), and evaluating different combinations of front-end and back-end modules, with the greyscale video and optical flow inputs on the LRW dataset, as presented in Fig. 2. 3D convolution networks can capture the short-term dynamics and be advantageous in visual lipreading, even when RNNs are deployed for the back-end. However, due to the huge number of parameters introduced by the 3D kernels, state-of-the-art methods in lipreading have only explored the shallow (under 3 layers) 3DCNNs. To explore these networks to their maximum, the authors present the first word-level lipreading pipeline using deep (over 3 layers) 3DCNNs.

The experiments show that: compared to the shallow 3D CNNs + deep 2D CNNs front-end, the deep 3D CNNs front-end with two-round pre-training on the large-scale image and video datasets can improve the classification accuracy;

using the optical flow input alone can achieve comparable performance as using the greyscale video as input; the two-stream network using both the greyscale video and optical flow inputs can further improve the performance.

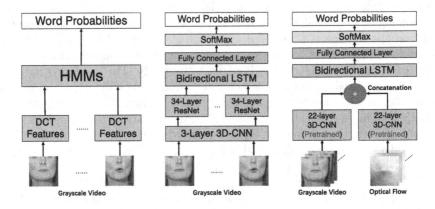

Fig. 2. The architecture of the framework proposed by [20].

Lu and Yan [21] propose a CNN and bidirectional LSTM (BLSTM) that uses hybrid neural network architecture for an automatic lip-reading system. The method first extracts key frames from each isolated video clip, uses five key points to locate the mouth region, extracts features from raw mouth images using an eight-layered CNN, and uses BLSTM to capture the correlation of sequential information among frame features in both directions in time, and uses the softmax layer to predict final recognition result. The limited number of key points reduces redundant information in consecutive frames, therefore the complexity of computation and processing. The CNN copes with image deformation, by translation, rotation, and distortion, hence strengthening the robustness and fault-tolerant capability, and a fully connected layer is used to get static features of a single mouth image. BLSTM improves both finding and exploiting long-time dependencies, from sequential data, so the relationship of the features among frames is built and strengthened.

The results show that the proposed DNN can effectively predict words from the mouth area, on a self-made database (6 speakers, 9 digits), compared to traditional algorithms that combine handcrafted features with a classification model.

Mesbah et al. [22] aimed to the development of a visual-only speech recognition system, proposing Hahn Convolutional Neural Network (HCNN), seizing their ability to represent images with less redundancy, and to be parameterized to retain the global or local characteristics of the image in the lowest orders. The proposed architecture consists of Hahn moments as a filter in the first layer, with its ability to hold and extract the most useful information in images effectively, and the performance of the CNNs in learning patterns and image classification.

The results show a reduction in processing time, normal to spatio-temporal modeling features, and visual features extraction with 3D CNN, ResNet, and Bidirectional LSTM.

Ma et al. [23] focus specifically on lip feature extraction under variant lighting conditions, since research has been mainly conducted for ideal conditions, therefore ideal lighting. The method consists of a pre-processing chain of illumination normalization and also improved local binary patterns (LBP) features. The first is applied to remove the influence of external illumination noise before the lip feature extraction in four steps: median filtering, gamma correction, multi-scale Retinex filtering, and contrast equalization. LBP is an illumination invariant descriptor of edges, which improves the recognition rate of lip-reading under variant lighting conditions.

Experiments show that the proposed algorithm has a lower recognition rate in natural than traditional pixel-based feature extraction method, but higher under variant lighting conditions.

Jeon et al. [24] address the homophemes as word ambiguity enablers, and words under 0,02s as "a", "an", "eight", and "bin", as they do not provide sufficient visual information to learn from. A novel lipreading architecture is presented, combining three different CNNs: 3D CNN, to efficiently extract features from consecutive frames; densely connected 3D CNN - to fully utilize the features; and multi-layer feature fusion 3D CNN with a pixel dropout layer and spatial dropout layer - to avoid overfitting and to extract shapes with strong spatial correlations with fine movements, while exploring the context information both in temporal and spatial domains. Then follows a two-layer bi-directional gated recurrent unit (GRU). The network was trained using connectionist temporal classification (CTC).

The results of the proposed architecture show character (5,681%) and word (11,282%) error rate reductions, for the unseen-speaker dataset, even when visual ambiguity arises.

Wang [25] also addresses the homophemes question, accumulating diverse lip appearances and motion patterns among the speakers, by capturing the nuances between words and different speakers' different styles respectively. As for the front-end, the method utilizes 2D (spatial only) and 3D (spatio-temporal) ConvNets to extract both frame-wise spatial fine-grained and short-term medium-grained spatio-temporal features, to capture both grained patterns of each word and various conditions in speaker identity, lighting conditions, and so on. Then fuses the different granularity features with an adaptive mask (bidirectional ConvLSTM, augmented with temporal attention, which aggregates spatio-temporal information in the entire input sequence), to obtain discriminative representations for words with similar phonemes, as a multi-grained spatio-temporal novel modeling of the speaking process, as depicted in Fig. 3.

The proposed model demonstrates state-of-the-art performance on two challenging lip-reading datasets. In future work, the authors propose to simplify the front-end and extract multi-grained features with a more lightweight structure.

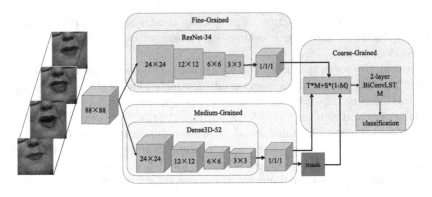

Fig. 3. The architecture of the framework proposed by [25].

Viseme-based lip-reading systems do not require pre-trained lexicons and can be used to classify both unknown words and different languages. Fenghour et al. [26] explore this fact to classify visemes in continuous speech, uses visemes as a classification schema for reading sentences, and use perplexity analysis for visemes to word conversion, stating that all contributions improve sentence-level lip reading. The proposed method uses visemes as a very limited number of classes, a unique deep learning model for classification, and perplexity analysis for recognized visemes to possible word conversion, resorting to purely visual cues from the LRS2 dataset and being robust to varying levels of lighting.

Results demonstrate a significant improvement in the classification accuracy of words compared to state-of-the-art works. For future research, the authors hint towards a more suitable architecture to further enhance the generalization capability and a higher training/test number of samples ratio.

Fenghour et al. [27] focus on viseme-based lipreading systems has been well suited to decoding videos of people uttering entire sentences. As the paper points out, the high classification accuracy of visemes (e.g., over 90%) contrasts with a comparatively low classification accuracy of words (e.g., just over 60%), due to the homovisemes phenomenon which leads to a one-to-many problem (e.g., "I Love You" = "Olive Juice" = "Elephant Shoes"). Aiming for a more efficient viseme-to-word conversion method to tackle this accuracy decline, the authors developed a DNN model with an Attention-based Gated Recurrent Unit and compared it against three other approaches (Perplexity-Iterator, Feed-Forward Neural Network, and Hidden Markov Model) through the LRS2 and LRS3 corpora.

Results show that the proposed model is effective at discriminating between words sharing visemes that are either semantically or syntactically different, and at modeling long and short-term dependencies, therefore being robust to incorrectly classified visemes.

Intending to learn strong models that recognize speech in silent videos, Prajwal et al. [9] focus on challenges in lip reading and propose tailored solutions, contributing to lip movement representations aggregation, robustness improvement to ambiguity by sub-word units based modeling, and to a Visual Speech Detection (VSD) model proposal. The paper proposes an end-to-end trainable attention-based pooling mechanism that learns to track and aggregate the lip movement representations, a sub-word (word-pieces) tokenization that not only matches with multiple adjacent frames but also with those which are semantically meaningful for learning a language easily, therefore greatly reducing the run-time and memory requirements, and a model for VSD trained on top of the lip-reading network since there is no automated procedure for cropping out the clips where the person is speaking.

The results show state-of-the-art Word Error Rate (WER), outperforming work trained on public data, even industrial models trained on orders of magnitude more data. Also, the designed Visual Speech Detection obtains state-of-the-art results, on this task and even outperforms audio-visual baselines.

Martinez et al. [28] address the limitations of the Bidirectional Gated Recurrent Unit (BGRU) and propose corresponding improvement proposals. First, the mouth region was extracted, and DCT was used to feature transform and then fed to HMM for modeling of the temporal dynamics. To address the limitations of the model and the authors proposed: that to improve the overall performance, BGRU layers are replaced with Temporal Convolutional Networks (TCN); to reduce training time (from 3 to 1-week GPU-time), and avoid relying on a cumbersome 3-stage sequential training, a cosine scheduler was adopted; to improve the generalization capabilities, variable-length augmentation was proposed. As each TCN receptive field is defined by kernel and stride sizes, several temporal convolutional blocks are achieved and stacked sequentially to act as a deep feature sequence encoder. Next, a dense layer is applied to each time-indexed feature vector, and a simple averaging consensus function is used. With different-sized kernels and multiple temporal scales, long and short-term information can be mixed up during the feature encoding.

Results on the largest publicly available datasets for isolated word recognition in English and Mandarin, LRW and LRW1000, show that a new state-of-the-art performance was achieved.

Huang et al. [5] propose a novel lip reading model using a transformer network, to achieve higher accuracy. The method makes use of the pre-trained neural network VGG16 to extract the lip features from the GRID corpus, adopts dimensionality reduction towards the originally high dimensions extracted features, and processes the features through the author's proposed Transformer network for training. The transformer adopts a self-attention mechanism instead of CNN and RNN, as is commonly used in deep learning. RNN tends to be slow in some sequential processing tasks. On the other hand, transformers' parallel processing greatly improves training speed.

The experiment shows a significant reduction in training costs, without compromising the enhancement of the lip-reading accuracy of the model.

In [29], the authors tackle the difficulty of meeting the requirements of practical applications for ALR, due to the complexity of image processing, hard-to-train classification, and long-term recognition processes, in three steps. Firstly they extract keyframes from their own established independent database. Secondly, they use the Visual Geometry Group of Oxford University and the Google DeepMind (VGG) network to extract the lip image features. Then, as an attention-based RNN, they compare two lip-reading models: a fusion model with an attention mechanism; and a fusion model of two networks.

The results of the proposed hybrid neural network architecture of CNN and attention-based LSTM, show an increase of 3.3% to the general CNN-RNN. The authors manifested the future intention to train the model on datasets of real-time broadcast videos.

"No Data, no Deep Learning", is a common hearing among AI researchers. Petridis et al. [7], focus on lip-reading for isolated word recognition training on small-scale datasets. The proposed method consists of two streams (each consisting of an encoder and a BLSTM): one stream encodes static information, using raw mouth RoIs as input; the other stream encodes local temporal dynamics, taking as input the difference between two consecutive frames. Each stream's temporal dynamics are modeled by a BLSTM, and stream fusion is done by another BLSTM. Four benchmark datasets were used, before the usage of very large lip-reading datasets.

The proposed method learns simultaneously to extract features and perform classification using LSTM networks. Results demonstrate that the proposed model achieves state-of-the-art performance, outperforming all other approaches reported in the literature, on all datasets.

Afouras et al. [30] aim to boost lip reading performance, by training strong models learning from ASR strong models, and not requiring human-annotated ground truth data. The proposed method distills (transfers knowledge/weights from a large model to a smaller one) from an ASR model, trained on a large-scale audio-only unlabelled corpus, with a teacher-student approach (the teacher's prediction is used to train the student). The cross-modal distillation combines CTC with a frame-wise cross-entropy loss, minimizing the KL-divergence between the student and teacher posterior distributions. The method and paper's contributions show that: ground truth transcriptions are not essential to train a lip-reading system; arbitrary amounts of unlabelled video data can be leveraged to improve performance; distillation significantly speeds up training; state-of-the-art results on (publicly available) LRS2 and LRS3 datasets can be obtained.

Results demonstrate effectiveness in training strong models for VSR by distilling knowledge from a pre-trained ASR model, and more generally from any available video of talking heads, e.g. from YouTube, therefore from any arbitrarily large amount of data.

Deep Learning methods have been used for developing ALR systems. As DL is vulnerable to adversarial attacks, so will ALR DL-based systems. Gupta et al. [31] proposed Fooling AuTomAtic Lip Reading (FATALRead), a method to perform adversarial attacks on state-of-the-art word-level ALR systems, conducted on a publicly available dataset, in view of making model design more robust and resilient against engineered attacks. Adversarial attacks toward video classification consist of adding a well-crafted minimal and imperceptible perturbation to the input, such that its classification is incorrect. The proposed model aims to replace the target output for another, by adding perturbations that alter the classification prediction.

FATALRead attacked successfully fools state-of-the-art ALR systems based on sequential and temporal convolutional architectures. The results show the vulnerability of the sequential and temporal convolutional network (TCN) architectures, to an adversarial attack in the domain of ALR.

Table 1 presents a resumed overview of the previously mentioned methods.

Table 1. Summary of the study analysis for Automatic Lipreading.

Study	Year of publication	Location	Focus	Method
Lopez et al. [15]	2017	Pompeu University, Barcelona, Spain	Study upper limit in Speech Recognition	Constructed database, compared hearing-impaired and non-hearing-impaired performances.
Zhang et al. [16]	2020	UCAS, Beijing, China	Rethinking the RoI - extraoral relevance	Study done with word-level and sentence-level VSR models, including extraoral parts, trained on in-the-wild dataset.
Lu et al. [17]	2019	NCUT, Beijing, China	Lip segmentation improvement	Each pixel of each layer is QTS structured, the probability of a branch is derived, a MAP-MRF is obtained, then the unsupervised segmentation turns in labelling optimization.
Lu and Liu [18]	2018	NCUT, Beijing, China	Lip segmentation improvement	Active contour model based, with a rhombus and a semi-ellipse as initial contours. Illumination equalization to RGB images, then combination of U (CIE-LUV) and DHT, resulting on 4 key points to adjust initial shape.
Das et al. [2]	2017	NIT, Nagaland, India	Lip contour extraction refinement	Pixel-based segmentation, mouth region k-means extracted on R/G ratio threshold, and refinement by binary classification of G and RGB planes, and by processing of combined lip partial areas.
Radha et al. [19]	2020	Chennai, India	Static and dynamic (s&d) visual features selection	Three viseme models comparison: one as control; one fusing s&d at features level; one fusing s&d at model level. MHI with DCT, Wavelet, and Zernike. Fusion models built by GMM L-R HMM.
Weng and Kitani [20]	2019	Carnegie Mellon, Pittsburgh, USA	Visual clues only word-level lip-reading	Deep 3DCNN two-stream I3D, instead of a shallow 3DCNN and a deep 2DCNN. Different combinations of front-end and back-end, greyscale, optical flow on LRW dataset.
Lu and Yan [21]	2020	NCUT, Beijing, China	Comparing DNN with traditional algorithms	Extraction of 5 key frames, then 5 key points of mouth region, CNN to extract features and BLSTM to extract both directions correlations.
Mesbah et al. [22]	2019	USMBA, Fez, Morocco	Visual-only speech recognition system	Hahn moments as a filter, and CNN as classifier.
Ma et al. [23]	2017	HIT, Shenzhen, China	Feature extraction under variant lighting	Pre-processing chain of illumination normalization, and improved LBP features.

(continued)

Table 1. (*continued*)

Study	Year of publication	Location	Focus	Method
Jeon et al. [24]	2021	GIST, Korea	Homophemes disambiguation; Character and word recognition	New architecture combining 3DCNN, densely connected 3DCNN, multilayer feature fusion 3DCNN, then GRU and CTC. Pixel dropout layer and spatial dropout layer.
Wang [25]	2019	UCAS, Beijing, China	Homophemes disambiguation capturing multi-grained spatiotemporal features	2D and 3D CNNs as front-end, for frame-wise fine spatial and short-term medium spatio-temporal features. Then fuses by Bi-ConvLSTM, with temporal attention.
Fenghour et al. [26]	2020	LSBU, London, UK	Visemes for unknown words in speech	Lexicon-free visemes as a very-limited classification schema and perplexity analysis for word conversion, using LSR2 and visual clues only.
Fenghour et al. [27]	2021	LSBU, London, UK	Viseme-to-word conversion	DNN with Attention-based GRU, compared to Perplexity-iterator, FFN and HMM, using LSR2 and LSR3.
Prajwal et al. [9]	2021	Oxford, UK	Learn strong models of ALR in silent videos	End-to-end trainable attention-based pooling mechanism, sub-word tokenization, and propose a visual speech detection mechanism.
Martinez et al. [27]	2020	SAIRS, Cambridge, UK	Limitations of BGRU	BGRU layers are replaced with multi-scale TCN, reducing 3 weeks to 1 week GPU-time, on LRW and LRW1000 datasets.
Huang et al. [28]	2022	SWUN, Chengdu, China	End-to-end model	Transformer network adopting a self-attention mechanism instead of CNN and RNN, on GRID corpora.
Lu and Li [29]	2019	NCUT, Beijing, China	Requirements of practical ALR applications	Extract key frames, use VGG for features extraction and compare a fusion model with attention mechanism to a fusion model of two networks. Apply in own independent database.
Petridis et al. [7]	2019	Imperial College London, UK	Isolated word recognition, with small-scale datasets	Two streams consisting of an encoder and a BLSTM, one encoding static information, the other local temporal dynamics. Four datasets are used.
Afouras et al. [30]	2020	Oxford, UK	Dismissing human-labelled data	Transfer of knowledge (weights) from large model to a smaller one, teacher-student approach. Cross-modal distillation, combining CTC with a frame-wise cross-entropy loss function.
Gupta et al. [31]	2021	IIT Indore, India	Robustness to adversarial attacks	Adversarial attacks on sequential and temporal convolutional architectures based ALR systems, and on publicly available datasets.

4   Conclusions

In many of the referenced papers, statements reinforce the idea of a lack of consensus, which only acts as a catalyst for more research and more work. The evolution has been so swift that decade-old methods are most likely to be obsolete, and derivations are so diversified that it is as unpredictable what will happen in the next decade as the movement of a simple magnetic pendulum subjected just to 3 magnetic fields beside the gravitational one.

Although uncertain, in the author's point of view the future will be based on: continuing the application of newer methods, followed by the simplification of the same; simplifying parts of the process, as attention narrows inputs' processing target; complicating parts of the process, weighing other data as visual or emotional contextualization.

Answering the Research Questions: RQ1 - End-to-end deep learning, resorting to Attention-based LSTM or Transformers appear to be more suitable for visual clues for automatic lip-reading.; RQ2 - The same answer as in RQ1.; RQ3 - No specific methods are studied with the available datasets; Although some datasets are more commonly explored in the presented papers, namely LRS2; RQ4 - As mentioned, many challenges are still open, e.g., how effective is recurrent training, resorting to parallel and in-series training?

Acknowledgements. This work is funded by FCT/MEC through national funds and, when applicable, co-funded by the FEDER-PT2020 partnership agreement under the project UIDB/00308/2020.

References

1. Huang, X., Acero, A., Hon, H.-W.: Spoken Language Processing: A Guide to Theory, Algorithm, and System Development. Prentice Hall PTR, Upper Saddle River (2001)
2. Das, S.K., Nandakishor, S., Pati, D.: Automatic lip contour extraction using pixel-based segmentation and piece-wise polynomial fitting. In: 2017 14th IEEE India Council International Conference (INDICON), Roorkee. IEEE, pp. 1–5 (2017). https://ieeexplore.ieee.org/document/8487538/
3. Bauman, N.: Speechreading (Lip-Reading) (2011). https://hearinglosshelp.com/blog/speechreading-lip-reading/
4. Petajan, E.D.: Automatic lipreading to enhance speech recognition. In: Degree of Doctor of Philosophy in Electrica l Engineering, University of Illinois, Urbana-Champaign (1984)
5. Huang, H., et al.: A novel machine lip reading model. Procedia Comput. Sci. **199**, 1432–1437 (2022). https://linkinghub.elsevier.com/retrieve/pii/S187705092200182X
6. Assael, Y.M., Shillingford, B., Whiteson, S., de Freitas, N.: LipNet: end-to-end sentence-level lipreading (2016). arXiv:1611.01599
7. Petridis, S., Wang, Y., Ma, P., Li, Z., Pantic, M.: End-to-end visual speech recognition for small-scale datasets (2019). arXiv Version Number: 4. https://arxiv.org/abs/1904.01954
8. Fung, I., Mak, B.: End-to-end low-resource lip-reading with maxout Cnn and Lstm. In: 2018 IEEE International Conference on Acoustics, Speech and Signal Processing (ICASSP), Calgary, AB. IEEE, pp. 2511–2515 (2018). https://ieeexplore.ieee.org/document/8462280/

9. Prajwal, K.R., Afouras, T., Zisserman, A.: Sub-word level lip reading with visual attention (2021). arXiv:2110.07603

10. Fenghour, S., Chen, D., Guo, K., Li, B., Xiao, P.: Deep learning-based automated lip-reading: a survey. IEEE Access, **9** 121184–121205 (2021). https://ieeexplore.ieee.org/document/9522117/

11. Hao, M., Mamut, M., Ubul, K.: A survey of lipreading methods based on deep learning. In: 2020 2nd International Conference on Image Processing and Machine Vision, Bangkok Thailand. ACM, pp. 31–39 (2020). https://dl.acm.org/doi/10.1145/3421558.3421563

12. Alam, M., Samad, M., Vidyaratne, L., Glandon, A., Iftekharuddin, K.: Survey on deep neural networks in speech and vision systems. Neurocomputing **417**, 302–321 (2020). https://linkinghub.elsevier.com/retrieve/pii/S0925231220311619

13. Bhaskar, S., Thasleema, T.M., Rajesh, R.: A survey on different visual speech recognition techniques. In: Nagabhushan, P., Guru, D.S., Shekar, B.H., Kumar, Y.H.S. (eds.) Data Analytics and Learning. LNNS, vol. 43, pp. 307–316. Springer, Singapore (2019). https://doi.org/10.1007/978-981-13-2514-4_26

14. Fernandez-Lopez, A., Sukno, F.M.: Survey on automatic lip-reading in the era of deep learning. Image Vis. Comput. **78**, 53–72 (2018). https://linkinghub.elsevier.com/retrieve/pii/S0262885618301276

15. Fernandez-Lopez, A., Martinez, O., Sukno, F.M.: Towards estimating the upper bound of visual-speech recognition: the visual lip-reading feasibility database. In: 2017 12th IEEE International Conference on Automatic Face & Gesture Recognition, Washington, DC, USA. IEEE, pp. 208–215 (2017). http://ieeexplore.ieee.org/document/7961743/

16. Zhang, Y., Yang, S., Xiao, J., Shan, S., Chen, X.: Can we read speech beyond the lips? Rethinking RoI selection for deep visual speech recognition (2020). arXiv Version Number: 2. https://arxiv.org/abs/2003.03206

17. Lu, Y., Zhu, X., Xiao, K.: Unsupervised lip segmentation based on quad-tree MRF framework in wavelet domain. Measurement **141**, 95–101 (2019). https://linkinghub.elsevier.com/retrieve/pii/S0263224119302180

18. Lu, Y., Liu, Q.: Lip segmentation using automatic selected initial contours based on localized active contour model. EURASIP J. Image Video Process. **2018**(1), 7 (2018). https://jivp-eurasipjournals.springeropen.com/articles/10.1186/s13640-017-0243-9

19. Radha, N., Shahina, A., Khan, N.: Visual speech recognition using fusion of motion and geometric features. Procedia Comput. Sci. **171**, 924–933 (2020). https://linkinghub.elsevier.com/retrieve/pii/S1877050920310760

20. Weng, X., Kitani, K.: Learning spatio-temporal features with two-stream deep 3D CNNs for lipreading (2019). arXiv:1905.02540. http://arxiv.org/abs/1905.02540

21. Lu, Y., Yan, J.: automatic lip reading using convolution neural network and bidirectional long short-term memory. Int. J. Pattern Recog. Artif. Intell. **34**(01), 2054003 (2020). https://www.worldscientific.com/doi/abs/10.1142/S0218001420540038

22. Mesbah, A., Berrahou, A., Hammouchi, H., Berbia, H., Qjidaa, H., Daoudi, M.: Lip reading with Hahn convolutional neural networks. Image Vis. Comput. **88**, 76–83 (2019). https://linkinghub.elsevier.com/retrieve/pii/S0262885619300605

23. Ma, X., Zhang, H., Li, Y.: Feature extraction method for lip-reading under variant lighting conditions. In: Proceedings of the 9th International Conference on Machine Learning and Computing, Singapore. ACM, pp. 320–326 (2017). https://dl.acm.org/doi/10.1145/3055635.3056576

24. Jeon, S., Elsharkawy, A., Kim, M.S.: Lipreading architecture based on multiple convolutional neural networks for sentence-level visual speech recognition. Sensors **22**(1), 72 (2021). https://www.mdpi.com/1424-8220/22/1/72

25. Wang, C.: Multi-grained spatio-temporal modeling for lip-reading. arXiv Version Number: 2 (2019). https://arxiv.org/abs/1908.11618

26. Fenghour, S., Chen, D., Guo, K., Xiao, P.: Lip reading sentences using deep learning with only visual cues. IEEE Access, **8**, 215 516–215 530 (2020). https://ieeexplore.ieee.org/document/9272286/

27. Fenghour, S., Chen, D., Guo, K., Li, B., Xiao, P.: An effective conversion of visemes to words for high-performance automatic lipreading. Sensors **21**(23), 7890 (2021). https://www.mdpi.com/1424-8220/21/23/7890

28. Martinez, B., Ma, P., Petridis, S., Pantic, M.: Lipreading using temporal convolutional networks. arXiv Version Number: 1 (2020). https://arxiv.org/abs/2001.08702

29. Lu, Y., Li, H.: Automatic lip-reading system based on deep convolutional neural network and attention-based long short-term memory. Appl. Sci. **9**(8), 1599 (2019). https://www.mdpi.com/2076-3417/9/8/1599

30. Afouras, T., Chung, J.S., Zisserman, A.: ASR is all you need: cross-modal distillation for lip reading (2020). arXiv:1911.12747 [cs, eess]. http://arxiv.org/abs/1911.12747

31. Gupta, A.K., Gupta, P., Rahtu, E.: FATALRead - fooling visual speech recognition models: put words on lips. Appl. Intell. (2021). https://link.springer.com/10.1007/s10489-021-02846-w

An Analysis of Usage and Reporting Patterns in a Mobile Health Application

Ana González Bermúdez[✉] and Ana M. Bernardos

Information Processing and Telecommunications Center, ETSI Telecomunicación, Universidad Politécnica de Madrid, Madrid, Spain
{ana.gonzalezb,anamaria.bernardos}@upm.es

Abstract. The use of mobile applications (apps) as a tool to monitor health-related parameters is now a common practice. Connected to wearables or stand-alone, these apps usually track the user by retrieving relevant information from mobile embedded sensors but also may serve to get self-reported data. To make sense, these apps require that the user remains active in the use of the application, to get the most complete data records. Different aspects may affect the user's adherence level to the app, both personal characteristics (personality, motivation, etc.) and app design and technical features (attractiveness, usability, perceived usefulness, etc.). The aim of this paper is to explore user's adherence by analyzing users' behavior on the use case of an app which aims at helping track emotional states by using emoticons. The adherence analysis focuses on evaluate the real impact of notifications, which is the main strategy to incentive adherence in this case. The study analyzes four weeks of data from 20 young users, that have volunteered to use the app within the framework of a study on mental health. Based on a selected set of behaviour-related features, a clustering analysis shows two well differentiated adherence groups: the first one that use the app several times a day, while the second is less regular. Regarding notifications, they reveal to have different impact depending on the user group, being much more effective for very active users. Other adherence incentives must be designed to improve the continuous use of the application.

Keywords: Mobile Health · personal health · application · adherence · reminders · notifications · behaviour

1   Introduction

The World Health Organization defines mobile health (mHealth) as "medical and public health practice supported by mobile devices" [1]. Apps are a common and important component of mHealth systems; they have the potential of adding value to patient care, help improve the awareness on health status, promote behavior change to healthier lifestyles, etc. In the second quarter of 2022, there were around 54,600 and 52,400 medical apps (excluding wellness and fitness ones) in Google Play and App Store respectively [2, 3], after having increased significantly over the last seven years. Industry experts believe

© ICST Institute for Computer Sciences, Social Informatics and Telecommunications Engineering 2023
Published by Springer Nature Switzerland AG 2023. All Rights Reserved
A. Cunha et al. (Eds.): MobiHealth 2022, LNICST 484, pp. 196–206, 2023.
https://doi.org/10.1007/978-3-031-32029-3_18

that by 2030, mobile apps will be embedded within standard treatment protocols for most diseases and conditions, and widely used in preventative care [4]. Mobile health applications can effectively support diagnosis and clinical decision making, make predictions on risk or detect a normal patters, provide support towards healthy behavior change, provide information to handle chronic diseases, etc.

How to improve apps' user experience and increase perceived usefulness is key to enhance adherence and leverage mHealth services. In this context, the aim of the paper is twofold: to understand how to optimally measure application adherence from usage features and analyze the impact of reminders/notifications as a tool to promote adherence, depending on the user profile and the context of application use. To do so, we will analyze usage data of a mobile application designed for youngsters to track their emotions (which is thought to be an enabler of a mHealth system that supports psychological tuition). The structure of the article is as follows. Section 2 contains a review of the state of the art on adherence techniques for mobile applications and their effectiveness. Section 3 describes the supporting technology that has been developed to provide the mHealth service for mental health. Section 4 compiles relevant details regarding the user study, the resulting data collection, and the chosen adherence-related features. Also, this section gathers results and its analysis. Section 5 concludes the paper and shows the future work.

2   State of the Art

Technology acceptance is related to perceived usefulness and perceived usability (Technology Acceptance Model, Davis, 1989). Particularized to mHealth [5], perceived usefulness is related to the fact that the use of the mobile application brings real and noticeable benefits to the user's health, and perceived usability refers to the effort needed to use the app. Therefore, acceptance is linked to the app being free of effort for the user to use it, and to provide functionalities and usage targets for the application that can achieve tangible health benefits for the user. Adherence can be thus understood as a consequence of both the application perceived usefulness (and motivation) and usability (in [6], 22 studies on apps usability are reviewed, concluding that usability is one of the main barriers to the adoption of mHealth systems). Bidirectionally, it will also be an enabler to perceived usefulness: the user adheres to the app because he/she finds it useful, and the mHealth can provide meaningful feedback and advanced features on continuous data thanks to the regular app usage. In [7], frequency of use is perceived to be an important fact in user satisfaction. In [8], 69% of people who use a health app several times a day or more strongly agreed on its effectiveness.

Mobile health apps seem to be able to bring huge value to users and patients when integrated as part of a clinical pathway, but there is still room to scientifically demonstrate this hunch. Some studies have tried to measure the impact of mHealth (in many different fields, e.g. [9] for patients with Covid-19, [10] for patients with coronary heart disease, or [11] for pregnant women with urinary incontinence) by comparing a control group (using traditional treatment methods) and a test group using an app; apps provide monitoring, reminders, feedback, motivational messages, personalized goals, etc. In general, studies' conclusions show improved health results in the test groups, pointing out that mHealth may improve standard care. Nevertheless, the usefulness of these apps is not always perceived by their users. According to [8], where 46 apps were analyzed, almost 20% of the surveyed users disagreed or strongly disagreed that health apps help them with their healthcare.

Usually, adherence is studied by exploring motivation for app use, frequency of usage, perceived effectiveness and abandonment rate and reason (whether and why a health app was installed but its usage discontinued). How to improve adherence is still a challenge: it is not enough for an app to provide a great functionality; it is also important to guarantee usability while preventing app abandonment through adequate techniques. mHealth applications make use of a variety of design incentives to engage the user [8, 12]. They may include notifications and reminders, personalized goals and performance feedback. Existing literature is scarce with respect to the analysis of the effectivity of adherence mechanisms. In this article, we aim at summarizing the different strategies to apply, which include:

- *M1 - Provide relevant information:* Delivery of relevant information about health or disease.
- *M2 - Personalized goals:* Ensure motivation strategies to improve habits and health condition.
- *M3 - Performance evolution:* Provide feedback about the progress through motivational messages and other communication pills aimed to encourage the patient to keep improving.
- *M4 - Comprehensive data visualization:* Show evolution of self-data through graphs, notes, etc. In some cases, it is also allowed to export data.
- *M5 - Delivery of notifications/reminders:* Used to remind the user to input data, take medication, etc.
- *M6 - Community:* Social statistics, which may include rankings against a 'group' of interest (e.g., other users with similar circumstances) to show whether performance is over the average.

Moreover, we aim at providing some insights on the real impact of reminders in a specific use case, in order to gain knowledge on how to improve design for the users to better adhere the application.

3   Use Case: Emotions Tracking for Mental Health Support in Youngsters

Nowadays, young people reveal an increasing demand (and acceptance) of mental health-care support. For a diagnosis, the time-to-doctor can take time, thus automated and semi-automated systems may be tools to facilitate and accelerate this process. Once under treatment, the digital phenotype collected by an app may serve to build personalized models of digital and physical lifestyles that may help identify anomalous behaviors on patients at risk, e.g., to trigger assistance alerts, modify the application workflow.

In this service context, we want to analyze users' adherence towards a mental health app, which is a key component on a digital health service for mental healthcare support for youngsters. The complete system is described below.

3.1 Context and System Architecture Overview

The technology solution has two main components. The first one is a mobile application for patients, which monitors their condition through passive data (information about their activity, collected directly from the digital device's sensors) and active data (emoticons representing feelings, directly reported by the users on the 'patient' side). The second component is a practitioner dashboard, that provides relevant information to the therapist during the sessions with the patient. The system is designed to provide full data sharing control through the app, i.e., patients must actively award access to their data during the therapy session and the access permission is kept ephemeral, only granted only during the session itself.

Through the mobile application, users can send reports (ideally several times a day) which consist of a simple choice of an emoticon that represents their mood, and information about where and with whom are they. Also, they can check on their history and get some complementary information about their activity data. Passive data (transparently gathered once consent is given) serve to generate a digital phenotype for users, considering their daily habits making use of the device sensors. For example, to monitor daily activity, we made use of the accelerometer and gyroscope measures, which allow us to analyze the number of steps taken by the patient. To calculate an estimation of the patients' circadian rhythm, we also use other information collected by the phone, such as the screen unlocking events (to determine interactions with the mobile phone) or the ambient light detected. Other characteristics analyzed with passive data are, for example, GPS locations or daily mobile phone usage.

The system backend provides storage, processing, and securitization features. Figure 1 shows the architecture of the mHealth system, with the three components stated above: the mobile application, for the user to register and send data; the dashboard for the therapist and the backend with storage for user personal information, emoticons and sensors data. A notification module is the one in charge of dispatching app prompts to applications users. Finally, a digital phenotype module oversees feeding the dashboard with relevant information for therapy.

3.2 User App and Adherence Mechanism

Figure 2 gathers some views of the mobile application interface in which the user reports an emoticon, also attaching context-based information on with whom and where the user is when reporting. The use of standard emoticons facilitates the identification of moods, although personal biases can apply on the choice of emoticons. The application design aims at being intuitive and easy to use. To incentive adherence, the application implements some of the adherence mechanisms stated above, in particular:

- *Performance evolution (M3)*. For physical activity data, the app provides comparative information along the time. This feedback is very simple and not related to mental health as clinical related feedback and derived analysis are extremely sensitive.
- *Comprehensive data visualization (M4)*. The patient can access a history of the emoticons sent and statistics of the digital fingerprint collected in the last 24 h.

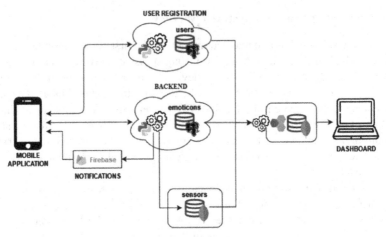

Fig. 1. Architecture system.

- *Delivery of notifications/reminders (M5).* Notifications are the main mechanism chosen to keep the user active in the app. The system sends several daily notifications to encourage users to report their emotional state. In this implementation, five prompts are delivered as shown below (Table 1).

Table 1. Hours when users receive notifications.

Notification	N1	N2	N3	N4	N5
Hour	9:00	11:00	14:00	17:00	20:00

3.3 User Study

Between October 2020 and March 2021, 20 young users (between 16 and 24 years of age, M = 20.06, SD = 2.54, 78% were female) seeking for mental healthcare assistance volunteered to use the beta app for a trial period of one month thanks to the call of a European organization providing services for youth. Users were people without any specific diagnosis on mental health diseases, but with interest in being able to access tools for their self-management and with standard skills on mobile devices usage.

4 Data Analysis

On these data, we carried out a general analysis on the generated data volume per user during a period of maximum 4 weeks, computing the number of records (a record is a timestamp with a sensor id and its value). Apart from volume and frequency (how many

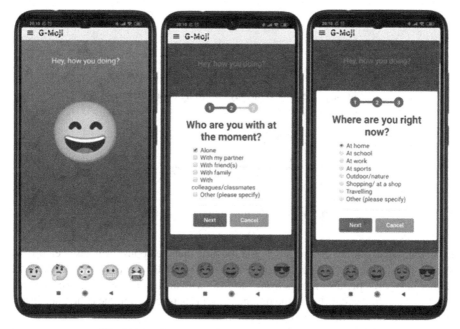

Fig. 2. Emoticons reporting interface of the application.

and how often), we also processed information about where, with whom and when emoticons reports were provided. And, being interested on the effect of notifications, we divide the day into slots (Fig. 3) to calculate the number of emoticons sent within each. We also computed the time difference between the notification was received and the user time to send a subsequent emoticon (average reaction time to the five notifications), as can be seen in Fig. 4. We following analyze the different user profiles in terms of app usage, the context in which users were reporting active data and some analysis on the notifications' effectiveness. To sum up, the data collected for the analysis can be grouped as follows.

- *Adherence data:* total emoticons sent, total active days, maximum consecutive active and maximum consecutive inactive days.
- *Context of sending emoticons:* total reports from home, total reports outside, total reports alone and total reports with company.
- *Hours of sending emoticons:* total reports sent in the following time slots.
- *Notifications feedback data:* Average reaction time to the five notifications and its standard deviations

4.1   Analyzing App Usage Patterns: Are There Different Types of User Profiles?

The average number of passive data per user was $\eta = 107{,}262$ records ($\sigma = 91{,}257$). This large difference of data volume among users is due to the explicit permissions to

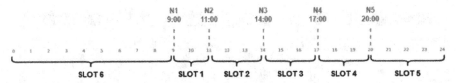

Fig. 3. Time slots in the day according to notifications

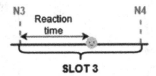

Fig. 4. Reaction time to the notifications

sensor data access on the Android/iOS and the time that the application has been up and running. The volume of active data (emoticons) is much lower, as expected. The total number of records per user ranges from 9 to 115 (with an average of $\eta = 65$ records per user, $\sigma = 50$). This variability in the number of reports is related to the adherence itself, i.e., the frequency for the user to report emoticons.

Taking as a basis both volume and frequency of reports, we can distinguish two different types of users. On the one hand, a group of 7 users (U0–U6) who report emoticons every day of the trial, not showing any period of inactivity (days with not even a single emoticon reported), and with a high average number of daily emoticons ($\eta = 4.74$ emoticons/day, $\sigma = 0.24$). On the other hand, the rest of users (U7–U19), who are less methodical, show inactivity periods (even of a week time) and report less emoticons in the active days than the first group ($\eta = 1.10$ emoticons/day and $\sigma = 0.47$). This split was confirmed by a cluster analysis carried out after a Recursive Feature Elimination on 29 features from each user, summarized previously.

4.2   In What Context Do Youngsters Use the Application?

As mentioned above, and as shown in Fig. 2, when users send an emoticon, they are asked two questions: where and with whom they are. Thanks to these questions we can evaluate the influence of the environment on the emoticons reporting. In addition, the context of use is generally not significantly different between the two groups. As shown in Table 2, emoticons reported from home 63.5% in the first group and 50.6% in the second. Work stands out as the next most common location, representing 15% of the emoticons registered, but with differences between groups: 7.8% for first group and 29.6% for second group. In addition, most emoticons were sent when users were alone, 56.3% and 40.8% respectively. The rest were recorded with family, partners, friends, or work colleagues. For example, the reports with co-workers are very similar with percentages of emoticons sent at work, 7.8% for first group and 21.4% for second group (Table 3). The schedule for notifications may justify the registered data, although in that sense, it is needed to have a look to the responsiveness of the users towards the notifications.

Table 2. Percentage of answers about where they are when they send the emoticon.

Users	Home	School	Work	Travelling	Outdoor	Other
U0–U6	63.5%	1.7%	7.8%	4%	2.4%	20.4%
U7–U19	50.6%	1.4%	29.6%	2.6%	3.7%	12.2%

Table 3. Percentage of answers about who they are with when they send the emoticon.

Users	Alone	Family	Co-workers	Partner	Friends	Other
U0–U6	56.3%	15,3%	7.8%	3.2%	3.9%	13.5%
U7–U19	40.8%	15.9%	21.4%	8.5%	5.5%	7.7%

4.3 Are Notifications an Effective Mechanism to Encourage Application Adherence?

The application sends 5 daily reminders for a user to report an emoticon, at: 9:00, 11:00, 14:00, 17:00 and 20:00. We analyzed the percentage over the total of emoticons sent in each time slot between notifications (Table 2). We observed clear differences between users who report emotions every day and those who do not do it. Users showing greater adherence have a uniform distribution of emoticons throughout the day (with almost no night-time sending). Meanwhile, users with more irregular adherence send more emoticons in the first half of the day and their interaction decreases as the hours go by. In addition, these users send more emoticons at night (Table 4).

Table 4. Percentage of emoticons sent in each time slot.

Users	9:00–11:00	11:00–14:00	14:00–17:00	17:00–20:00	20:00–24:00	24:00–9:00
U0–U6	18%	20%	20%	21%	19%	2%
U7–U19	26%	25%	22%	11%	7%	8%

Secondly, we analyzed the average time difference between a reminder and the next emoticon, to analyze the reaction time towards a notification, to correlate both reminder-emoticon (even if no cause-effect event can be directly inferred). As can be seen in Table 3, U0–U6 users send emoticons about 30 min after receiving the notification, while the rest of the users usually take more than twice that time. Then, the recording pattern in the first group could be therefore associated with a better response to notifications. Moreover, in the second group of users we perceive better feedback to notifications in the morning. For the notifications later in the day, users almost never respond within half an hour time (Table 5).

Table 5. Average reaction time to notifications and its standard deviations.

Users	N1	N2	N3	N4	N5
U0–U6	27 min. (σ = 25 min)	27 min. (σ = 34 min)	28 min. (σ = 33 min)	26 min. (σ = 27 min)	29 min. (σ = 41 min)
U7–U19	45 min. (σ = 32 min)	83 min. (σ = 69 min)	61 min. (σ = 38 min)	62 min. (σ = 32 min)	84 min. (σ = 31 min)

4.4 Determining Behaviour Types on Application Usage

The clustering analysis was only able to discriminate between two groups: users showing a high adherence to the application (group 1) and those reporting a more irregular use (group 2). Group 2's users reported fewer emoticons per day on average that Group 1's users, being more intense in the app usage during mornings/midday. Additionally, they registered periods of inactivity (e.g. not using the application over the weekends). Regarding company, both groups agree on the context in which they tend to use the app, with all of them being more active when they are at home and/or alone. Regarding the generation of notifications as an effective mechanism for application adherence, we found that users have responded to prompts in a 70% of cases (with a threshold of a maximum average of 60 min to determine the notification as effective), thus "typically" responding to notifications. Moreover, 30% of users responded to notifications in less than 30 min. Group 1's users almost always react to notifications and quite quickly. But Group 2's users do not always react (they apparently are more reactive for notifications delivered early in the day) and take longer to input data.

Although we explored the effect of fatigue over the weeks and the value of notifications for this, these results were not relevant because the second group of users did not have enough data and usually did not complete the four weeks of the study.

5   Conclusions

Although, from the retrieved data, users in our experiment can be classified into two main different groups, this short analysis shows the variability of usage patterns over the same application. Observing that periods of inactivity may differ between users, user profiling could be useful to model activity and usage intensity. The objective would be to design specific measures to foster adherence during inactivity periods and to guarantee timely reporting along the day. In this direction, notifications have been shown to be a key mechanism for their adherence: they do help to keep users active, but unfortunately seem to be more efficient with those users already showing higher adherence. For the more inactive user, notifications reveal to be useful but not sufficient. Corrective measures may include a) to facilitate notifications customization, thus their frequency, delivery context and timing is better for each specific user (adaptive and automated customization is also an option to consider); b) to better model the user motivation and expectations when starting the app, to enrich the operation context by adapting interfaces and adherence mechanisms; c) to include other adherence mechanisms that may explore rewards, group performance advice, etc.

In addition to the problems concerning users who did not complete the four weeks of data reporting, the study is limited by the number of users and the difficulties to directly communicate with them during the study and the limited amount of data. Within the study, there is also a weakness due to the lack of social data about users, which prevents analysis along these lines. Nevertheless, the study reveals that rough clustering and posterior classification can be enough for setting up a first strategy for notifications handling. In any case, it would be interesting to carry out a broader study with better access to users' demography and social data.

In this study we have not been able to measure the impact of using data as a support for clinical treatment, thus it is in our roadmap to conduct a study in a use case in which the app, in practice, is integrated in a clinical pathway. The fact of using the app for clinical follow up may substantially influence how adherence is considered from the design viewpoint.

Acknowledgment. This work has been supported along the time by the UPM RP180022025 grant and REACT-CM MadridDataSpace4Pandemics Project. The authors would like to thank volunteer users for their contribution to the work.

References

1. Ryu, S.: Book Review: mHealth: New Horizons for Health through Mobile Technologies: Based on the Findings of the Second Global Survey on eHealth (Global Observatory for eHealth Series, Volume 3) (2016). Healthc. Inform. Res.
2. Statista: Number of mHealth apps available in the Google Play Store from 1st quarter 2015 to 2nd quarter 2022 (2022). https://www.statista.com/statistics/779919/health-apps-available-google-play-worldwide/%0AGoogle
3. Statista: Number of mHealth apps available in the Apple App Store from 1st quarter 2015 to 2nd quarter 2022 (2022). https://www.statista.com/statistics/779910/health-apps-available-ios-worldwide/
4. Heyen, N.B.: mHEALTH 2030. EHealthCom, Organisation for the Review of Care & Health Applications (2016)
5. Deng, Z.: Understanding public users' adoption of mobile health service. Int. J. Mob. Commun. **11**, 351–373 (2013). https://doi.org/10.1504/IJMC.2013.055748
6. Zapata, B.C., Fernández-Alemán, J.L., Idri, A., Toval, A.: Empirical studies on usability of mHealth apps: a systematic literature review. J. Med. Syst. **39**, 1–19 (2015). https://doi.org/10.1007/s10916-014-0182-2
7. Research2Guidance: mHealth app economics. https://research2guidance.com/wp-content/uploads/2017/11/R2G-mHealth-Developer-Economics-2017-Status-And-Trends.pdf
8. de Korte, E., Wiezer, N., Roozeboom, M.B., Vink, P., Kraaij, W.: Behavior change techniques in mhealth apps for the mental and physical health of employees: systematic assessment. JMIR mHealth uHealth **6**, e167 (2018). https://doi.org/10.2196/mhealth.6363
9. Un, K.C., et al.: Observational study on wearable biosensors and machine learning-based remote monitoring of COVID-19 patients. Sci. Rep. **11**, 4388 (2021). https://doi.org/10.1038/s41598-021-82771-7
10. Ni, Z., Wu, B., Yang, Q., Yan, L.L., Liu, C., Shaw, R.J.: An mHealth intervention to improve medication adherence and health outcomes among patients with coronary heart disease: randomized controlled trial. J. Med. Internet Res. **24**, e27202 (2022). https://doi.org/10.2196/27202

11. Jaffar, A., Mohd Sidik, S., Foo, C.N., Muhammad, N.A., Abdul Manaf, R., Suhaili, N.: Preliminary effectiveness of mHealth app-based pelvic floor muscle training among pregnant women to improve their exercise adherence: a pilot randomised control trial. Int. J. Environ. Res. Public Health **19**, 2332 (2022). https://doi.org/10.3390/ijerph19042332

12. Nicholas, J., Fogarty, A.S., Boydell, K., Christensen, H.: The reviews are in: a qualitative content analysis of consumer perspectives on apps for bipolar disorder. J. Med. Internet Res. **19**, e105 (2017). https://doi.org/10.2196/jmir.7273

Artificial Intelligence Based Procedural Content Generation in Serious Games for Health: The Case of Childhood Obesity

Eleftherios Kalafatis[1]([✉]), Konstantinos Mitsis[1], Konstantia Zarkogianni[1], Maria Athanasiou[1], Antonis Voutetakis[2], Nicolas Nicolaides[2], Evi Chatzidaki[2], Nektaria Polychronaki[2], Vassia Chioti[2], Panagiota Pervanidou[2], Konstantinos Perakis[4], Danae Antonopoulou[5], Efi Papachristou[5], Christina Kanaka-Gantenbein[2,3], and Konstantina S. Nikita[1]

[1] School of Electrical and Computer Engineering, Athens, Biomedical Simulations and Imaging Laboratory, National Technical University of Athens, Athens, Greece
leftkal@biosim.ntua.gr
[2] Childhood Obesity Unit, First Department of Pediatrics, Medical School, Agia Sophia Children's Hospital, National and Kapodistrian University Athens, Athens, Greece
[3] Division of Endocrinology, Diabetes and Metabolism, First Department of Pediatrics, Medical School, Agia Sophia Children's Hospital, National and Kapodistrian University Athens, Athens, Greece
[4] Research and Development Department, UBITECH, Chalandri, Greece
[5] Inspiring Earth, PEGNEON, Athens, Greece

Abstract. This paper presents a novel Procedural Content Generation (PCG) method aiming at achieving personalization and adaptation in serious games (SG) for health. The PCG method is based on a genetic algorithm (GA) and provides individualized content in the form of tailored messages and SG missions, taking into consideration data collected from health-related sensors and user interaction with the SG. The PCG method has been integrated into the ENDORSE platform, which harnesses the power of artificial intelligence (AI), m-health and gamification mechanisms, towards implementing a multicomponent (diet, physical activity, educational, behavioral) intervention for the management of childhood obesity. Within the use of the ENDORSE platform, a pre-pilot study has been conducted, involving the recruitment of 20 obese children that interacted with the platform for a period of twelve weeks. The obtained results, provide a preliminary justification of PCG's effectiveness in terms of generating individualized content with sufficient relevance and usefulness. Additionally, a statistically significant correlation has been revealed between the content provided by the proposed PCG technique and lifestyle-related sensing data, highlighting the potential of the PCG's capabilities in identifying and addressing the needs of a specific user.

Keywords: serious game · adaptive · procedural content generation · genetic algorithm · health · sensors · childhood obesity

A. Cunha et al. (Eds.): MobiHealth 2022, LNICST 484, pp. 207–219, 2023.
https://doi.org/10.1007/978-3-031-32029-3_19

1 Introduction

Serious games (SG) are games with a primary purpose other than entertainment and constitute a widely recognized and effective means for educating, raising awareness, and driving behavioral changes [1, 2]. Health interventions based on SGs benefit greatly from the ability to provide a safe virtual environment, enhance engagement [3], and deliver immediate feedback [4, 5]. Furthermore, SGs can potentially tailor game content according to player needs towards personalized health interventions [6]. A recent review study employs the term "individualization" to describe SGs with adaptive capabilities. Individualization can improve user experience and engagement, as well as promote knowledge acquisition. Delivery of individualized content can be achieved either through tailored game design or by algorithmically generating content to match the user's personalized needs [7].

PCG is a method of creating content algorithmically, often based on artificial intelligence (AI) techniques, and is commonly employed to produce a large amount of novel content (i.e., game maps, dungeons, Non-Player Characters - NPC). Two main approaches to PCG exist, one that relies on random generation of content and a second that takes into consideration player interaction data [8]. Data gathered from a variety of sensors can also be integrated into PCG techniques. With the integration of such types of data in the PCG workflow, the content provided is usually relevant to the desired SG target, maximizing user engagement and thus adherence to the intervention.

SGs for health benefit greatly from the incorporation of state-of-the-art sensing technology [9]. PCG techniques employing sensing data can produce patient-tailored and clinically relevant content, resulting in a smart personalized health intervention. More specifically, the availability of real-time sensing data providing information regarding the user's lifestyle, behavioural habits and health status, makes feasible the development of sensor-based adaptive SGs with increased capacity to address important challenges in self-health management [10]. Moreover, current research on PCG in SGs for health highlights the potential of the technology to generate game content automatically and on-demand, thus reducing the time and effort needed for design purposes and increasing replayability [11, 12].

A few publications on SGs for health incorporating PCG techniques that employ sensing technology have been identified in the relevant literature. "The Emotional Labyrinth" tracks physiological signals (e.g. heart rate, electrodermal activity, breathing rate) to assess user emotion and create PCG environments to help the player achieve emotional self-awareness [13]. Another PCG based SG intervention focuses on stimulating motor movement in stroke patients through utilizing basic gesture expressions captured by applying Kinect and Myo [14]. In a recent study, the importance of a PCG-based SG in improving user-experience has been highlighted. Focusing on training individuals with sleep apnea in self-disease management, the SG includes a card game where the player faces procedurally generated opponents. The opponents are created by a PCG method employing a genetic algorithm (GA), taking into consideration the player's performance through their interaction with the SG [15]. GA is a AI-based heuristic approach that falls into the category of evolutionary algorithms.

The present study focuses on the generalization of this PCG methodology towards its integration in the ENDORSE platform [16]. In particular, the method has been enhanced to receive and analyze data from lifestyle and clinically relevant sensors in real-time. Preliminary results from the integration of the proposed methodology in the ENDORSE platform are presented for the case of childhood obesity.

2 Materials and Methods

2.1 The ENDORSE Platform

The ENDORSE project introduces a novel integrated platform to promote self-health management in T1DM and childhood obesity. The target group involves ages within the range of 6 to 14 years. The platform comprises a mobile SG for children, as well as mobile applications for parents and healthcare professionals, enabling remote health monitoring while providing personalized content. The ENDORSE platform leverages data collected from a multitude of sources that include sensors (Fitbit Ace 2 physical activity tracker, Freestyle Libre continuous glucose measurement sensors), IoT devices (Insulclock smart insulin pen), as well as interaction with the SG and the mobile applications. Personalization is achieved through the incorporation of a recommendation system able to deliver individualized content. Content generated by the ENDORSE recommendation system consists of two distinct parts: game missions and messages. The messages are made available to the children through the SG interface and to the parents through the mobile application.

The ENDORSE SG consists of a variety of mini-games in the form of missions of two types: educational and action. Healthcare professionals have been intensively involved in the SG design activities in order to assure the validity and efficiency of the SG's educational and behavioral goals. Through gameplay, the user collects in-game currency and food ingredients. The currency can be spent in avatar customization, whereas food ingredients can be used in a meal preparation mini-game to collect further rewards. In addition, educational and progress messages appear daily in a predefined game space. The messages selected by the ENDORSE recommendation system come from a pool of messages created by the healthcare professionals. Educational messages include tips and advice about healthy lifestyle and disease self-management. Progress messages are motivational and provide positive reinforcement based on the progress monitored by the platform's sensors. Aiming at minimizing the SG's impact on total daily screen time, only two game missions, an educational and an action, are available each day.

In the pre-pilot phase of the ENDORSE platform, four total missions have been included. "Cross the Swords" (Fig. 1a) and "Dive and Rise" (Fig. 1c) are action missions and "Fruit Ninja" (Fig. 1d) and "Balance Beam" (Fig. 1b) are educational missions. In "Dive and Rise" the player is incentivized to collect as many healthy foods as possible while controlling a swimming avatar. "Fruit Ninja" is a mission that requires the player to slice different kinds of food that follow a random parabolic path across the screen. A designated bar fills as the mission progresses. The mission is successful if the sliced food ingredients are considered ideal snack options. "Balance Beam" presents a narrow bridge that the avatar has to cross while maintaining balance by using a paddle. A random food appears on one side of the paddle and the player has to pick its quantity (correct portion). While choosing the right portions the avatar maintains its balance. "Cross the Swords" places the avatar in a reflex contest against a creature. The player has to react quickly and pierce different kinds of snacks. The daily missions are accessible through an in-game map (Fig. 2a).

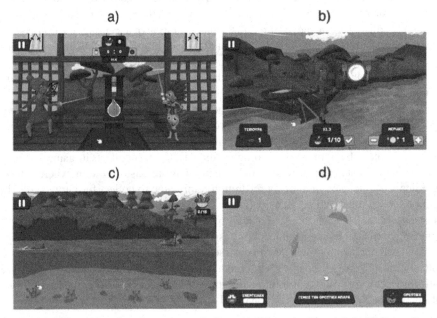

Fig. 1. Gameplay screenshots from game missions. (a) "Cross the Swords" (b) "Balance Beam" (c) "Dive and Rise" (d) "Fruit ninja"

Finally, a meal preparation mini game ("balanced meal" or "lunch box") is always accessible in the game lobby (Fig. 2b). All the ingredients that the player collected in the missions are available there for use. The player places the various food ingredients in the "lunch box" for evaluation. They are rewarded with coins based on their ability to create balanced meals.

The ENDORSE mobile application that is available to the parents serves four purposes. Firstly, it hosts a section that displays the messages delivered by the ENDORSE recommendation system on a daily basis. In addition, it provides a portal, where the parents can communicate with the healthcare professionals in the form of message exchange. It also gives the opportunity to the parents to enter the weekly weight of their children as well as their dietary options on a daily basis. Lastly, the application serves as a means of distributing the required questionnaires to the parents, such as the Post-Intervention Feasibility Study Questionnaire.

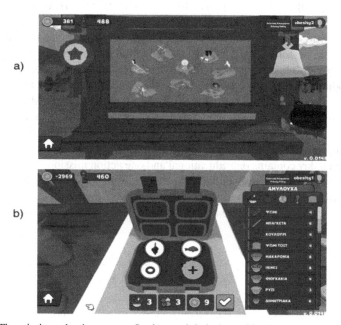

Fig. 2. (a) The mission selection screen. On the top right is the notification bell that rings whenever the user has an available message delivered by the ENDORSE recommendation system. (b) The meal preparation screen. On the right, the available ingredients are shown.

2.2 Genetic Algorithm

The proposed PCG technique generates SG content based on a Genetic Algorithm (GA). This technique has been initially incorporated into a card SG aiming to promote self-health management and raise awareness for obstructive sleep apnea through simulated debates against NPCs [15]. The ENDORSE Recommendation System utilizes an extended version of the GA that procedurally generates personalized content, taking into consideration sensor data collected by the ENDORSE platform.

For the integration of the PCG technique in the ENDORSE platform, SG missions and displayed messages have been encoded in binary gene values, with "1" representing content presence. A collection of genes constitutes a chromosome, while each gene is represented by a designated chromosome position. As depicted in Fig. 3, chromosomes have been split into two parts. The first part (MG) includes genes that determine the daily availability of missions for the SG. The second part (RG) is responsible to select tailored messages that will be displayed to the end-users. The GA is initialized with a population of chromosomes, each characterized by a selection of genes that correspond to either the availability of a mission or the display of a particular message. A total of 380 GA's chromosomes are generated for the initial population to provide adequate diversity among the chromosome population. Each gene has a 5% probability to mutate in order to adjust for chromosomes with limited diversity. Furthermore, the length of the chromosomes has been significantly enlarged compared to the original approach [15], containing 103 genes in order to accommodate 28 of them for mission content and 75 for messages. Constraints have been applied to the chromosomes to limit the availability of daily game missions. No chromosome is allowed with more than two missions per day, while each day contains one educational and one action mission. A chromosome is selected randomly as a representative and generates initial content for the ENDORSE platform. Based on data collected from sensors and user interaction, a fitness function (see Eq. 1) is applied to determine the fittest chromosomes from the initial population.

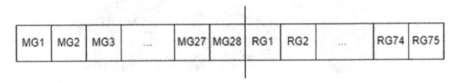

Fig. 3. Chromosome layout. MG refers to Mission Genes, RG to Recommendation Genes

$$FS = W_{MG1} * MG1 + \ldots + W_{MG28} * MG28 + W_{RG1} * RG1 + \ldots + W_{RG75} * RG75 \tag{1}$$

The fitness function employs weights (W_{gene}), assigned to each gene, representing the desirability of the gene's presence in the next GA state. These weights are trained according to the content they control which defines constants a_x and b_x, based on relevant data collected by the ENDORSE platform. Weights for game missions are trained based on SG interaction data as seen in Eq. 2.

$$W_{MG} = \begin{cases} W_{MG} + a_1, & \text{if mission score is low} \\ W_{MG} - a_2, & \text{if mission score is high} \\ W_{MG} - a_3, & \text{if mission is played} \end{cases} \tag{2}$$

Weights controlling the display of messages are trained based on multimodal data collected from the platform's sensors. Specific thresholds have been applied on the obtained sensing data towards classifying every day as good, medium, or bad, in terms of recognition of healthy lifestyle habits and self-health management. For educational messages, Eq. 3 is applied.

$$W_{RG} = \begin{cases} W_{RG} - b_1, & \text{for each good day} \\ W_{RG} - b_2, & \text{for each medium day} \\ W_{RG} + b_3, & \text{for each bad day} \end{cases} \tag{3}$$

For progress messages the weight training follows Eq. 4.

$$W_{RG} = \begin{cases} W_{RG} + b_1, & \text{for each good day} \\ W_{RG} - b_2, & \text{for each medium day} \\ W_{RG} + b_3, & \text{for each bad day} \end{cases} \tag{4}$$

This weight training ensures that the GA promotes content that is linked to identified player needs, replicating it further and passing it on to new generations. SG missions where the player scores poorly are promoted over missions that are either played frequently or are completed with high game scores. Educational messages linked to healthy behaviors monitored by the platform's sensors have a lower chance of appearing. Progress messages are more likely to appear to progress healthy habits or remind about identified unhealthy tendencies.

At the end of each GA iteration, the fittest chromosomes are paired to produce the new generation. The 20 highest scoring chromosomes are selected, based on the score provided by the fitness function, to create a next generation of chromosomes that has the same population as the original, through the crossover. One of those is also chosen to be the representative, responsible for providing the system's content.

Crossover (see Fig. 4) occurs separately for the mission content and the messages (MGs and RGs) to ensure the structural integrity of the offspring and its compliance with the constraints. For each pair of chromosomes, the MGs and RGs are split independently (Fig. 4a) into two segments at a random point (i.e., MGA1 -MGA2, RGA1 – RGA2 for

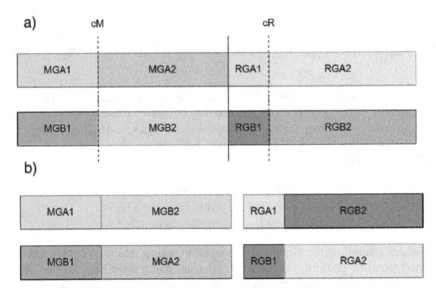

Fig. 4. Chromosome crossover. (a) Two random markers, cM and cR, split the chromosomes. (b) Two new gene sequences for MG and two for RG are generated. Their combinations produce four offspring.

chromosome A). Then each segment of the chromosomes is combined with another to create two sets of new MGs and RGs (Fig. 4b). Finally, the MGs and RGs are combined in four ways resulting in four total offspring.

Algorithm 1 presents a summary of the process of updating the GA for a new generation. The algorithm accepts as input a collection of data from the previous GA state for each user as well as data from their interaction with the platform and data gathered by the activity tracker. Its output is the generation's representative chromosome. As described, the crossover happens separately for MG and RG (lines 6 and 15) and takes into account the previous generation's fittest chromosomes. In case the newly selected representative RG or MG is exactly the same as the previous generation's one, the chromosome population is deemed saturated and is reinitialized while keeping the same weights (lines 9–11 and 18–20). Then the representative is redrawn out of the newly created fittest chromosomes. This process acts as a way of adding genetic diversity to the population, in case the gene mutation isn't enough. Lastly, the function saves the current GA state that will be retrieved in the following iteration's update.

Algorithm 1: Genetic Algorithm Update		
Data:		Previously selected chromosome CH
		Previous generation Gen, its difficulty D and its weights W, user interaction with the platform UI and data from activity tracker UD
Result:		Newly selected chromosome CH

```
1    function NewGeneration(CH, Gen, D, W, UI, UD)
2        previous MG, previous RG ← split CH
3        # region Serious Game
4        D ← CalculateNewDifficultyMG(MG, D, UI)
5        W ← CalculateNewWeightsMG(MG, W, UI, UD)
6        Gen ← CrossoverMG(Gen, W)
7        Gen ← MutationsMG(Gen)
8        new MG ← SelectChromosomeMG(Gen, W)
9        if new MG same as previous MG
10           Gen ← InitialisePopulationMG(W)
11           new  MG ← SelectChromosomeMG(Gen, W)
12       # endregion
13       # region Messages
14       W ← CalculateNewWeightsRG(RG, W, UI, UD)
15       Gen ← CrossoverRG(Gen, W)
16       Gen ← MutationsRG(Gen)
17       new RG ← SelectChromosomeRG(Gen, W)
18       if new RG same as previous RG
19           Gen ← InitialisePopulationRG(W)
20           new  RG ← SelectChromosomeRG(Gen, W)
21       new RG ← ApplyRGMask(new RG)
22       # endregion
23       CH ← concatenate new MG and RG
24       CreateNewSave(CH, Gen, D, W)
25       return CH
```

2.3 Validation Framework

The PCG technique as part of the ENDORSE recommendation system was validated in terms of user acceptance, and accuracy of the delivered personalized content during the ENDORSE pre-pilot obesity study. Twenty (20) obese children (aged 6–14) participated in the pre-pilot study for 12 weeks. The ENDORSE game and a Fitbit Activity Tracker [17] were used by the participating children, while the ENDORSE mobile application was used by their parents. The ENDORSE pilot trial has been approved by the national and ethical committee.

The intervention included 12 iterations, each lasting one week. During each iteration, data regarding the children's physical activity were gathered and fed into the GA's fitness functions. Simultaneously, data accounting for the children's interaction with the content and missions of the SG were collected. One of the GA's highest-scoring chromosomes was designated representative and was responsible for providing the weekly content.

The report produced by the Fitbit activity tracker included the daily number of steps, sedentary time and sleep time. For each participant, the average steps per day were calculated excluding those days with less than 2000 steps. This cutoff was set as an indicator of applying the Fitbit Activity Tracker. Similarly, the average sleep duration was measured, taking into consideration those days with greater than 0 recorded minutes of sleep. The thresholds for classifying the days as good, medium or bad were decided according to relevant literature [18, 19].

The integration of the PCG technique was evaluated in two directions. Within the first direction, a post-intervention questionnaire was drafted including questions relevant to the acceptance (Q1, Q2) and usefulness (Q3) of the tailored content [16]. The parents could answer each question with an integer score ranging from 1 to 5. The questionnaires were filled by the parents following the completion of the intervention plan. In the second direction, Pearson's Correlation test was performed on the data gathered from the activity trackers and the messages provided by the GA in order to assess PCG's ability to provide content relevant to the child's lifestyle status. Messages controlled by the GA were split into the following categories: "Physical Activity", "Sedentary Time" and "Sleep Duration". "Physical Activity" and "Sedentary Time" were correlated with average daily steps per participant and "Sleep Duration" with average sleep duration. Each of these categories was represented in the GA by two genes, one designated for educational messages and the other for progress messages. Pearson's correlation was calculated for these genes both separately and in combination, with the relevant data collected from sensors.

3   Results

The scores obtained from questions relevant to the acceptance of individualized content are presented in Table 1. Overall, a positive score was awarded to all three questions. The highest score was achieved in Q2, investigating the usefulness of the displayed messages towards the achievement of their personal goals (Q2: 4.13 points). The weakest score was reported in Q1, regarding the relevance of the displayed messages to the child's needs, (Q1: 3.07 points). A statistically significant difference (1.04 points, p = 0.0217) was identified by applying the Student's t-test between questions Q1 and Q2, regarding the relevance and the usefulness of the messages displayed through the SG.

Table 1. Post-Intervention Questionnaire

Questions	Scores	
	Mean Value	Standard Deviation
Q1: How relevant to your child's needs did you find the messages shown through the game?	3.07	1.38
Q2: How useful did you find the daily messages you received to achieve your goals?	4.13	1.06
Q3: How useful did you find the game's ability to display educational messages?	3.40	1.50

Pearson's correlation results are presented in Table 2. Among all participants, the average steps per day were 9840.6 and the average sleep duration was 458.6 min. Out of the 20 participants, 2 were dropouts and 3 didn't respond to the post-intervention questionnaires. Negative correlations were observed in all the investigated combinations. Statistical significance was revealed between the number of "Physical Activity" messages sent to the average steps ($p = 0.042$) and the number of combined "Physical Activity" and "Sedentary Time" messages to the average steps ($p = 0.030$).

Table 2. Pearson's Correlation

Category	Correlation		
	Gene 1	Gene 2	Combination
Physical Activity	−0.20	−0.30	**−0.45**
Sedentary Time	−0.17	−0.25	−0.29
Physical Activity and Sedentary Time	-	-	**−0.48**
Sleep Duration	−0.23	−0.11	−0.19

4 Discussion

Answers to the post-intervention questionnaires indicate overall acceptance regarding the individualized content provided by the GA. However, a statistically significant difference was found between message relevance and usefulness. Based on the answers to Q1 and Q2, the messages sent by the GA were regarded by the participants as more useful than relevant. This may rely on the fact that the messages were designed by healthcare professionals specifically for the SG intervention and thus inherited general usefulness to the health condition of the recipients. On the other hand, the message's inclusion in the SG content was defined by the GA. Despite its ability to recognize and promote relevant messages, a comparatively lower score on Q1 is to be expected, as one of the

GA's primary directives is the diversification of content. Both scores, though, indicate that the messages had a positive effect in the SG setting.

The negative correlations presented in Table 2 show GA's sensitivity to trends regarding lifestyle and self-health management habits captured by the platform's sensors. When users displayed high levels of physical activity, the frequency of related messages declined and vice versa. The fact that this same pattern was observed in every category, in some cases even with statistical significance, shows the general success of GA's functionality. The fitness functions managed to translate user trends into appropriate changes in gene weights, thus enabling the GA to perform the natural selection of the most suitable genes for its chromosomes. Furthermore, the GA avoided reaching very high values of negative correlations, which would be a sign of content saturation. The non-deterministic selection of content performed by the GA provided the ENDORSE recommendation system with the capability to occasionally omit certain categories with high weights in favor of others with lower. Such behavior highlights the difference between a rule-based system and the GA, in terms of providing varying personalized content.

Results from this preliminary analysis were collected within the pre-pilot phase of the ENDORSE project. The ENDORSE pilot studies, which feature a SG version with additional game missions and enhanced functionalities in the ENDORSE recommendation system, have been recently concluded. Analysis of the newly acquired data is expected to provide further insight regarding the GA's capabilities to produce individualized content.

5   Conclusion

In this study, we presented the integration of a novel GA-based PCG approach into the ENDORSE platform which harnesses the power of Artificial Intelligence, m-health and gamification mechanisms, towards implementing a multi-component intervention for the management of childhood obesity. The PCG approach automatically provides the platform with SG content and educational messages by collecting data from physical activity sensors and interaction with the SG. Post-intervention analysis revealed the potential of the proposed PCG methodology to adapt to user data and provide relevant content. The impact of the individualized content on the users will be analyzed in a future study.

Acknowledgments. This research was supported within the framework of the ENDORSE project, which is funded by the NSRF. Grant agreement: T1EΔK-03695.

References

1. Djaouti, D., Alvarez, J., Jessel, J.-P.: Classifying serious games: the G/P/S model. In: Handbook of Research on Improving Learning and Motivation Through Educational Games: Multidisciplinary Approaches. IGI global (2011)
2. Chow, C.Y., Riantiningtyas, R.R., Kanstrup, M.B., Papavasileiou, M., Liem, G.D., Olsen, A.: Can games change children's eating behaviour? A review of gamification and serious games. Food Qual. Prefer. **80**, 103823 (2020)

3. Mitsis, K., Zarkogianni, K., Dalakleidi, K., Mourkousis, G., Nikita, K.S.: Evaluation of a serious game promoting nutrition and food literacy: experiment design and preliminary results. In 2019 IEEE 19th International Conference on Bioinformatics and Bioengineering (BIBE) (2019)

4. Sterkenburg, P.S., Vacaru, V.S.: The effectiveness of a serious game to enhance empathy for care workers for people with disabilities: a parallel randomized controlled trial. Disabil. Health J. **11**(4), 576–582 (2018)

5. Lievense, P., Vacaru, V.S., Liber, J., Bonnet, M., Sterkenburg, P.S.: "Stop bullying now!" Investigating the effectiveness of a serious game for teachers in promoting autonomy-supporting strategies for disabled adults: a randomized controlled trial. Disabil. Health J. **12**(2), 310–317 (2019)

6. Orji, R., Vassileva, J., Mandryk, R.L.: Modeling the efficacy of persuasive strategies for different gamer types in serious games for health. User Model. User-Adap. Inter. **24**(5), 453–498 (2014). https://doi.org/10.1007/s11257-014-9149-8

7. Sajjadi, P., Ewais, A., De Troyer, O.: Individualization in serious games: a systematic review of the literature on the aspects of the players to adapt to. Entertain. Comput. **41**, 100468 (2022)

8. Togelius, J., Kastbjerg, E., Schedl, D., Yannakakis, G.N.: What is procedural content generation? Mario on the borderline. In Proceedings of the 2nd International Workshop on Procedural Content Generation in Games. Association for Computing Machinery, New York (2011)

9. Ahmad, S., Mehmood, F., Khan, F., Whangbo, T.K.: Architecting intelligent smart serious games for healthcare applications: a technical perspective. Sensors **22**(3), 810 (2022)

10. Mitsis, K., et al.: A multimodal approach for real time recognition of engagement towards adaptive serious games for health. Sensors **22**(7), 2472 (2022)

11. Pereira, Y.H., Ueda, R., Galhardi, L.B., Brancher, J.D.: Using procedural content generation for storytelling in a serious game called orange care. In: 2019 18th Brazilian Symposium on Computer Games and Digital Entertainment (SBGames) (2019)

12. Carlier, S., Van der Paelt, S., Ongenae, F., De Backere, F., De Turck, F.: Empowering children with ASD and their parents: design of a serious game for anxiety and stress reduction. Sensors **20**(4), 966 (2020)

13. Bermúdez i Badia, S., et al.: Toward emotionally adaptive virtual reality for mental health applications. IEEE J. Biomed. Health Inform. **23**(5), 1877–1887 (2019)

14. Esfahlani, S., Thompson, T.: Intelligent Physiotherapy through procedural content generation. In: Proceedings of the AAAI Conference on Artificial Intelligence and Interactive Digital Entertainment, vol. 12, no. 2, pp. 27–30 (2016)

15. Mitsis, K., Kalafatis, E., Zarkogianni, K., Mourkousis, G., Nikita, K.S.: Procedural content generation based on a genetic algorithm in a serious game for obstructive sleep apnea. In: 2020 IEEE Conference on Games (CoG) (2020)

16. Vasilakis, I.A., et al.: The ENDORSE Feasibility pilot trial: assessing the implementation of serious games strategy and artificial intelligence-based telemedicine in glycemic control improvement. In: Diabetes Technology & Therapeutics, vol. 24, MARY ANN LIEBERT (2022).

17. Dontje, M.L., de Groot, M., Lengton, R.R., van der Schans, C.P., Krijnen, W.P.: Measuring steps with the Fitbit activity tracker: an inter-device reliability study. J. Med. Eng. Technol. **39**(5), 286–290 (2015)

18. Shultz, S.P., Browning, R.C., Schutz, Y., Maffeis, C., Hills, A.P.: Childhood obesity and walking: guidelines and challenges. Int. J. Pediatr. Obes. **6**(5–6), 332–341 (2011)

19. Hirshkowitz, M., et al.: National Sleep Foundation's sleep time duration recommendations: methodology and results summary. Sleep Health **1**(1), 40–43 (2015)

Building Digital Health Systems to Support Treatment Administration: A Preliminary Case Study

Ana González Bermúdez[(✉)] and Ana M. Bernardos

Information Processing and Telecommunications Center, ETSI Telecomunicación, Universidad Politécnica de Madrid, Madrid, Spain
{ana.gonzalezb,anamaria.bernardos}@upm.es

Abstract. The emergence of Digital Health Systems (DHS) has had an impact on the understanding of the diagnosis, treatment and cure of diseases. In the case of chronic or long-term illnesses, these systems may improve the disease follow-up. However, these target scenarios also raise specific challenges. For example, due to the long-term nature of treatments, it may be harder for patients to maintain active use of the technology assets, being this aspect key to leverage DHS potential. From a review of the literature, this article analyzes the aspects surrounding patient adherence, to compile a concept model to drive DHS design. The concept model is applied over a DHS focused on patients under a specific health condition (kidney disease) that implies a long-term treatment (peritoneal dialysis). Under this treatment, clinical follow-up and medication adjustment require patients to track daily practical aspects and register health status, to dynamically manage daily life and disease. The availability of granular information also helps clinicians to optimize the judgement of treatment's effectiveness and counter effects. The result is a DHS that relies on a mobile application and a secure backend server accessible to the professionals in charge of patient management. It is focused on simplifying patient's data gathering, data continuity and completeness, and meaningful data retrieval and visualization for the parties involved (patient and clinician). The article explains the design process, with adherence in mind, and, as partial validation, an analysis of the user experience of four 'lead' users (volunteer patients and practitioners), with a review of the adherence results on the patients' side.

Keywords: Digital Health · Mobile Health · patient · application · adherence · usability · usefulness · abandonment

1 Introduction

The management of health conditions has changed with the emergence of digital health systems. Worldwide regulatory agencies are approving digital strategies to diagnose, monitor and support the treatment of diseases [1]. Digital Health Systems (DHS) are designed to improve consumer health and disease management through the use of digital

© ICST Institute for Computer Sciences, Social Informatics and Telecommunications Engineering 2023
Published by Springer Nature Switzerland AG 2023. All Rights Reserved
A. Cunha et al. (Eds.): MobiHealth 2022, LNICST 484, pp. 220–232, 2023.
https://doi.org/10.1007/978-3-031-32029-3_20

technologies. These tools have the potential to impact strongly on the management of chronic or long-term conditions, both for patients and clinicians. Chronic diseases are defined broadly as conditions that last several months (>3) or longer, and require ongoing medical attention or limit activities of daily living or both. Cancer, heart disease, stroke, diabetes, and arthritis are some of the most frequent chronic conditions.

To maximize the benefit of DHS, it is important to assess their impact, as well as the barriers and enablers to adoption. Over the last decade, research has tried to show the potential of digital healthcare systems. For example, a number of proposals, [2–7], focused on managing heart disease (arterial hypertension, cardiometabolic diseases, etc.) through sensors and apps tailored to incentivize behavioral change, compile different studies on how these technologies impact on patients' health status. These studies include traditional trials with control and intervention groups that shows the second group (the one using the application) overperforming the first one (with regular management) in terms of health outcomes.

This article explores how to design a DHS to provide a sound value proposition, both for patient and clinician, when managing a long-term condition. The main objective is to understand the specific needs that DHS for chronic disease management should tackle, to support patients in their treatment and practitioners in their follow-up and accompanying processes. Although DHS may be built on different tools, in this case we will center on DHS involving, in brief, a mobile application for the patient, a backend for data storage and processing, and a dashboard for the practitioners to access data. Then the mobile health (mHealth) component is a cornerstone of the system. The diversity of chronic conditions will undoubtedly modify the type of functionalities and goals that the DHS must address, but the objective includes abstracting and generalizing some main design guidelines that may be horizontally applicable.

The paper structure is as follows. First, in Sect. 2, gathers a review of key concepts, state of the art, and cause-effect elements related to adherence and mHealth systems, as patient-oriented mobile tools are the ones guaranteeing data input. On this analysis, we present a concept model to drive design of DHS and exemplify it through the system presented in Sect. 3, which is focused on peritoneal dialysis treatment management for kidney disease patients. This type of patient must record the volumes of infusions and drains they perform daily, apart from recording health indicators such as weight or blood pressure to manage e.g., food and liquid intakes. In Sect. 4, the proposed DHS has been built and validated with a small group of users. Being a preliminary work, Sect. 5 analyzes conclusions and further steps.

2   Understanding Adherence in mHealth

A key issue in mobile health is adherence to mobile applications enabling data gathering; the workings of Digital Health Systems assume that users will provide an adequate amount of data, that will be as recommended and intended by clinicians [8, 9]. If the application on the patient side does not collect the expected amount of data, the system will not achieve the optimal results. Obviously, adherence should not be the same on a stand-alone mHealth system (only relying on an app and an automated service) than on a system counting on clinicians' feedback on the other side. But trying to isolate the app from the rest of the system, in general, adherence can be understood because of perceived usefulness and usability. If the application causes fatigue, the user may be less eager to use it or even abandon it (therefore, improved usability is conceptually correlated to better adherence). Moreover, if the user perceives benefits from using an application (perceived usefulness), s/he will have an incentive not to abandon it. Ideally, it will also be an enabler to perceived usefulness: the user adheres to the app because s/he finds it useful, and the DHS can provide meaningful feedback and advanced features because complete personal data logs are available due to the regular app usage.

How to improve adherence to a health mobile app is still a challenge. Mobile health apps make use of a variety of design incentives to engage the user. Some of the main mechanisms are user status tracking and performance feedback [3, 4, 6, 10, 11]. Also, there are popular mechanisms to adhere users such as personalized goals set-up, reminders and prompts or gamification with rewards delivery, as it can be seen in [12–15]. Additionally, strategies aiming at behavior change, such as motivational messaging or social sharing functionalities are common [14, 15]. Table 1 summarizes the list of strategies/design features in literature that may be considered. The mechanisms from 1 to 4 are mainly related with adherence in its literature. On the other hand, from 5 to 17 are mainly related with usefulness, but most of these are also associated with adherence (e.g., community support, gamification or performance feedback) or usability (e.g., data personalization or connection to devices). The mechanisms more related with usability are 18–27 and these are rarely mentioned as such in the development of the applications, although they are present in almost all the proposals.

It is not just important to get to know the existing mechanisms, but also the way users rate them. As show at [12, 14, 15], the mechanisms most highly valued by patients are mainly monitoring, personalized goals set up, access to health information and notifications/reminders. On the other hand, the lowest rated mechanisms are rewards and social comparison (nevertheless, the prevalence of these techniques in this type of system is very common). In the next Section, we will organize mechanisms into an adherence concept model.

3   Adherence Concept Model to Build a Patient-Oriented App

As previously stated, adherence, usefulness and usability are closely related, impacting one over the others. We can assume that, to foster high adherence, the application on the patient side must be perceived as a valuable tool (being able to provide the promised benefits) effortless to use [16]. The same requirements can be posed for clinicians-oriented tools, as the DHS is at least a two-sided platform, but patients' data are key to activate the full system. So, the model next is focused on identifying key aspects when designing the patient app side of the DHS, which will oversee obtaining data from the user to provide the right service.

The adherence strategies compiled in Table 1 have been organized into four non-exclusive groups, depending on its objective:

O1) Incentivize Data Entry. In this group, we refer to all the strategies to get as many data as possible, such as notifications and reminders delivery (to remind of pending

Table 1. Adherence strategies considered in literature for mHealth.

ID	Strategy	Short description	Studies
1	Send personal data	Allow the sending of data related to the Patient's health status or experience with the application	[2–4, 6, 10–12, 14, 15]
2	Display personal data	Display simple views of collected patient data, allowing the patient to access them whenever s/he wants	[2–4, 6, 10–12]
3	Communication with the sanitary	To create a simple communication channel between the patient and the healthcare staff	[2, 6, 11, 13]
4	Reminders, notifications	Use of alerts to remind the patient to interact with the application, submit data, keep an appointment, etc.	[2–4, 11–13, 18]
5	Health information	Provide access to information about the targeted health problem that is useful to the patient	[2, 4, 6, 12, 14, 18]
6	Community support	Creation of channels of communication between patients to share experiences and support each other	[13–15]
7	Social comparison	Show data from other patients (with the possibility to establish a ranking) to motivate the user to improve	[4, 14, 15]
8	Personalized goals	The application or the user can set goals to be achieved with the intention of motivating the user	[3, 4, 12, 14, 15]

(*continued*)

Table 1. (*continued*)

ID	Strategy	Short description	Studies
9	Motivational messages	Texts aimed at encouraging the user to continue to improve and get involved in their health	[14, 18]
10	Gamification	Use of game elements to motivate and engage patients in health-related contexts	[12, 13]
11	Performance feedback	Provide patients feedback and data about their progress, to motivate to improve or to change behaviors	[3, 4, 10, 11, 13–15, 19]
12	Risk assessment	Establish indicators to measure and report on the patient's condition. Then, process the data collected to detect risk and alert the patient and practitioner	[2, 3, 7, 10, 11, 19]
13	Data personalization	To be able to adjust the data requested or displayed to users' preferences	[3, 7, 11, 14]
14	Emergency button	Button that allows the patient to call emergency services with a single click	[2]
15	Relaxation exercises	Used to enable the patient to assist in the process of lifestyle change	[14]
16	Export personal data	Option of downloading a document with the data history	[19]
17	Connection to devices	The application can be connected to a health measuring device for easy data collection	[2, 7, 10, 11]

(*continued*)

Table 1. (*continued*)

ID	Strategy	Short description	Studies
18	Minimalist design	Avoid displaying large information on the same screen, avoiding empty information and trying to avoid scrolling	[17]
19	Intuitive design	E.g., buttons that look like buttons, that the flow between windows is understood	[6, 17]
20	Coherent order	In a view it is recommended to order the displayed information from most to least important	[17]
21	Language adapted	Avoid technical terms, language adapted to all types of patients, using vocabulary that they understand. It is recommended to use the second person, to take a friendlier tone	[6, 17]
22	Clarity of instructions	Provide guidelines for using the application, in the form of an information menu and/or a video tutorial at the beginning of its use	[2, 3, 17]
23	Accelerators, shortcuts	Enable fast application interaction	[17]
24	Undo actions	For example, allow the user to delete data sent in case of a mistake	[17]
25	Error prevention	Try to prevent the user from making a mistake, for example by using confirmation messages to avoid pressing a button by accident	[17]

(*continued*)

Table 1. (*continued*)

ID	Strategy	Short description	Studies
26	Avoid free text entries	If used, given the option to delete everything with a single click	[17]
27	Appropriate colors	For example, excessive use of black tends to cause rejection, or the components shown should contrast with the background	[17]

tasks, to alert of inactivity or to directly request to send data) or connection to electronic measurement devices (thus, encouraging the user to retrieve data by simplifying the collection procedure). By collecting the maximum amount of user data, the system will be able to offer an optimal service. Regular and timeliness data collection is key to apply, in general, machine learning techniques that enable personalized models and detect anomalies or even predict risky states. When dealing with chronic conditions, these functionalities may be part of the value proposition of the DHS system.

O2) Facilitate the Application Use. We group together those strategies mainly related to enhance usability. In mHealth terms, usability refers to the effort required to use the application (greater usability also allows for greater perceived usefulness). Among others, we include traditional principles, such as using a simple language, tracking system status, avoiding errors and facilitate their management (indicating how to solve them, allowing undoing actions, etc.), quick interaction, minimalism or no empty information [17]. These mechanisms prevent user fatigue and the user from abandoning the application because it takes too much effort. Additionally, for long-term users, specific short cuts and customizable views may coexist with learnable functionalities.

O3) Extend Information. They are basically strategies related to enhance usefulness perception through information (e.g., displaying personal data or curated information about the disease) or to create a security context for the storage of their data and the way they are handled (e.g., allowing data export, risk assessment or communication with doctors). In the case of chronic conditions, the system should support reliable information retrieval in different stages of the disease evolution, from getting familiar to it, to learning to detect changes and risk, while also optimizing contact with practitioners.

O4) Support Behaviour Change. These are strategies which aim at changing the pattern of behaviour, such as: motivational messages, personalized targets, social comparison (encouraging healthy competition among users) or task reminder techniques. Achieving changes in self-behavior increases perceived usefulness of the technology. Chronic disease therapies may require specific training for patients, and interactive guidance to reach targets to improve their health condition.

As mentioned above, the identified objectives are not exclusive one against other, which means that, in many cases, each strategy is not only supporting a single objective. In most cases they can be related to two or more objectives, as shown in Fig. 1.

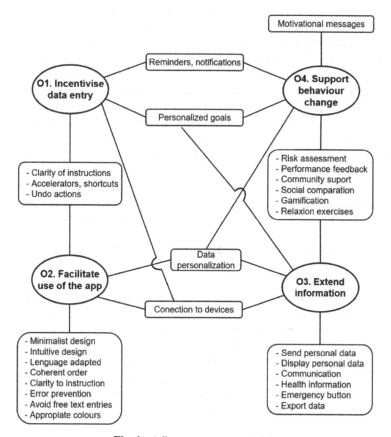

Fig. 1. Adherence concept model.

4   Preliminary Use Case: A DHS for Kidney Disease Patients

4.1   Design Stage

The concept model for adherence proposed in the previous section has been applied to build a DHS for patients with kidney failure following peritoneal dialysis. This dialysis is performed introducing a fluid into the peritoneal cavity through a catheter placed in the abdomen. To avoid the excess of fluids in the abdomen, patients need to carefully control the amount of fluid infused and drained throughout the day. Therefore, patients must record information about their treatment guidelines several times per day. Additionally, they must take note of some specific health status data, such as daily weight and blood pressure. This information is used by clinicians to adjust therapy, when necessary, e.g., due to hypertension or fluid retention issues. Many patients decide to use standard notes apps or traditional notebooks to track their evolution and to explain the records to their doctors at regular check-ups. So, the objective of the designed DHS is, initially, to facilitate treatment follow-up and health status awareness, while making it easier for the clinician to perform data-driven disease monitoring. In technical terms, the system has the following components: a mobile application, a backend server and two databases and a professional dashboard.

At the design stage, we aimed at understanding how patients performed data collection, what kind of language they used and what specific needs they had. To get better understanding on the disease and its management, we initially hold several conversations with clinicians. On these conversations, clinicians underlined that patients often adopt a very specific vocabulary to refer about their condition.

Prior to the DHS implementation, two volunteer patients under treatment were asked to complete a questionnaire to learn about their habits, and determine what needs they wanted to satisfy with the app. Their main concerns were forgetting to save data, losing data, saving data incorrectly and getting the wrong therapy (e.g., wrong time or dialysis fluid).

Thus, with this information, we used our concept model to better determine the DHS adherence strategies supporting patients' needs:

- The principal mechanism used to incentivize data entry (O1) would be notifications. Those are to be used to remind patients to send data and avoid inactivity. Patients also receive an alert for a new message from their doctor.
- To facilitate the use of the app (O2), we would try to embrace all the guidelines of the concept model: minimalist design (avoiding unnecessary information), coherent order (according to the most relevant data for the patient), language adapted to patients, intuitive, avoiding errors (using confirmation request to send data and indicating the type of error to help solve it), avoiding free text entries, reporting the status of the system (e.g., data saved correctly or loading), etc.
- Regarding extended information (O3), we would implement the capability of sending and displaying personal data (using simple and adapted questionaries, graphs, and tables), the capability to communicate with clinicians and the access to health information about peritoneal dialysis.
- To encourage behavioral change (O3, O4), we carried out a data analysis to obtain indicators of the patient's condition to report their evolution and to alert the doctor in case their therapy needs to be reviewed. The main calculations are the pressure variations or the total fluid in the abdomen variations.

We also followed an iteratively procedure to co-design the practitioner's dashboard.

4.2 Toward Validation: Some Early Usage Data

The developed system has been under validation during a short period of time, in two different stages. This validation should be considered preliminary due to the limited number of subjects involved, but it has enabled us to get some valuable feedback to determine next steps to take. In the first stage, the two volunteer patients and doctors were using the resulting DHS for a week time. Right after, they evaluated the usability and the usefulness of the functionalities under an adapted mHealth App Usability Questionnaire (MAUQ), from University of Pittsburgh [20, 21]. This questionnaire asks about how they feel about using the application, how challenging it is, if they would continue using it, or if they would recommend it. Overall, the scores for the 4 individuals were favorable, usability obtained on average 4.15/5 and functionalities obtained 4.625/5.

However, there were differences between clinicians and patients. The former's perceived usability scored on average 4.6, while the latter scored only 3.6. The main difference in the questionnaires is that patients rate the safety and reliability of the application lower. This may happen mainly because initially patients did not have the option of downloading the app from traditional app marketplaces. Additionally, patients complain about the inability to recover from certain errors, since the data sent cannot be modified. The following table shows the evaluation of the functionalities, distinguishing between patients (P1, P2) and doctors (D1, D2). As expected, users differ in their interests (Table 2).

Table 2. Surveys of functionalities.

Functionality	P1	P2	D1	D2
Save personal data	4	5	4	5
Display personal data	4	5	4	5
Therapy information	3	5	5	5
Communication from patient to doctor	5	5	5	5
Communication from doctor to patient	5	4	5	5
Notifications	5	5	4	4
Automatic filling of the data to be sent	4	5	5	5
Request sending confirmation	5	5	3	5

For both doctors, notifications are rated lower than other functionalities, while for patients it is one of the most highly rated mechanism for the application. The patient showing more criticism considers that displaying therapy guidelines is not that important, while both doctors (and the other patient) agree on its importance. We can also observe that one of the doctors (D1) does not perceive the usefulness of requesting confirmation on sending in the same way as the rest. These small discrepancies confirm the importance of considering both stakeholders (patients and clinicians) in the design of the system, as they may have different viewpoints over the same functionality.

After this initial pre-evaluation, certain styles were adjusted and new adherence strategies were included, such as the possibility of customizing personalized notifications. With this, a trial has been launched with 6 users, to carry out a more complete analysis of the benefits of the system. The information related to adherence collected during the trial from each user is shown in the following table (Table 3).

Table 3. Analysis of users indeed the trial.

Users	Total days	Active days	Dialysis days	General data	Msg to doctor	Msg to patient
U1	177	156	168	165	6	10
U2	115	115	117	266	3	3
U3	90	81	85	192	0	0
U4	82	82	85	111	1	1
U5	36	36	108	38	0	0
U6	25	16	17	18	0	1

As can be seen in the previous table, the levels of use of the application by patients are favorable. The average percentage of days those users have submitted data on their therapy is 90.36% (with a standard deviation of almost 14%). This shows that the patients of this small trial have been using the application almost constantly, which indicates very high levels of adherence. In contrast, it is observed that messaging is rarely used by almost any of them.

5   Conclusions

The concept model presented in the article is a summary of our experience when dealing with DHS patient adherence in a specific chronic condition, but it is still obviously a work in progress. The results obtained from the limited user trial show reasonable adherence, but the trial has an evident limitation in terms of scope, as few users have served as testers. In any case, the collaboration of lead users has made the system's design smoother. We are following compile some design guidelines that may be helpful for facing future designs:

1) Assuming a patient-centered design approach, that enable the designer to understand the management difference among patients' profiles (e.g., those that have been under treatment for a long time and those that are initiating it). We have concluded the importance of establishing a design procedure starting with the retrieval of relevant information about the patients' health situation and their specific data needs (e.g., type and frequency). Additionally, it is important to understand the current patient's practices, as it may be beneficial to mimic them and translate them into digital means, instead of creating a new methodology from scratch (e.g., for information logging). It is desirable to adapt language, vocabulary and even give specific customization mechanisms for patients, as patients on long-term treatments tend to develop their own terminology to refer to procedures, drugs and symptoms, and taking this into account in the app design can make it more friendly. Additionally, we have detected those patients on the same treatment can understand the application requests differently, thus it is crucial to support data gathering with accurate

and sufficient explanation. This information can disappear over time (or be hidden), together with newcomers training tips.

2) Devoting time to achieve a proper understanding of the disease evolution and its stages, in order to analyze the implication over the tools' features. The objective is to effectively translate this into dynamic application features both for the patient and the doctors.

3) Dynamic redesign with clinicians is needed to incrementally include tools that can get the most from the retrieved data taking their experience and practices as a base. For example, to make the dashboard acceptable for clinicians, it is helpful to conduct design reviews and consider their specific visualization requests and how to support them (e.g., data to show, key performance indicators, type of preferred visualization – tables vs. charts, risk detection, communication flow).

4) Analyze how the DHS is going to be integrated into the clinical pathway. This may lead to identify new administration features and user profiles. For example, in our case, the DHS enables asynchronous communication between patient and clinicians. This implies a dealing with the extra interaction in organizational terms.

5) The serious need of highly committed clinicians to promote the use of the service among their patients and colleagues. Clinicians' adherence is also important, as being a two-sided system, patients will only perceive full usefulness whether their health providers are paying attention to their data and requests and the communication is fluid.

A pending issue that we have not addressed in this version of the DHS is how to smooth or simplify data gathering by using connected sensors or even treatment machines data (e.g., in the case of ambulatory dialysis, the cyclers). Being desirable, the fragmented vendor ecosystem and the bundle with proprietary software platforms is always a hindrance. In any case, manual and continuous input of key data can increase patient awareness over the disease and health status, so it is important to find creative ways to leverage this continuous interaction. The DHS is a tool that may behave as an open window to the patient and the disease, so it may serve for multiple uses and evolve over time to provide support to the patient, always taking into consideration the preservation of data protection regulations.

Acknowledgment. Authors gratefully acknowledge the design feedback and participation on trials of volunteer clinicians and patients of Hospital 12 Octubre in Madrid, Spain, and sponsorship from REACT-CM MadridDataSpace4Pandemics Project and UPM Project RP180022025.

References

1. Pillay, R.: Digital Health Trends 2021: Innovation, Evidence, Regulation, and Adoption (2021)
2. Gong, K., et al.: Mobile health applications for the management of primary hypertension: a multicenter, randomized, controlled trial. Medicine (Baltimore) **99**, e19715 (2020)
3. Debon, R., et al.: Effects of using a mobile health application on the health conditions of patients with arterial hypertension: a pilot trial in the context of Brazil's Family Health Strategy. Sci. Rep. **10**, 6009 (2020)

232 A. G. Bermúdez and A. M. Bernardos

4. Paldán, K., et al.: Supervised exercise therapy using mobile health technology in patients with peripheral arterial disease: pilot randomized controlled trial. JMIR mHealth uHealth **9**, e24214 (2021)
5. Devi, B.R., et al.: MHealth: an updated systematic review with a focus on HIV/AIDS and tuberculosis long term management using mobile phones. Comput. Methods Programs Biomed. **122**, 257–265 (2015)
6. Wiljen, A., et al.: The development of an mHealth tool for children with long-term illness to enable person-centered communication: user-centered design approach. JMIR Pediatr. Parent. **5**, e30364 (2022)
7. Bonini, N., et al.: Mobile health technology in atrial fibrillation. Expert Rev. Med. Devices **19**, 327–340 (2022)
8. Kelders, S.M., Kok, R.N., Ossebaard, H.C., Van Gemert-Pijnen, J.E.W.C.: Persuasive system design does matter: a systematic review of adherence to web-based interventions. J. Med. Internet Res. **14**, e152 (2012)
9. Sieverink, F., Kelders, S.M., Gemert-Pijnen, V.: Clarifying the concept of adherence to eHealth technology: systematic review on when usage becomes adherence. J. Med. Internet Res. **19**, e402 (2017)
10. Wong, C.K., et al.: Artificial intelligence mobile health platform for early detection of COVID-19 in quarantine subjects using a wearable biosensor: protocol for a randomised controlled trial. BMJ Open (2020)
11. Johansson, L., Hagman, E., Danielsson, P.: A novel interactive mobile health support system for pediatric obesity treatment: a randomized controlled feasibility trial. BMC Pediatr. **20**, 1–11 (2020)
12. Murnane, E.L., Huffaker, D., Kossinets, G.: Mobile health apps: adoption, adherence, and abandonment. In: UbiComp ISWC 2015 (2015)
13. Amagai, S., Pila, S., Kaat, A.J., Nowinski, C.J., Gershon, R.C.: Challenges in participant engagement and retention using mobile health apps: literature review. J. Med. Internet Res. **24**, e35120 (2022)
14. Michie, S., Ashford, S., Sniehotta, F.F., Dombrowski, S.U., Bishop, A., French, D.P.: A refined taxonomy of behaviour change techniques to help people change their physical activity and healthy eating behaviours: the CALO-RE taxonomy. Psychol. Heal. **26**, 1479–1498 (2011)
15. Munson, S.A., Consolvo, S.: Exploring goal-setting, rewards, self-monitoring, and sharing to motivate physical activity. In: 2012 6th International Conference on Pervasive Computing Technologies for Healthcare (PervasiveHealth) and Workshops. PervasiveHealth (2012)
16. Deng, Z.: Understanding public users' adoption of mobile health service. Int. J. Mob. Commun. **11**, 351–373 (2013)
17. Nielsen, J.: Usability Heuristics (1995)
18. Carrasco-Hernandez, L., et al.: A mobile health solution complementing psychopharmacology-supported smoking cessation: randomized controlled trial. JMIR mHealth uHealth **8**, e17530 (2020)
19. World Health Organization: Monitoring and Evaluating Digital Health Interventions: A practical guide to conducting research and assessment (2016)
20. Zhou, L., Bao, J., Setiawan, I.M.A., Saptono, A., Parmanto, B.: The mHealth app usability questionnaire (MAUQ): development and validation study. JMIR mHealth uHealth **7**, e11500 (2019)
21. mHealth App Usability Questionnaire (MAUQ) for Standalone mHealth Apps Used by Patients. https://doi.org/10.2196/11500

eSleepApnea - A Tool to Aid the Detection of Sleep Apnea

Rui Alves[1(✉)], Paulo Matos[1,2], João Ascensão[1], and Diogo Camelo[1]

[1] Polytechnic Institute of Bragança, Bragança, Portugal
{rui.alves,pmatos}@ipb.pt, {a34505,a36739}@alunos.ipb.pt
[2] Research Centre in Digitalization and Intelligent Robotics (CeDRI),
Instituto Politécnico de Bragança, Campus de Santa Apolónia,
5300-253 Bragança, Portugal

Abstract. Nowadays, the appearance of chronic respiratory diseases is something increasingly common. A good example is sleep apnea, a respiratory disease characterized by recurrent episodes of pharyngeal collapse. It's a disease unknown by one part of the population, but when not controlled in time allows the emergence of other diseases. The complexity of symptoms, which are often diseases that arise as a consequence of apnea (e.g. arterial hypertension), makes its diagnosis difficult to be made, leading, in the long term, to a considerable reduction in the quality of life of patients. This paper presents an IoT solution for detecting sleep apnea signals, without the need to place auxiliary devices in the patient's body.

Keywords: Sleep Apnea · Sensors Network · Microwave Sensor · Arduino · IoT

1 Introduction

Identifying some of the key symptoms of the different pathologies (e.g., chest pain in cases of myocardial infarction) is often the key to the patient's full recovery because it enables medical help to be activated in a timely manner [1]. However, whether it's due to ignorance of the existence of various diseases [2] or because the symptoms do not affect the quality of life of patients, usually, medical help is only sought at a later stage of symptoms, delaying its diagnosis and leaving the chances of cure seriously compromised. However, for certain problems, such as sleep apnea, a full recovery is not always possible, but an early diagnosis greatly reduces its consequences.

Sleep apnea [3] is a respiratory sleep disorder described by momentary but frequent obstruction of the airways, causing total or partial interruptions in breathing. The total lack of knowledge of the disease and its long-term complications, associated with a lack of clear perception of interruptions in the respiratory flow by patients, leads to the diagnosis being confirmed long after the

This work has been supported by FCT - Fundação para a Ciência e Tecnologia within the Project Scope: UIDB/05757/2020.

A. Cunha et al. (Eds.): MobiHealth 2022, LNICST 484, pp. 233–240, 2023.
https://doi.org/10.1007/978-3-031-32029-3_21

occurrence of the first episodes of respiratory block, so that the consequences of the disease already affect the quality of life of patients.

Using a mobile application, the Microwave sensor for capturing breathing patterns, an Arduino MKR NB 1500 board for sending data to the cloud and a set of intelligent algorithms for detecting breathing stops in the received data, This article proposes a solution that will help in the identification of signs of sleep apnea without the need to place external devices in the patient's body. The remaining paper is organized as follows: Sect. 2 provides a brief description of sleep apnea; technical details of the proposed solution are described in Sect. 3; in Sect. 4 are presented the conclusions of the work and objectives for future work.

2   Sleep Apnea

Sleep apnea [4] is a pathology that causes momentary blockage of breathing during sleep, resulting mostly in snoring and constant daytime sleepiness. It can also cause symptoms [5] such as difficulty concentrating, headache, irritability, etc. Blockage phenomena occur due to a narrowing of the airways, in the region of the nose and throat, something that happens mainly deregulation in the activity of the muscles in the throat region, which may be excessively relaxed or narrowed during breathing. This deregulation often results from factors such as: the existence of a narrow throat, thick neck and round head, low levels of thyroid hormones (hypothyroidism), and in some cases, the history of stroke.

This pathology can be classified into 3 types [6]: obstructive sleep apnea - occurs most often, due to obstruction of the airways, caused by relaxation of the breathing muscles; central sleep apnea - arises after some pathology that causes a brain injury (ex: brain tumor, post-stroke) and changes the ability of the patient to regulate the respiratory effort during sleep; mixed apnea - is caused by the presence of both obstructive apnea and central apnea. In addition to these 3 types, in people with inflammation of the tonsils, tumor or polyps in the region, the appearance of temporary apnea is frequent.

Despite the characteristic symptoms of the disease, the definitive diagnosis of sleep apnea syndrome [7] is made with polysomnography, which is an examination that analyzes the quality of sleep, measuring brain waves, movements of breathing muscles, the amount of air that enters and leaves during breathing, in addition to the amount of oxygen in the blood. It is through this examination that it is possible to classify the severity of sleep apnea by counting the number of breath stops during sleep. When stops are less than 5 per hour, the test is considered normal, but depending on the number of stops per hour the severity varies between: mild (5 to 15), moderate (15 and 30) and severe (more than 30). In parallel, this examination also makes it possible to understand, if there is a predominance of apnea with position (Positional Sleep Apnea), what happens in many cases and can be improved simply by sleeping sideways. The performance of this examination can be done in the hospital or in an outpatient clinic, however, in any of the cases implies the placement of devices in the patient's body, which in situations where patients reject the presence of the disease can be complicated to perform.

Thus, the search for alternative means, such as that presented in this paper, that allow to identify signs of the disease without the need for the placement of auxiliary devices or a trip to the hospital, It can work as a first line of screening and as a counseling, for patients who reject the presence of the disease, to perform polysomnography for final confirmation of the diagnosis.

3   Proposal Solution

In Fig. 1 it's possible to observe the architecture of the proposed solution. Briefly, the solution is composed of two parts. The first part of the solution corresponds to the microwave sensor [8,9] and Arduino board, and is placed in the patient's home, while the second part corresponds to the services, stored in the cloud, that process the data coming from the sensors.

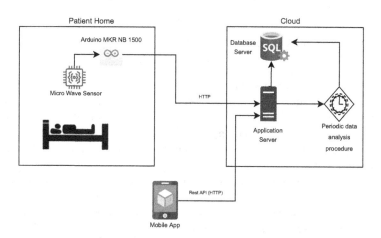

Fig. 1. Overview of proposal solution architecture.

In general, the functioning of the solution involves capturing the patient's breathing pattern. Captured data is sent to the cloud for processing and storage. The processing tasks of this data perform once a day, usually at the beginning of the day, where they try to obtain the number of anomalies in the breathing pattern of each patient. The results produced by the background tasks can be consulted by the doctor or caregiver of the patient, where it is possible to see the number of anomalies detected each night. In the following sections, each component of the solution will be detailed.

3.1   Microwave Sensor and Arduino

The Microwave Sensor is a sensor that uses high-frequency radio waves operating at 360°. The sensitivity in the change of reflected waves, makes the operation of these sensors very similar to that of radars. Continuous monitoring enables changes in return waves to be quickly identified.

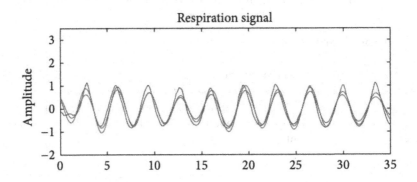

Fig. 2. Comparison of respiration belt signal versus Doppler Radar signal [10]

In Fig. 2, analyzing the red line, this represented a normal pattern of breathing captured by the microwave sensor. Analyzing the waves represented is possible to clearly identify the process of inhalation/expiration of air. The time of a respiratory arrest in cases of sleep apnea can vary between 10 s and 2 min, thus, the sensitivity that this sensor possessed, allows such stops to be identified in the data collected. In the proposed solution, this sensor, together with the Arduino, is positioned and centered with the patient's chest at a height of 90 cm. The frequency of sending data, which are sent using Narrowband-IoT (NB-IoT), is minute by minute and begin to be sent by Arduino to the cloud, from the time defined by care, as will be detailed in section refma. The use of NB-IoT is justified by the fact that there is no stable connection to the internet in the homes of users, and the simplicity in configuration that is, so that the solution works as expected is not necessary a connection to home networks. In addition, one of the key points of this technology is to enable the ease of connection that exists in smartphones can be used in the IoT world, namely ultra-low consumption communications, allowing to remove the need for battery recharges by its users. The selection of the Arduino MKR 1500 [11,12] is due to the fact that it is the first and only one of the Arduino family compatible with LTE Cat M1 and NB-IoT [13–15].

Listing 1.1. Example of JSON string sent by Arduino board to cloud

```
{
    "user_id":123,
    "data":[0,0,1,0,1,1,0,0,0,0,0,0,0,0,0,0,0,0,0,0,0,0,0,0,0,0,1,1,1,1],
    "timestamp": 1662887046
}
```

Another point that supports the use of NB-IoT is the size of the transmitted data. In the Listing 1.1, you can see the data frame that is sent to the Cloud. The field *user_id* represents the user identification and can be changed via mobile application. In the field *data* it is possible to analyze the data collected from the sensor, and represent the variation of the reflection waves of the previous 30 s. It is by processing the data in this field that background tasks (see Sect. 3.2) can detect possible stops. Finally, the *timestamp* represents the Unix time of the actual message sending.

3.2   Background Tasks

The background tasks are composed by two components:

- A model that is responsible to identify the number of respiratory arrests that a person has in a night of sleep.
- A process that is responsible for the diagnosis of people by analysing the values returned by the model.

For a model to be trained, a dataset is needed. But, since the authors of this paper didn't find a dataset that could be used to be applied to this solution, before this model can be trained, a dataset needs to be generated using the system of this solution. When the system of this solution generates enough data, a dataset will be built with data of people who have been diagnosis with sleep apnea and people who have not. With this dataset built, the model will be trained using this data to identify the number of respiratory arrests that a person has in a night of sleep. Then, the model will be fine-tuned and tested in order to increase the capacity of generalization and the accuracy rate of it. When the performance of this model is satisfactory, it will start to be used to process data generated by the system. The model will process this data, once per day, when everyone finishes this exam.

When the model [16] has just processed the data of all the people who took the examination in the current day, the process is called. Depending on the values returned by the model, the process will give a diagnosis of the people who took the examination in the current day. The result of the diagnosis can be positive mild, positive moderate, positive severe or negative. The process reaches these results using the algorithm that has been mentioned in the Sect. 2. When the number of respiratory arrests is less than 5 per hour, then the test is considered negative. If the number of respiratory arrests is more than 5, the test is considered positive, but depending on this value, the result can be a positive mild (5 to 15), positive moderate (15 and 30) and positive severe (more than 30).

When the results of the examinations of everyone are calculated, the resulted data is then saved on the database of the system. This will allow this data to be accessed by the mobile application.

3.3   Mobile Application

In Fig. 3 it is possible to analyze the layout of the built mobile application. This application has an important role in the built architecture, since, through it, caregivers/doctors can consult the results of the data processing from the sensors.

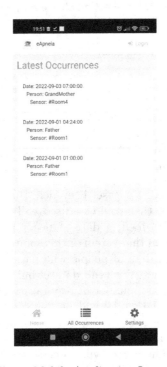

Fig. 3. Mobile Application Layout

Although it is not represented, the Arduino is connected to a BLE sensor [17], allowing care to change the time that the readings of the sensor values start. In addition, it is using the mobile application that it is possible to obtain the *user_id* field. This field is the serial number of Arduino and is necessary to then request the result of data processing to the existing restfull API [18]. This process is only performed once at the time of system configuration.

4   Conclusion

At the current stage, the solution is already at an advanced stage of development and testing. As mentioned, detection of sleep apnea is often a complicated process given the lack of perception of symptoms by patients. The simplicity of configuration, the need not to place devices external to the body of patients, makes the solution presented a solution with some potential to function as a first line of screening in the detection of sleep apnea. In addition, one of the secondary objectives of this solution is to make the results produced, only in cases where stops are detailed, lead the patient to do the diagnostic confirmation tests of apnea.

However, although the solution is well underway and necessary to recognize that there are several contexts that have not been validated. The initial context of tests, emphasizes on the assumption that the person under evaluation sleeps all night on his stomach, however, this assumption is not transversal to all people, but you can be cautioned in this solution by placing more microwave sensors to monitor other sleeping positions. Another context that has not been validated and in the opinion of the authors it is necessary to validate is the amount of bed linen that patients use daily, because this quantity can have a negative influence on the data produced by the sensors, making it difficult to detect respiratory stops.

4.1 Future Work

Despite the great potential, the solution still has a long way to go. The following points have been left for future work:

- Validate the solution built for scenarios where patients do not sleep on their stomach.
- Optimize the sending of data by Arduino, in order to ensure the best balance between the number of submissions and the captured information.
- Confirm the impact on data collection with the presence of large amounts of bed linen on the patient.
- Perform studies to understand the difference between the results produced by this solution and the diagnostic tests for sleep apnea (e.g. polysomnography).

References

1. Fang, J., Luncheon, C., Ayala, C., Odom, E., Loustalot, F.: Awareness of heart attack symptoms and response among adults - united states, 2008, 2014, and 2017. MMWR Morb. Mortal. Wkly Rep. **68**(5), 101–106 (2019)
2. Rosendal, M., Jarbøl, D.E., Pedersen, A.F., Andersen, R.S.: Multiple perspectives on symptom interpretation in primary care research. BMC Fam. Pract. **14**(1), 167 (2013)
3. Abbasi, A., et al.: A comprehensive review of obstructive sleep apnea. Sleep Sci. **14**(2), 142–154 (2021)
4. Javaheri, S., et al.: Sleep apnea: types, mechanisms, and clinical cardiovascular consequences. J. Am. Coll. Cardiol. **69**(7), 841–858 (2017)
5. Slowik, J.M., Sankari, A., Collen, J.F.: Obstructive sleep apnea. In: StatPearls [Internet]. StatPearls Publishing (2022)
6. Aldahasi, M.A., et al.: An overview on obstructive sleep apnea diagnosis and management in primary health care centre. J. Biochem. Technol. **11**(4), 93–97 (2020)

7. Foroughi, M., Razavi, H., Malekmohammad, M., Naghan, P.A., Jamaati, H.: Diagnosis of obstructive sleep apnea syndrome in adults: a brief review of existing data for practice in Iran. Tanaffos **15**(2), 70–74 (2016)

8. Microwave sensors- how do they work? https://www.ledlights4you.co.uk/microwave-sensors-how-do-they-work/. Accessed 05 June 2022

9. Microwave sensor vs pir sensor. https://www.martecaustralia.com.au/microwave-sensor-vs-pir-sensor/. Accessed 05 June 2022

10. Lee, Y.S., Pathirana, P.N., Evans, R.J., Steinfort, C.L.: Noncontact detection and analysis of respiratory function using microwave doppler radar. J. Sens. 2015, 548136 (2015)

11. Arduino MKR NB 1500. https://dev.telstra.com/iot-marketplace/arduino-mkr-nb-1500. Accessed 05 June 2022

12. MKR family. https://store.arduino.cc/arduino/mkr-family. Accessed 05 June 2022

13. GSA. Narrow band IoT & M2M - global narrowband IoT - LTE-M networks - March 2019. https://gsacom.com/paper/global-narrowband-iot-lte-m-networks-march-2019/. Accessed 01 Mar 2021

14. GSMA. Mobile IoT deployment map. https://www.gsma.com/iot/deployment-map/. Accessed 01 Mar 2021

15. GSMA. Security Features of LTE-M and NB-IoT Networks, 2019. https://www.gsma.com/iot/wp-content/uploads/2019/09/Security-Features-of-LTE-M-and-NB-IoT-Networks.pdf. Accessed 07 Mar 2021

16. Hands on signal processing with python. https://towardsdatascience.com/hands-on-signal-processing-with-python-9bda8aad39de. Accessed 05 June 2022

17. Nikodem, M., Slabicki, M., Bawiec, M.: Efficient communication scheme for Bluetooth low energy in large scale applications. Sensors **20**(21), 6371 (2020)

18. Payara platform community. https://www.payara.fish/products/payara-platform-community/. Accessed 08 May 2021

Exploring a Modular Approach for Deploying and Testing Cardiac Image Processing and Analysis Methods in the Clinical Workflow

João Abrantes[1], Nuno Almeida[1,2], and Samuel Silva[1,2]([✉])

[1] Institute for Electronics and Informatics Engineering of Aveiro (IEETA),
University of Aveiro, Aveiro, Portugal
`jgabrantes@ua.pt`
[2] Department of Electronic, Telecommunications, and Informatics (DETI),
University of Aveiro, Aveiro, Portugal
`{nunoalmeida,sss}@ua.pt`

Abstract. Cardiac health is a big concern, worldwide, with cardiovascular disease (CVD) being the most predominant cause of death, making early diagnosis a top priority in public health. The technology supporting the diagnosis of CVD, e.g., cardiac computerized tomography angiography (CTA), has been evolving at a fast pace providing a wide range of data on the anatomy and function of the heart. When developing novel processing and analysis methods to tackle this data, one important challenge concerns how to make them available for clinicians to test. The aim would be to enable full exploration of these methods in the clinical workflow, i.e., supporting all the standard image visualization and analysis features provided by clinical workstations, from early on, to foster insight over their features and usefulness to inform development. Additionally, with the advances of technology, mobile devices, beyond the traditional workstations, have gained importance, e.g., during consultation. However, they have limited processing resources. In this regard, this work explores a modular multiplatform solution to support the early deployment of cardiac analysis methods to the clinician's office. To this effect, we define the requirements for such a platform and present a first instance of its development exploring the Open Health Imaging Foundation resources. At its current stage, we demonstrate the feasibility of the approach and the integration of simple image processing modules in the pipeline.

Keywords: image processing and analysis · modular software architecture · multiplatform approaches · cardiac CT angiography

1 Introduction

According to the World Health Organization, cardiovascular diseases (CVDs) are the cause of death for an estimated 17.9 million people, every year, representing

A. Cunha et al. (Eds.): MobiHealth 2022, LNICST 484, pp. 241–254, 2023.
https://doi.org/10.1007/978-3-031-32029-3_22

32% of all deaths worldwide [19]. In this regard, it is important to continuously improve the capabilities of clinical diagnosis [11,14–16] since the detection of CVDs at an early stage grants a higher rate of success on treatment and cure of a cardiac patient. With the technological advances seen in recent years there was a significant improvement in medical imaging and software assisted diagnostic solutions, making them more precise, efficient, and increasingly noninvasive. In cardiac health specifically, these improvements lead to the capability of analyzing three dimensional images of the whole heart and even to simulate reconstructive and invasive procedures based on computerized tomography (CT) and magnetic resonance imaging (MRI) data. From the cardiac diagnosis perspective, important advances also entail the ability to acquire these images over time, providing data that can be used to analyze cardiac function, e.g., to assess the left ventricle movement and contractility.

The sheer amount of data provided by the imaging technologies and their complexity, along with the need to increasingly move into a quantitative framework supporting diagnosis, makes computer assisted diagnosis (CAD) tools a requirement [9]. In this regard, a strong body of work exists regarding the research of more advanced diagnosis methods, addressing ways to improve the data that is made available to clinicians, e.g., summarizing and characterizing, in a quantitative manner (e.g., calcium scoring [8]) cardiac function. However, the path for their validation and deployment faces some challenges. First of all, cardiac CT exams entail a considerable volume of data (approx. 1.5 GB), resulting in processing and analysis methods that require a fair amount of computational resources and, second, the proposed approaches are not easily deployed to be tested by the clinicians due to the fact that the existing cardiac workstations (mostly proprietary) do not allow enough versatility for integrating these new solutions. These aspects work as barriers for a more thorough assessment and exploration by clinicians for several reasons: (a) the developers often need to create a base platform that provides the full set of basic features to manipulate and visualize the imaging data, aligned with the current standard clinical workflow, so that they can be used by the clinicians profiting from their familiarity and training in using other tools; (b) obtaining feedback from clinicians is possible, but made harder and less informing, given that these novel systems are not integrated in their workflow, which entails a limited amount of data considered for testing and less space to freely explore the available features in novel ways; (c) even if a new workstation is placed at the cardiac service, adding and updating the available features to keep up with development is troublesome, particularly if it entails doing it locally, each time; and (d) mobile platforms have gained space in the clinical setting, given their portability, e.g., to bring into consultation with a colleague or to check exams while with a patient – which can boost the discussion around new methods—, but the current setting for cardiac analysis is limited to workstations and, given the complexity of the data, is computationally intensive, not making it compatible with a mobile approach.

thesIn the scope of improving CAD tools for cardiac diagnosis based on CT imaging of the heart, our team is proposing novel ways to assess coronary artery function through numerical simulations. In this context, and considering the challenges identified above, the work presented here starts by identifying major requirements to address them and explores the feasibility of a modular solution for clinical CT imaging processing that could serve the design and test of these novel methods. This should provide the grounds that both facilitate their deployment and exploration by the clinicians towards a more adequate setting to profit from their insights.

The remainder of this document presents the conceptualization of the required solution, in Sect. 2, resulting in the requirements that guide the design and development decisions. Then, Sect. 4 presents an overview of the current stage of the work describing a first proof of concept of our proposal built around the Open Health Image Foundation (OHIF) resources. Finally, some conclusions are presented, in Sect. 5, along with some routes for further work.

2   Background

In this section we start by briefly establishing the context for our work, particularly regarding the needs for the clinical side, and shortly overview common toolkits supporting the development of novel methods for image processing, analysis, and visualization. These help establish the overall scenario for the envisaged platform and define a first set of requirements guiding development.

2.1   Clinical Context

As computed tomography imaging evolved, two imaging protocols emerged for cardiac diagnosis: Coronary computed tomography angiography (CCTA) and Myocardial CT Perfusion (CTP). Coronary computed tomography angiography images the coronary arteries and allows evaluating the presence and severity of cardiac artery disease (CAD) by allowing the inspection to detect if plaque buildup has narrowed the coronary arteries. CCTA is performed by injecting contrast in the blood vessels and the image can be acquired throughout the cardiac cycle [1,4,7] using an acquisition technique that trigger scans during a specific interval of the cardiac cycle which provides higher-quality scans with no pulsation artifacts (ECG gated Angiography). Although CCTA can rule out the presence of obstructive CAD with a high degree of certainty, the morphologic information provided by this technique is still not sufficient to determine the downstream functional consequences of a given coronary lesion. The technological development in CT lead to the possibility to perform stress myocardial perfusion to evaluate coronary artery disease, providing not only anatomical information, but also covering the functionality of heart's stenosis [2,17]. Myocardial perfusion is based on the distribution of the iodinated contrast injected in the patient, during its first pass in the myocardium. The hypoattenuating areas containing less contrast material will determine myocardial perfusion defects [18]. The goal of Perfusion CT is to reconstruct and display the myocardium of the left ventricle as a volumetric perfusion map by enabling quantitative measures of myocardial perfusion as attenuation of this region over time [6]. A number of requirements have to be fulfilled for these techniques to work as intended, after the acquisition of a CT exam, the image dataset needs to be reconstructed, processed and prepared for the following diagnosis process. In CCTA multiple reconstruction parameters will dictate the quality of the reconstructed axial image. For post-processing CCTA uses different methods as: curved multiplanar reformats, shaded-surface display (SSD), maximum intensity projection (MIP), and volume rendering [12].

With any of these types of exams there are a few steps and tools that compose a common workflow of the clinicians while exploring them to gather information supporting the diagnosis, as depicted in the diagram of Fig. 1. Data is acquired from the CT exam and is automatically sent to the PACS server, which is connected to a viewer where a clinician can browse the patients and associated studies. By selecting one study, the viewer will load the CT image from the PACS server. Then, the clinician adjusts the viewing configuration to position the different viewing planes to obtain the best possible orientation to examine, for example, the left ventricle. To improve viewing, the way the pixels are displayed can be adjusted to enhance ranges of intensity. At this point, the clinician can take measures of particular structures of interest or apply any processing to extract notable information, e.g., computing the amount of blood inside the left ventricle, over time.

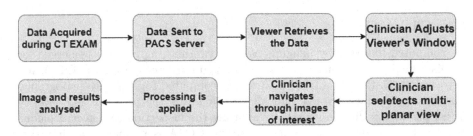

Fig. 1. Overall steps taken by a clinician to access and examine a cardiac CT exam and gather information to support diagnosis.

By analyzing the overall depiction of the clinician's workflow, when working with the cardiac images, it is relevant to note that there are several features to adjust the viewing for the intended diagnosis goals and image type that need to be present. These are important because they allow setting optimal viewing conditions for the anatomy of interest and according to the clinician's preference for interpreting the data. Being able to set particular conditions for visualization of the anatomy is paramount to harness the clinician's experience and reach views that are comparable with, e.g., other cases, and abide, for instance, to recommended practice. Therefore, to bring novel processing and analysis methods into the clinician's workflow, it is vital to ensure all the steps that precede their application and allow proper visualization and analysis of the outcomes.

While the existing workstations, at the clinical setting, provide these tools (e.g., syngo.CT[1]), they are mostly proprietary and integration of novel processing and analysis methods is not possible or in a very limited manner. Additionally, mobile devices, such as tablets, have gained prominence, in the clinical setting, and being able to provide at least a simplified version of the workflow in these devices, e.g., to support bedside consultation can expand its usage scope. Therefore, having a platform that could ensure the required workflow for different platforms and devices, and an easy integration and evolution of novel processing and analysis methods is a key resource to advance research in this topic.

2.2   Tools for Medical Image Processing and Visualization

There is a great volume of tools and packages commonly used by researchers to develop novel methods to visualize, process, and analyze medical images for a wide range of applications [10]. There are powerful tools such like OpenCV[2] and ITK[3] that offer a range of features for image manipulation, processing and analysis. Other tools offer useful solutions for image visualization such as VTK, Cornerstone, SCIRun and Volview. Additionally there are more complex tools such as MevisLab[4] or even Matlab that provide a mixture of features from simple image manipulation up to powerful processing solutions for data and information visualization. This reflects different architectures, approaches, and languages that are quite suitable for fast prototyping of novel methods, but this heterogeneity creates a challenge on how to integrate solutions by there tools into the same platform. This is one additional reason for our aim for modularity as explained in the next sections.

3   Conceptual Vision and Requirements

The end goal for the development of this software is to support not only current imaging-based diagnosis methodologies but, most importantly, to integrate the features that support the test of new ones. In our envisaged scenario (see Fig. 2 for an illustrative diagram), researchers are developing new tools to support diagnosis, at their lab, and using a small set of anonymous imaging data for testing. When the methods reach a stage where a number of features is already usable, the researchers decide that they require the methods to be tested and validated by clinicians to inform further development. At this time, the researchers make the method available in the platform.

At the cardiology service, a clinician loads a recent CCTA exam from the PACS server and uses the newly deployed method to analyze the data, e.g., to extract the coronary arteries. This can be performed both at a workstation or while using a tablet, e.g., to check some detail about a particular patient when discussing the case with a colleague.

---

[1] syngo.CT.
[2] OpenCV: https://opencv.org/.
[3] ITK: https://itk.org/.
[4] MevisLab: https://www.mevislab.de/.

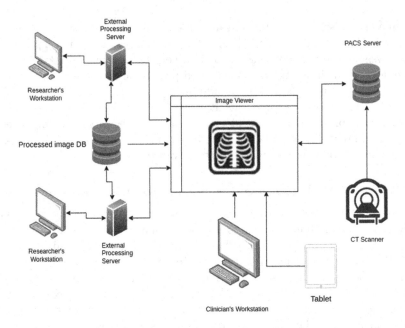

Fig. 2. Diagram depicting the overall scenario envisaged for supporting a faster translation from research to the clinical office supporting a faster cycle for exploration and test of novel processing, analysis, and visualization methods.

3.1   Requirements

To support the vision described above and depicted in Fig. 2, it is important that the proposed platform provides the clinician with a set of tools that are common to the cardiac workflow (see Table 1). It needs to include: (a) access to a DICOM Image Archive to retrieve patient's data and images; and (b) a user interface that will combine a number of essential features, e.g., Image Visualizer (the canvas itself) , window level adjustment, viewer layout customization (where images can be displayed in different quadrants of the canvas, aimed to display different image planes). Overall, it is important to note that the researchers will profit from all the requirements identified for the clinician side, since it will also provide them with ways of testing their methods inserted into the clinicians' workflow. Additionally, from the researchers' perspective, the platform needs to enable using different tools for developing novel methods and fast ways to deploy and update these methods.

Since one major goal for the platform is to be extensible and dynamic, having a modular approach is paramount since each component can be developed independently. This is a major concern, because it grants a higher consistency to the application, since changing or updating one feature will not modify the system as a whole. If a new processing methodology is needed or was developed and it needs to be tested, it can be easily added to the features by creating a new service or modifying an existing one without major compromises with the whole

Table 1. Overview of main requirements considering the perspective of the researcher and clinician for the envisaged system.

Researcher-side	Clinician-side
	DICOM data Retrieval
Fast Image Data Retrieval and Sending	Multi-planar View
Agile deployment of new processing functions	Viewer Layout customization
	Measurement tools
Abstraction from the viewer complexity	Window levels adjustment
Technological independence from the remaining components	Annotation tools
	Study and Series Browser and Lister
	DICOM Metadata access

project. It was also deemed important to prioritize open-source solutions when choosing an approach. Within the scientific research context, it is important that there is transparency with the process of result acquisition – as opposed to a black box solutions –, since it grants the possibility to critically analyze the results and reproduce them, something that is hampered when the source code is not available [5]. Furthermore, modularity should also consider an approach that enables their remote execution, e.g., in a remote server, instead of needing to run locally. This is important to enable using the system in devices with less computational resources, e.g., tablets, by offloading the processing operations.

4 Design and Development

Based on the modularity aspect required it was decided to explore a Micro-Kernel or Micro-Service Software architecture, where each component is independent of each other and inter-operate through an API or having a core system where each component acts as a plugin. The data storage service should work independently of the viewer, and more complex processing operations should be hosted in external services, removing any limitation in the language and framework that the image viewer might impose, making it possible for someone to develop new processing units without needing to know how the core system works, creating an abstraction layer from this service to the core system. Based on the requirements previously listed our system will consist of a PACS Server, a DICOM Image Viewer and one or more image processing services.

We decided on starting with the Image Viewer, since it will be the central component of the platform. It is the viewer which loads images from the PACS, provides access to the basic imaging manipulation tools, and where the most complex imaging processing features will be triggered. In this regard, we endured some research on current existing open-source image viewers.

4.1   Selection of Image Viewer Core Framework

Based on the conceptualized approach and requirements, the literature was surveyed regarding existing solutions that could serve as the core framework for our work. While a few exist, e.g., PostDicom[5], Horos[6], MANGO[7], and DICOM Web Viewer[8], two deserved particular attention for their considerable range of features and were tested more thoroughly.

Weasis. The first open source project that was taken in consideration was Weasis [13]. It is a standalone and web-based DICOM viewer with a modular architecture based on OSGI (Java). It is multi-languague and has a flexible integration with various imaging information systems as PACS, RIS (Radiological Information System), PHR (Personal Health Record) and HIS (Hospital Information System). This viewer allows high-rendering with OpenCV library. Its architecture is based on plugins which are organized in Plugin Type bundles and are in the form of Maven Archetypes. However, since this project has little code-level documentation and is organized as a Java Enterprise project it was found to have a steep learning curve to start developing for it, making it an unrealistic solution for the time constraints of this project.

OHIF. The second open source viewer that was considered was OHIF [3] an open source, web-based, medical imaging platform running as a node.js application. Originally build for radiology it is designed to load large volumes of data in a short period of time, retrieving metadata and pixel data ahead of time. It uses cornerstone.js, a Javascript library for visualization of medical images in web browsers that support the HTML5 for rendering, decoding and annotation of medical images. Works out-of-the-box with Image Archives that support DICOMWeb (DICOM Standard for web-based medical imaging using RESTful services). Provides a plugin framework for creating task-based workflow modes which can re-use the core functionalities. This web-based software includes an extensible user interface (UI) containing various components available in a reusable component library built with React.js and Tailwind CSS. OHIF is currently at its third version OHIF-v3 with which is the current stable version, however since version 3 still lacks a multi-dimensional image handler, it was decided to move to the previous version 2 which includes certain frameworks not yet implemented in version 3. We have found this solution more adequate for the needs of this project, it has an extensive documentation, and several guidelines on the development process. It is a fully web-based application, with an active open-source development community with new features and extensions in sight to be released, and built to be extendable, adaptable and customizable for different workflows and scenarios. With that in mind, OHIF would be our

---

[5] PostDICOM: https://www.postdicom.com/.

[6] Horos: https://horosproject.org/.

[7] Mango: https://ric.uthscsa.edu/mango/.

[8] Dicom Web Viewer: https://ivmartel.github.io/dwv/.

viewer component that will then be extended with the features required to integrate with external processing and analysis methods. In light of our choice, it is important to understand how OHIF is structured. To this effect, a synthesis of its main architectural aspects is covered in what follows.

4.2 OHIF Architecture

The OHIF project [3] is maintained as a mono-repo, mainly divided in two directories, with /platform containing the business logic, component, and application libraries that, combined, make this medical viewer and the/extensions directory containing different packages that can be registered in the core of the application at the/platform directory by an Extension Manager module. The business logic consists of pre-packaged features that are common to different medical image Viewers needs as Hotkeys, DICOM Web requests, hanging protocols, managing study's measurements and metadata and many more while being decoupled from any view library and rendering logic. It uses React as the front-end framework but it can be used with any other front-end frameworks. The extension layer serves as the ohif instance specification where the needed functionalities for specific uses, ui components and new behaviors are located. This layer allows to wrap and integrate functionalities of 3rd party dependencies in a reusable way, to change how application data is mapped and transformed, to display a consistent/cohesive UI and to inject custom components to override build-in components. Several extensions are already maintained by the Viewer itself i.e.. Cornerstone.js[9], a JavaScript library for displaying medical images in modern web browsers and VTK.js, another browser-based medical image framework which supports 3D Images and advanced renderings like multi-planar reconstruction.

4.3 Overall System Architecture

Figure 3 depicts the overall components of the architecture devised for the platform. At its core, it has the OHIF viewer. Since OHIF has a flexible policy with which data archive to choose to inter-operate with. Any data archive can be integrated with the viewer. As a PACS solution, we adopt the dcm4chee-arc-lite DICOM archive running in a Docker container connected to the node.js application of the viewer. For managing the integration of external processing methods from custom image processing servers, represented in Fig. 3, and without loss of generality, by a Flask[10] server, two OHIF extensions are added to the OHIF viewer for the communication with the server. Extensions in OHIF are the considered "plug-ins" in this project's context. The *Data Selector and Sender* extension module filters data from the retrieved DICOM data, transforms it in a way to be sent to the image processing server with a POST Request (via XmlHttprRequest). The *DisplaySet Builder* module is responsible for taking the

---

[9] Cornerstone.js: https://www.cornerstonejs.org/.

[10] Flask: https://flask.palletsprojects.com/en/2.2.x/.

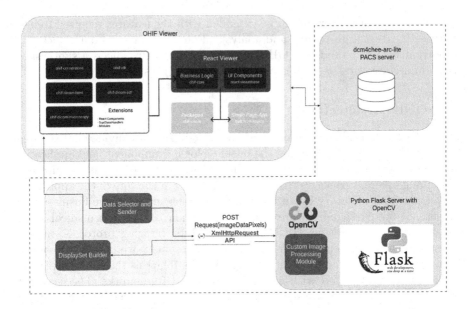

Fig. 3. Overall System Architecture. Adopting OHIF at its core, several components are considered to extend functionality towards the desired requirements. The components inside the dashed region result from the proposals in this work.

processing outcome of the external method and making it available for inspection, on the viewer. Those two modules are triggered by a new button added in the Viewer's toolbar.

4.4   Proof-of-Concept Instantiation

To test the current stage of the proof of concept we adopted a simple use case entailing opening a CT exam from a PACS server, applying a Gaussian smoothing using a method deployed in the cloud and visualizing the outcomes of this processing back in the image viewer. This would allow demonstrating the feasibility of our proposal by instantiating it for a particular purpose. In what follows we provide a brief description of the concrete roles played by each of the contributed modules in this use case scenario.

PACS Server. As said before, Dcm4chee Dicom was the chosen DICOM archive. It was easily integrated with OHIF since there is already a DICOM Query retrieval component which was configured to point to the new image archive. From that step on, it was then possible to browse patients and their studies stored at the PACS server.

Data Selector and Sender retrieves the pixel data of the current image by using the image loader provided by the cornerstone.js extension CornerstoneWadoImageLoader, which loads an image object using its imageID URL scheme. At its current stage of development, OHIF supports reading 3D exams, but an iteration through the slices of the CT exam is needed to load the full volume and populate a three-dimensional array with the data loaded by *cornerstone*. Having a three-dimensional structure with the pixel data of the volume, this module serializes it to a JSON object and sends it to the processing server via XmlHttpRequest.

DisplaySet Builder is responsible for the deserialization of data received from the processing server and loading the data to a three-dimensional structure which will feed a new ImageSet, the object responsible for organizing images in its respective series, listing them in the study list, and making them available for visualization in the image viewer.

Image Processing Method. As depicted in the architecture diagram, in Fig. 3, we adopted a Flask Server and developed a small Python script that uses openCV to apply a Gaussian smoothing filter. The server receives a POST request sent by the Data Selector and Sender module, loads the JSON object and consumes a *numpy* array with the data which will then be processed by a Gaussian filter implemented in OpenCV. After the processing is done, the processed array is serialized and sent back to the viewer as the POST response.

Overall Viewer Interface. Figure 4 shows different screenshots of the user interface from the listing of exams available at the PACS server, the overall disposition of elements on screen, multiplanar views and, in the last row, a sample image slice before and after the application of Gaussian smoothing – by integration with our custom module—to illustrate the successful implementation of the processing pipeline.

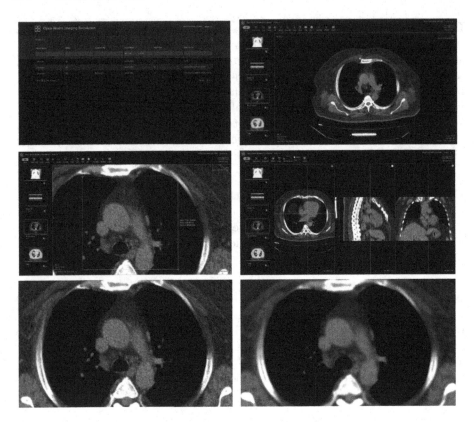

Fig. 4. Representative examples of the current state of the graphical user interface showing, from left to right, and top to bottom: (a) list of exams retrieved from the PACS server; (b) exam slice visualization; (c) region of interest selection; (d) orthogonal planes view; and (e) and (f) a detailed view of an exam before and after being smoothed through the implemented modules.

5   Conclusions

In light of challenges identified for improving how research on novel methods for cardiac analysis from CT can be deployed for evaluation and testing, in clinical environments, we identify a set of requirements that should contribute to address these challenges. The work presented here demonstrates the suitability of our proposal to support the application and development of novel diagnosis techniques for Cardiac CT, offering a modular solution for clinical analysis and at the same time being a shared environment between the researcher and the clinician. To this effect, we show that it is possible to profit on the OHIF resources and develop custom modules to integrate processing features into the viewer. In this regard, the researcher has a layer of abstraction from the core system not limiting the technologies and frameworks used for development and, as so, skipping completely any stage of adaption or learning curve of the system that would be involved. From the clinician perspective, while our proof-of-concept can still evolve, a basic set of common tools is already showcased and should provide the grounds for addressing their common workflow while dealing with cardiac CT. The devised approach can be accessed through any device or platform and its modular nature allows offloading the computationally intensive processing to the cloud, enabling the use of smaller devices, such as tablets.

The current stage of our proof-of-concept opens routes for several advances in two main fronts. The chosen core framework, the OHIF viewer, is in constant development with many new features on the horizon to be released, such as segmentation support, DICOM image upload to PACS and MPR view with the integration of Cornerstone3D.js. Since our approach involved proposing extensions to the OHIF framework, and no core code has been touched, we can easily profit from its evolution.

Additionally, this proof-of-concept opens routes for further exploring the development and integration of new functionalities, the most prominent being: (a) the integration of (semi-)automated segmentation of the left ventricle, a central anatomical landmark for the processing and analysis of these exams; (b) a multi-profile feature so that different clinicians can access a varying set of functionalities of the viewer depending, for instance, on the device (e.g., less features on a tablet); and (c) deal with processing outputs that are not an image volume (as in our use case), e.g., a polygonal mesh generated from an image.

Acknowledgements. This research is supported by National Funds, through FCT, in the scope of project CAD-FACTS (PTDC/EMD-EMD/0980/2020) and by IEETA - Institute of Electronics and Informatics Engineering of Aveiro Research Unit funding (UIDB/00127/2020).

References

1. Chang, H.J., et al.: Selective referral using CCTA versus direct referral for individuals referred to invasive coronary angiography for suspected CAD: a randomized, controlled, open-label trial. JACC: Cardiovasc. Imaging **12**(7 Part 2), 1303–1312 (2019)
2. Danad, I., Szymonifka, J., Schulman-Marcus, J., Min, J.K.: Static and dynamic assessment of myocardial perfusion by computed tomography. Eur. Heart J. - Cardiovasc. Imaging **17**(8), 836–844 (2016). https://doi.org/10.1093/ehjci/jew044
3. Erik Z., et al.: Open health imaging foundation viewer: an extensible open-source framework for building web-based imaging applications to support cancer research. JCO Clin. Cancer Inf. **4**, 336-345. https://doi.org/10.1200/CCI.19.00131. https://github.com/OHIF/Viewers
4. Hoffmann, U., Ferencik, M., Cury, R.C., Pena, A.J.: Coronary CT angiography
5. Ince, D.C., Hatton, L., Graham-Cumming, J.: The case for open computer programs. Nature **482**(7386), 485–488 (2012)
6. Nieman, K., Balla, S.: Dynamic CT myocardial perfusion imaging
7. Marano, R., et al.: CCTA in the diagnosis of coronary artery disease. Radiol. Med. (Torino) **125**(11), 1102–1113 (2020)
8. Mu, D., et al.: Calcium scoring at coronary CT angiography using deep learning. Radiology **302**(2), 309–316 (2022)

9. Noack, P., Jang, K.H., Moore, J.A., Goldberg, R., Poon, M., et al.: Computer-aided analysis of 64-and 320-slice coronary computed tomography angiography: a comparison with expert human interpretation. Int. J. Cardiovasc. Imaging **34**(9), 1473–1483 (2018)

10. Nolden, M., et al.: The medical imaging interaction toolkit: challenges and advances. Int. J. Comput. Assist. Radiol. Surg. **8**(4), 607–620 (2013)

11. Nowbar, A.N., Gitto, M., Howard, J.P., Francis, D.P., Al-Lamee, R.: Mortality from ischemic heart disease: analysis of data from the world health organization and coronary artery disease risk factors from NCD risk factor collaboration. Circ.: Cardiovasc. Qual. Outcomes **12**(6), e005375 (2019)

12. Rankin, S.: CT angiography. Eur. Radiol. **9**(2), 297–310 (1999)

13. Roduit, N.: Weasis medical viewer : Weasis documentation (2021). https://nroduit.github.io/en/

14. Roth, G.A., Mensah, G.A., et al.: Global burden of cardiovascular diseases and risk factors, 1990–2013;2019. J. Am. Coll. Cardiol. **76**(25), 2982–3021 (2020). https://doi.org/10.1016/j.jacc.2020.11.010

15. Sun, W., Zhang, P., Wang, Z., Li, D.: Prediction of cardiovascular diseases based on machine learning. ASP Trans. Internet Things **1**(1), 30–35 (2021)

16. Tzoulaki, I., Elliott, P., Kontis, V., Ezzati, M.: Worldwide exposures to cardiovascular risk factors and associated health effects: current knowledge and data gaps. Circulation **133**(23), 2314–2333 (2016)

17. Van Assen, M., et al.: Prognostic value of CT myocardial perfusion imaging and CT-derived fractional flow reserve for major adverse cardiac events in patients with coronary artery disease. J. Cardiovasc. Comput. Tomogr. **13**(3), 26–33 (2019)

18. Varga-Szemes, A., Meinel, F.G., Cecco, C.N.D., Fuller, S.R., Bayer, R.R., Schoepf, U.J.: CT myocardial perfusion imaging. Am. J. Roentgenol. **204**(3), 487–497 (2015). https://doi.org/10.2214/ajr.14.13546

19. World-Health-Organization: Cardiovascular diseases (CVDs) (2021). www.who.int/news-room/fact-sheets/detail/cardiovascular-diseases-(cvds)

Getting Contact to Elderly Associates Through the ICT: An Exploratory Study

Guilherme Martins[1]([✉]) [iD], Violeta Carvalho[1,2,3] [iD], Carlota Afecto[1] [iD],
Senhorinha Teixeira[1] [iD], and Cristina S. Rodrigues[1] [iD]

[1] Algoritmi, Minho University, Guimarães, Portugal
`guissmartins.work@gmail.com`, `violeta.carvalho@dps.uminho.pt`
[2] MEtRICs, Minho University, Guimarães, Portugal
[3] CMEMS, Minho University, Guimarães, Portugal

Abstract. Information and Communication Technologies - ICT has become a crucial element in the daily life of modern societies. Nevertheless, the elderly population does not follow the evolution of this new digitized world at the same pace. Thus, is necessary to ICT answer the digital demands of older adults. For this purpose, their literacy issues, physical limitations, and motivation have to be understood. This work presents an exploratory study into how the members of the association of former students of the commercial school of Braga – AAAEICBraga, interact with ICT, such as the use of mobile phones, smartphones, computers, and the Internet in order to improve the dissemination of activities. 14 answers to the questionnaire were obtained from participants aged over 60. The results showed that most of the respondents demonstrate a good competence regard to the use of ICT. This conclusion is a proof that the AAAEICBraga associates are prepared to be informed through social networks of the new association activities. These activities can improve the social contact between associates (and other people) and provide them a healthier and more active lifestyle.

Keywords: Digital divide · Older adults · ICT · technological literacy

1 Introduction

In recent years, the population has been facing remarkable technological advances and young people have easily followed them. However, the same does not apply to the elderly population. Although some of them have tried to adapt to new technologies, there is still an age-related digital divide, also called as "grey divide" [1, 2]. Many show resistance and prefer to keep the old-fashioned methods [3–5]. This can be related to several reasons, for instance, they think that do not have the abilities/literacy to use or lack interest and motivation to learn about novel Information and Communication Technologies – ICT [6–9]. In addition, it has been shown that manifold factors contribute to the digital divide such as education, monthly income, quality of life, technical interest, prior computer use, religion, marital status, and also friends and family [1, 10–12]. However, it is interesting

A. Cunha et al. (Eds.): MobiHealth 2022, LNICST 484, pp. 255–270, 2023.
https://doi.org/10.1007/978-3-031-32029-3_23

to note that some authors have verified that, in terms of gender the differences in internet usage are not significant [1, 10]. Neves et al. [13] observed that education was related to the mobile phone, computer, and Internet usage of the elderly in Lisbon. Furthermore, the authors verified that although many of them use mobile phones, the use of computers and the internet is reduced. In another study [14], these authors investigated the social capital of a group of adults (18+) and verified that this decreased with age. Another issue that can thwart older adults to interact with ICT is the applications' layout, as explored by Czaja and co-workers [15]. Moreover, Morris et al. [9] have observed that many older people are unaware of the advantages that ICT can provide, and this has to be urgently overcome. Despite the many advantages of ICTs, these can play an important role in home-based healthcare [19]. Findings showed that attitudes towards technology use and smartphone utilization ability have significant effects on older adults' disposition to use those tools. It was also found that older adults with a higher education level and financial power were more prepared to use healthcare ICT at home [19].

On the other hand, Gascón et al. [16] evaluated the perception of the Catalonia elderly about the use of ICTs but with the same social, economic, and geographical background and observed that in general, they shared the same opinions and that complexity was not pointed out as the main problem.

In addition to the previous factors that can influence the interaction of older people with ICT, the results presented by Moore et al. [17] showed a negative correlation between computer literacy and increasing age. Thus, efforts have to be done to fight these differences and reduce digital exclusion based on age since ICTs play a vital role in social involvement, well-being, and education for the elderly [4]. For all these reasons, the creation and improvement of different user-friendly interaction methods are needed to answer the digital demands of elderly people [6, 16, 18].

In the present exploratory work, the members of the association of former students of the industrial and commercial school of Braga – AAAEICBraga, were surveyed to understand how they perceive the use of mobile phones, smartphones, computers, and the Internet. The AAAEICBraga emerged in 1975, at the centenary of the school. Since then, several members joined the association and today count with about 360 active members with an average age of over 60 years aged. Currently, the association informs its members about the planned activities using social media (Facebook), email, or in person at the association headquarters. However, many members do not have email or social media, so the only way they are aware of the activities is when they go to the association and see the flyers. In light of this, the present work aims to explore the technological literacy of AAAEICBraga members, mostly 3rd age (+60 years), to understand their opinion and openness regarding the new technologies and thus improve and implement more efficient methods of contact between the association and its members.

2 Methods and Data Source

As previously explained, the present work explores the technology literacy of the members of the association of former students of the industrial and commercial school of Braga – AAAEICBraga. More specifically it is intended to answer the following question: "Are the elderly AAAEICBraga members using mobile phones, smartphones, computers, and Internet?".

The data collection was done through a self-administered questionnaire (which is given directly to the respondents, without intermediaries, and the answers are marked by the respondents, avoiding any type of influence). Therefore, a pre-test of the questionnaire was carried out with five potential respondents in the target age group to detect doubts or omissions, and to assess the clarity and accessibility of the language, the coherence and understanding of the questions, and the suitability of the different options presented. Minor corrections were necessary and after its implementation, the design of the questionnaire was considered finished.

The final questionnaire had six parts of questions. The first part considered the characterization of the respondent, such as gender, age, and education level. From the second to the fifth part, respondents were questioned about cell phone use, smartphone use, computer use (fixed or portable), and internet use. The sixth part assesses the technological profile of each respondent.

Since the majority of the members of the association were retired, the team thought of easy ways for the inquiry process, considering the paper preference of this age group and those members with low levels of technological knowledge. Therefore, there were available two ways of answering the questionnaire:

- on paper (available to fill out in on the association's building);
- an online questionnaire, created through the *Google Forms* software.

The questionnaire was made available for response in the second half of July 2022 and members were invited to participate in the study through an announcement from the Association's Facebook webpage: https://www.facebook.com/AAAEICBraga/ and an email (those with email contact). A total of 17 answers were obtained from AAAE-ICBraga's members (8 of them were answered on paper and 9 online). This low response rate can be explained by the fact that the association's activities are on a summer break, with most of its members supporting their grandchildren on school holidays. Recognizing the advantage of using online questionnaires (it provides full databases convertible to Spreadsheets (Excel) and .csv files with all the respondents' answers), responses collected on paper were converted to online responses (including a note that they were originally collected on paper). After importing to SPSS, the database was edited and worked on in order to ensure adequate analysis of the answers (for example, in questions with several answer options, it was necessary to unfold each of the options in a new variable).

As the age of the respondents is a variable of interest in the present paper, the age distribution was studied, having identified 3 outliers with ages lower than 60 years (see Fig. 1).

Thus, it was decided to remove the responses of these outliers from the analysis, which resulted in a final sample of 14 valid elements. Results are presented through the next topic.

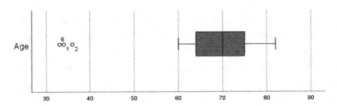

Fig. 1. Boxplot - Respondents' Ages.

3 Main Statistical Findings and Results

The characterization of respondents considered gender, age and education level. Respondents are equally represented in terms of gender, with 50% male and 50% female (see Table 1).

Table 1. Results – Respondents' Gender.

	Total	Male	Female
N	14	7	7
%	100.0%	50.0%	50.0%

Respondents' ages range between 60 and 82 years, with an average of 71.43 and a standard deviation of 6.235 years (Fig. 2).

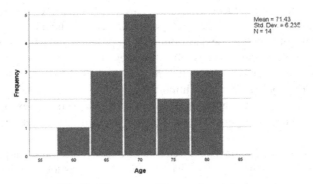

Fig. 2. Histogram of Respondents' Ages.

The education level was accessed through a direct question with the following options:

1. Preparatory education
2. Industrial education
3. Commercial Education

4. Female training course
5. High School
6. Industrial Institutes
7. Higher education
8. Other (please specify)

Following Anderberg, Eivazzadeh, and Berglund's study [21], each respondent was later classified into one of three levels of education:

(1) *Low* (those who did not finish secondary school);
(2) *Medium* (those who finish secondary school but no further education);
(3) *High* (those with some form of higher education) (Table 2).

Table 2. Results – Respondents' level of education.

	Total	Low	Medium	High
N	14	0	10	4
%	100.0%	0.0%	71.4%	28.6%

Table 3 presents the results for access to technology. All respondents have a cellphone and use the internet, 64.3% of them have a smartphone and 85.7% have a computer.

Table 3. Access to technology

	Total	Yes	No	Yes	No
Do you have a cellphone?	14	14	0	100.0%	0.0%
Do you have a smartphone?	14	9	5	64.3%	35.7%
Do you have a computer?	14	12	2	85.7%	14.3%
Do you use internet?	14	14	0	100.0%	0.0%

The next subsections present the type of usage and what are the perceived motivations or barriers in the use of each technology.

3.1 Cellphone Usage

The type of cellphone usage was accessed with two questions, one considering the reason for having a cell phone (5 options, including "other") and the frequency of use (4 options). As presented in Table 4, the main reasons to have a cell phone are "Talk to friends", "Being reachable when away from home" (both selected by 85.7% of respondents), and "Talk to family" (selected by 78.6% of respondents). The other option was mainly chosen to specify professional reasons (4 respondents).

The question "How often do you use your cell phone?" considered four possible options: (1) At least once a day; (2) At least once a week; (3) At least once a month; (4) Very rarely.

Table 4. Reasons for having a cell phone

The reasons for having a cell phone are: (you can choose more than one option)	Total	Selected option	Option not select	Selected option	Option not select
Talk to friends	14	12	2	85,7%	14,3%
Being reachable when away from home	14	12	2	85,7%	14,3%
Talk to family	14	11	3	78,6%	21,4%
Use in an emergency	14	9	5	64,3%	35,7%
Other (please specify)	14	7	7	50,0%	50,0%

All the respondents assumed using the cell phone "at least once a day" (100%).

3.2 Smartphone Usage

The type of smartphone usage was accessed with one question considering the reason for having a smartphone (7 options, including "other"). As presented in Table 5, the main reasons to have a smartphone are "Talk to family and friends", "Take photos", "Use apps like Whatsapp, Facebook,..." (each one selected by 88.9% of the respondents with a smartphone), and "Browse the internet" (selected by 77.8% of respondents). Only one respondent assumed using the smartphone to "play".

If the respondent did not have a smartphone, the questionnaire comprised a question regarding reasons for not having a smartphone (5 options, including "other"). The results are presented in Table 6. The main reason for not having one smartphone" is the option "No smartphone needed" (selected by 80.0% of the respondents with no smartphone).

Table 5. Reasons for having a smartphone.

The reasons for having a smartphone are: (you can choose more than one option)	Total	Selected option	Option not select	Selected option	Option not select
Talk to family and friends	9	8	1	88,9%	11,1%
Take photos	9	8	1	88,9%	11,1%
Use apps like Whatsapp, Facebook…	9	8	1	88,9%	11,1%
Browse the internet	9	7	2	77,8%	22,2%
Access online banking	9	6	3	66,7%	33,3%
Other (please specify)	9	2	7	22,2%	77,8%
Play	9	1	8	11,1%	88,9%

One respondent chose simultaneously the options "Doesn't know how to use a smartphone" and "Considers it expensive to have a smartphone". It is interesting to notice that no respondent considered to be too old to use a smartphone.

Table 6. Reasons for not having a smartphone.

If you don't have a smartphone, the reasons for not having a smartphone are: (you can choose more than one option)	Total	Selected option	Option not select	Selected option	Option not select
No smartphone needed	5	4	1	80,0%	20,0%
Doesn't know how to use a smartphone	5	1	4	20,0%	80,0%

(*continued*)

Table 6. (*continued*)

If you don't have a smartphone, the reasons for not having a smartphone are: (you can choose more than one option)	Total	Selected option	Option not select	Selected option	Option not select
Considers it expensive to have a smartphone	5	1	4	20,0%	80,0%
Considers to be too old to use a smartphone	5	0	5	0,0%	100,0%
Other (please specify)	5	0	5	0,0%	100,0%

3.3 Computer Usage (Fixed/Laptop Computer)

The type of computer usage was accessed with two questions regarding the reason for having a computer (8 options, including "other") and the frequency of use (4 options). All respondents with a computer selected as the main reason to have it "Use email" (100%). The other reasons presented in Table 7 are "Browse the internet" and "write texts" (both selected by 91.7% of respondents). The other option was mainly chosen to specify professional reasons (3 respondents). No respondent assumed to use the computer to "Play".

Table 7. Reasons for having a computer.

The reasons for having a computer are: (you can choose more than one option)	Total	Selected option	Option not select	Selected option	Option not select
Use email	12	12	0	100,0%	0,0%
Browse the internet	12	11	1	91,7%	8,3%

(*continued*)

Table 7. (*continued*)

The reasons for having a computer are: (you can choose more than one option)	Total	Selected option	Option not select	Selected option	Option not select
Write texts	12	11	1	91,7%	8,3%
Access online banking	12	9	3	75,0%	25,0%
Use Facebook, ...	12	8	4	66,7%	33,3%
Save photo albums	12	7	5	58,3%	41,7%
Other (please specify)	12	3	9	25,0%	75,0%
Play	12	0	12	0,0%	100,0%

The question "How often do you use your computer?" considered four possible options (see Table 8). The majority of respondents answered, "at least once a day" (83.3%).

Table 8. Computer frequency of use.

How often do you use your computer?	N	%
At least once a day	10	83,3%
At least once a week	1	8,3%
Very rarely...	1	8,3%
At least once a month	0	0,0%
Total	12	100.0%

If the respondent did not have a computer, the questionnaire comprised a question regarding reasons for not having a computer (5 options, including "other"). Of the two respondents with no computer, one selected the option "No computer needed" (50.0%), and the other respondent chose the "other" option, specifying "I have a tablet". The results are presented in Table 9.

Table 9. Reasons for not having a computer.

If you don't have a computer, the reasons for not having a computer are: (you can choose more than one option)	Total	Selected option	Option not select	Selected option	Option not select
No computer needed	2	1	1	50,0%	50,0%
Other (please specify)	2	1	1	50,0%	50,0%
Doesn't know how to use a computer	2	0	2	0,0%	100,0%
Considers it expensive to have a computer	2	0	2	0,0%	100,0%
Considers to be too old to use a computer	2	0	2	0,0%	100,0%

3.4 Internet Usage

The type of internet usage was accessed with two questions regarding the frequency of use by day (3 options) and by week (4 options) and a third one to specify which online activities are performed. Considering the internet use frequency, the majority of respondents use the internet "Less than 2 hours a day" (92.9%), with the week frequency ranging from "More than 5 days a week" (42.9%) to "Less than 3 days a week" (35.7%) (see Table 10 and Table 11).

Table 10. Internet frequency of use by day.

How many hours per day do you use the internet? (choose only one of the options)	N	%
Less than 2 h a day	13	92.9%
Between 2 to 5 h a day	1	7.1%
More than 5 h a day	0	0.0%
Total	14	100.0%

Table 11. Internet frequency of use by week.

How many days per week do you use the internet? (choose only one of the options)	N	%
More than 5 days a week	6	42.9%
Less than 3 days a week	5	35.7%
Between 3 to 5 days a week	3	21.4%
Total	14	100.0%

Comprising the online activities, the questionnaire presented 7 possible activities, including the "other" option to specify. The respondents selected as their main online activities "Read the news" (71.4%), "Search for information on health topics" (50%), and "Chat online" (42.9%). The other option was mainly chosen to specify professional activities (2 respondents). Only two respondents assumed to use the computer to "Play" or "Shop online" (each option selected by one respondent only). Results are presented in Table 12.

Table 12. Online activities.

What activities do you usually do online? (you can choose more than one option)	Total	Selected option	Option not select	Selected option	Option not select
Read the news	14	10	4	71,4%	28,6%
Search for information on health topics	14	7	7	50,0%	50,0%
Chat online	14	6	8	42,9%	57,1%
Watch videos and listen to music	14	4	10	28,6%	71,4%
Other specify please	14	4	10	28,6%	71,4%
Play	14	1	13	7,1%	92,9%
Shop online	14	1	13	7,1%	92,9%

3.5 Technology Profile

The technology profile was accessed with two questions. The first question invites respondents to rate their technology competence: "*On a scale from 1 (minimum) to 10 (maximum), how do you rate your competence when it comes to using a smartphone or a tablet?: _____(write the numerical value that best characterizes your competence)"*. Respondents' answers range from 3 to 10, with an average of 6.79 and a standard deviation of 1.718. Results are presented in Fig. 3.

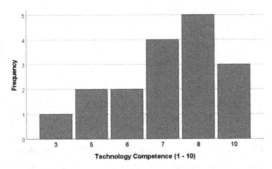

Fig. 3. Technology competence (self-assessment).

The second question was adapted to Portuguese from the TechPh scale developed by Anderberg, Eivazzadeh, and Berglund's study [21]. Each respondent selected the level of agreement with the following six statements (Likert scale ranging from 1 (strongly disagree) to 5 (strongly agree):

1) I find the new technological devices fun
2) Using technology makes my life easier
3) I like to buy the latest models or updates
4) Sometimes I'm afraid of not being able to use the new technical things
5) Today, technological progress is so rapid that it's hard for me to keep up.
6) I would have dared to try new technical devices to a greater extent if I had more support and help than I have today.

The majority of respondents totally agree with "Using technology makes my life easier" (statement 2 with 85.7% of positive responses, that is, the sum of levels "agree" and "totally agree") and "I find the new technological devices fun" (statement 1, with 78.6% of positive responses). Respondents tend to disagree with "I would have dared to try new technical devices to a greater extent if I had more support and help than I have today" (statement 6 with 42.9% of negative responses, that is, the sum of levels "totally disagree" and "disagree"). Results are summarized in Table 13.

Table 13. Level of agreement with the TechPH statements.

How much do you agree with the following statements (scale from 1 (strongly disagree) to 5 (strongly agree): (for each statement, choose only one agreement option)	Totally disagree (1)	Disagree (2)	Neither agree nor disagree (3)	Agree (4)	Totally agree (5)	Positive answers
1. I find the new technological devices fun	0,0%	7,1%	14,3%	64,3%	14,3%	78,6%
2. Using technology makes my life easier	0,0%	7,1%	7,1%	57,1%	28,6%	85,7%
3. I like to buy the latest models or up-dates	7,1%	7,1%	42,9%	35,7%	7,1%	42,9%
4. Sometimes I'm afraid of not being able to use the new technical things	14,3%	21,4%	35,7%	21,4%	7,1%	28,6%
5. Today, technological progress is so rapid that it's hard for me to keep up	0,0%	35,7%	35,7%	14,3%	14,3%	28,6%

(*continued*)

Table 13. (*continued*)

How much do you agree with the following statements (scale from 1 (strongly disagree) to 5 (strongly agree): (for each statement, choose only one agreement option)	Totally disagree (1)	Disagree (2)	Neither agree nor disagree (3)	Agree (4)	Totally agree (5)	Positive answers
6. I would have dared to try new technical devices to a greater extent if I had more support and help than I have today	14,3%	28,6%	21,4%	21,4%	14,3%	35,7%

4   Discussion and Conclusion

In the present study, the adoption of new ICT by the AAAEICBraga members was explorated to understand their willingness and accessibility to use these tools. When compared to younger adults, older adults have a certain resistance that is related to several factors namely functional, attitudinal, and physical. As a consequence, some of them suffer from social exclusion that in a long term can negatively affect the wellbeing and social participation of the elderly in some activities.

Despite the fact of being a small sample, it was interesting to observed that the majority of respondents show a great level of use of the new technologies, contrary to the association´s perceptions and some society stereotypes. All respondents have cell phones and uses the internet. Also, the results show that most of them use their phone almost every day, at least 1 hour per day, access the computer at least once a week, and surf the internet 5 days per week. The answers suggest that ICT contributes with great benefits to their lives, like being contactable with family and friends, searching for useful information online, and using applications as *Facebook* and *WhatsApp*.

These results are a positive indicator that the AAEIC members has some familiarity with technologies. Are they prepared to be informed of the new association activities through social networks? If, by expanding the study to a more expressive sample, this predisposition is confirmed, this accessibility to ICT from the members can be a huge opportunity for AAAEICBraga to promore with more success their activities, reaching more members to have a healthier and more active lifestyle, to avoid isolation and social exclusion, contributing to the wellbeing of the elderly.

References

1. Friemel, T.N.: The digital divide has grown old: determinants of a digital divide among seniors. New Media Soc. **18**, 313–331 (2016). https://doi.org/10.1177/1461444814538648
2. Fang, M.L., Canham, S.L., Battersby, L., Sixsmith, J., Wada, M., Sixsmith, A.: Exploring privilege in the digital divide: implications for theory, policy, and practice. Gerontologist **59**, E1–E15 (2019). https://doi.org/10.1093/geront/gny037
3. Castells, M., Fernández-Ardèvol, M., Qiu, J.L., Sey, A.: Mobile Communication and Society: A Global Perspective. The MIT Press, USA (2006)
4. Miguel, I., Da Luz, H.A.: Internet use for active aging: a systematic literature review. In: Iberian Conference on Information Systems and Technologies (CISTI) (2017). https://doi.org/10.23919/CISTI.2017.7975697
5. Hauk, N., Hüffmeier, J., Krumm, S.: Ready to be a silver surfer? A meta- analysis on the relationship between chronological age and technology acceptance. Comput. Hum. Behav. **84**, 304–319 (2018). https://doi.org/10.1016/j.chb.2018.01.020
6. Agudo-Prado, S., Pascual-Sevillano, M.Á., Fombona-Cadavieco, J.: Uses of digital tools among the elderly. Revista Comunicar **20**, 193–201 (2012). https://doi.org/10.3916/C39-2012-03-10
7. Rebelo, C.: Utilização da Internet e do Facebook pelos mais velhos em Portugal: estudo exploratório. The use of the Internet and Facebook by the elders in Portugal: an exploratory study. Obs. J. **9**, 129–153 (2015). http://www.scielo.mec.pt/scielo.php?script=sci_arttext&pid=S1646-59542015000300008&lng=pt&nrm=iso&tlng=pt
8. Selwyn, N., Gorard, S., Furlong, J., Madden, L.: Older adults' use of information and communications technology in everyday life. Ageing Soc. **23**, 561–582 (2003). https://doi.org/10.1017/S0144686X03001302
9. Morris, A., Goodman, J., Brading, H.: Internet use and non-use: views of older users. Univers. Access Inf. Soc. **6**, 43–57 (2007). https://doi.org/10.1007/s10209-006-0057-5
10. Arroyo-Menéndez, M., Gutiérrez-Láiz, N., Criado-Quesada, B.: The digitization of seniors: analyzing the multiple confluence of social and spatial divides. Land **11**, 1–38 (2022). https://doi.org/10.3390/land11060953
11. Sun, X., et al.: Internet use and need for digital health technology among the elderly: a cross-sectional survey in China. BMC Public Health **20**, 1–8 (2020). https://doi.org/10.1186/s12889-020-09448-0
12. Rice, R.E., Katz, J.E.: Comparing internet and mobile phone usage: digital divides of usage, adoption, and dropouts. Telecomm. Policy **27**, 597–623 (2003). https://doi.org/10.1016/S0308-5961(03)00068-5
13. Neves, B.: Too old for technology? How the elderly of Lisbon use and perceive ICT. J. Commun. Inform. **8**, 1–12 (2012). https://doi.org/10.15353/joci.v8i1.3061
14. Neves, B.B., Fonseca, J.R.S., Amaro, F., Pasqualotti, A.: Social capital and Internet use in an age-comparative perspective with a focus on later life. PLoS ONE **13**, 1–27 (2018). https://doi.org/10.1371/journal.pone.0192119

15. Czaja, S.J., Lee, C.C.: The impact of aging on access to technology. Univers. Access Inf. Soc. **5**, 341–349 (2007). https://doi.org/10.1007/s10209-006-0060-x

16. Fondevila Gascón, J.F., Carreras Alcalde, M., Seebach, S., Pesqueira Zamora, M.J.: How elders evaluate apps: a contribution to the study of smartphones and to the analysis of the usefulness and accessibility of ICTS for older adults. Mob. Media Commun. **3**, 250–266 (2015). https://doi.org/10.1177/2050157914560185

17. Moore, A.N., Rothpletz, A.M., Preminger, J.E.: The effect of chronological age on the acceptance of internet-based hearing health care. J. Speech Lang. Hear. Res. **24**, 280–283 (2015). https://doi.org/10.1044/2015_AJA-14-0082

18. Neves, B.B., Waycott, J., Malta, S.: Old and afraid of new communication technologies? Reconceptualising and contesting the 'age-based digital divide.' J. Sociol. **54**, 236–248 (2018). https://doi.org/10.1177/1440783318766119

19. Jo, H.S., Hwang, Y.S., Dronina, Y.: Mediating effects of smartphone utilization between attitude and willingness to use home-based healthcare ICT among older adults. Healthc. Inform. Res. **27**, 137–145 (2021). https://doi.org/10.4258/HIR.2021.27.2.137

20. Seaborn, K., Sekiguchi, T., Tokunaga, S., Miyake, N.P.: Voice over body? Older adults' reactions to robot and voice assistant facilitators of group conversation. Int. J. Soc. Robot. **15**, 21–23 (2022). https://doi.org/10.1007/s12369-022-00925-7

21. Anderberg, P., Eivazzadeh, S., Berglund, J.S.: A novel instrument for measuring older people's attitudes toward technology (TechPH): development and validation. J. Med. Internet Res. **21**, e13951 (2019). https://doi.org/10.2196/13951

Harnessing the Role of Speech Interaction in Smart Environments Towards Improved Adaptability and Health Monitoring

Fábio Barros[1,2], Ana Rita Valente[1,2], António Teixeira[1,2],
and Samuel Silva[1,2(✉)]

[1] Institute of Electronics and Informatics Engineering of Aveiro (IEETA),
University of Aveiro, Aveiro, Portugal
{fabiodaniel,rita.valente,ajst,sss}@ua.pt
[2] Department of Electronics, Telecommunications and Informatics (DETI),
University of Aveiro, Aveiro, Portugal

Abstract. The way we communicate with speech goes far beyond the words we use and nonverbal cues play a pivotal role in, e.g., conveying emphasis or expressing emotion. Furthermore, speech can also serve as a biomarker for a range of health conditions, e.g., Alzheimer's. With a strong evolution of speech technologies, in recent years, speech has been increasingly adopted for interaction with machines and environments, e.g., our homes. While strong advances are being made in capturing the different verbal and nonverbal aspects of speech, the resulting features are often made available in standalone applications and/or for very specific scenarios. Given their potential to inform adaptability and support eHealth, it's desirable to increase their consideration as an integral part of interactive ecosystems taking profit of the rising role of speech as an ubiquitous form of interaction. In this regard, our aim is to propose how this integration can be performed in a modular and expandable manner. To this end, this work presents a first reflection on how these different dimensions may be considered in the scope of a smart environment, through a seamless and expandable integration around speech as an interaction modality by proposing a first iteration of an architecture to support this vision and a first implementation to show its feasibility and potential.

Keywords: speech interaction · nonverbal speech features · health monitoring · eHealth · multimodal architectures

1 Introduction

In a world where we are surrounded by technology, researchers have been using assistive technology to build intelligent environments around people aiming to

This work is partially supported by FCT grant 2021.05929.BD and by IEETA - Institute of Electronics and Informatics Engineering of Aveiro Research Unit funding (UIDB/00127/2020).

A. Cunha et al. (Eds.): MobiHealth 2022, LNICST 484, pp. 271–286, 2023.
https://doi.org/10.1007/978-3-031-32029-3_24

increase their quality of life and also provide a protected and secure ecosystem to assist them in their daily living (e.g. Smart Houses) [6,23,28]. This assistance can entail support for a wide variety of tasks, e.g., controlling equipment in the household or improve how interaction can be performed with different technologies to support communication with family and friends, and can also be complemented with the monitoring of the persons health condition informing, for instance, how the person might need to be motivated to perform more exercise or if attention from a health professional is warranted. There are several ways of monitoring the person's physical and cognitive state. However, approaches that are noninvasive and part of the environment, instead of equipment that needs to be worn are desirable, since they are less intrusive and do not depend on user adherence (or caregiver intervention) [34]. In this context, data that can be collected from normal user activity, during the day and night could play an important role. Examples of such data can be posture, mobility, gestures, facial expressions, and also speech.

Speech, our most natural and efficient form of communication, is currently one of the most promising modalities to interact with technologies and environments due to a strong development of speech technologies in recent years (boosted by the availability of services for speech recognition, e.g., from Google and Azure). In this context, most of the works applying speech technologies for interaction with smart environments have been including services that perform speech recognition, speech synthesis, or even dialog systems [33]. And speech can be an important and intuitive form of interaction for all, but its consideration may be particularly important in assistive scenarios, since it potentially improve adaptability to different audiences. Additionally, speech is more than just words and a strongly personal trait, and how it is produced can add to the communication, e.g., intonation, stress and prosody [12], and reflect aspects of our physical and mental condition. In this regard, it can be harnessed to understand the emotional and cognitive state of humans and, in recent years, it has been widely explored for the detection, prevention and follow-up of some diseases, disorders, and communication problems, such as Alzheimer's or bipolar disease, through the analysis of semantic [35] and acoustic features [15].

All this wealth of information that can be obtained from speech has motivated intense research on its different dimensions and the literature has been prolific in providing methods to do so [10,11,22,26]. Nevertheless, the nonverbal aspects of speech along with its value as a biomarker for several conditions, which could play a pivotal role in increasing system adaptiveness and adding to the monitoring capabilities of assistive environments, are still not widely considered. In this regard, solutions that provide these features as part of individual applications, as is often the case, while showcasing the value of these technologies, narrow the scope of their use, and bringing them to interactive environments in a way that fosters their utility to a broader set of services is strongly desired. Furthermore, all these methods entail a certain degree of complexity and, from a developer's perspective, having to master the integration and use of several of these methods may be troublesome. Therefore, it would be important to bring these methods into interactive assistive environments as off-the-shelf features that different services could just profit from, e.g., to improve adaptation, or understand more about the user's physical and mental status. Additionally, with the increased consideration of speech interaction, the analysis could be performed over the daily interactions with the system, adding to the naturalness and non-intrusiveness of how the monitoring is performed. In this context, the work presented here provides a first proposal of how this integration can be performed reflecting on an initial set of requirements, proposing the overall architectural aspects to serve this purpose, and describing a first proof-of-concept implementation showcasing our proposal.

2   Speech Communication and Interaction

In what follows we provide a short overview of the potential of speech data to improve both interaction and health-related monitoring. This does not aim to be a thorough account of all possibilities, but an illustration of the kind of features we aim to integrate.

2.1   Intrinsic Properties and Applications of Speech

Speech is a form of communication that is, often, closely associated with the spoken words. However, there are also nonverbal cues present in speech that provide more information than just the linguistic content [9,16,25].

By considering them we can, in fact, potentially make human-machine interaction easier and more satisfying, increasing its credibility and realism, and increasing feelings of empathy and affection [5]. Methods such as speaker emotion recognition [1], speaker verification/identification [2], and detection of language, age, and gender [14,20,31] are some examples illustrating how can speech contribute to a more adaptive human-machine interaction. Furthermore, several nonverbal speech cues, i.e., vocal sounds without speaking any word, can express important information for the communication process, for instance by informing we are paying attention or that we do not agree with what is being said.

In addition, the acoustic and linguistic resources of speech are also a valuable resource for healthcare. They become important in the detection, prevention and intervention of neurological and psychiatric disorders such as Autism, bipolar disorder, Schizophrenia, Alzheimer and others [16]. There are several studies indicating its importance, for example, Tanaka et al. [29], conducted a study of speech characteristics, such as pitch, intensity, speech rate, and voice quality for the detection of autism. Karam et al. [19] extracted a set of low-level features using the openSMILE toolkit [11] such as RMS energy, zero-crossing rate, pitch, voice activity detection, mel spectrum for a long-term monitoring of mood states for individuals with bipolar disorder. Sch-net, proposed by Fu, Jia, et al. [13], by extracting fluency, intensity-related and, spectrum-related features, achieved a deep learning architecture, for detection of schizophrenia. Additionally, voice tone alteration, speech rate alteration and speech speed alteration are features characterizing Alzheimer's disease according with Bertini et al. [4].

Overall, these works show a very recent, diverse, and active work on harnessing the richness of speech with a wide variety of approaches. Nevertheless, one relevant aspects is that these methods are often still not deployed in a wider application scope or they are made available through standalone custom applications, e.g., to support a specific clinical setting. Our vision is that if these can be brought to profit from the growing role of speech as an interaction modality, their applicability is widened and their potential is driven farther towards eHealth.

2.2 Supporting Speech Interaction

Considering that we are evolving towards interactive environments with am increasingly dynamic number of devices, applications, and interaction modalities, such as smarthomes, architectures that can support interaction in these transient environments are paramount. However, there is no standardization of these technologies and methods so that existing efforts to support multimodal interaction can be reused in different scenarios beyond those for which they were originally designed. To tackle these adversities, several efforts have been made supported on the recommendations of the W3C for multimodal interactive architectures [8], such as Mudra [17], and Cu-me [30]. Among these efforts, a representative example is the AM4I architecture and framework [3]. It is based on a modular design where interaction modalities (e.g., speech, gestures, touch) are decoupled from applications. Besides this decoupling, the provided framework also has the advantage of providing some modalities off-the-shelf. This is important since it means that a developer, when integrating a novel application, does not need to master any of the interaction technologies and if different modalities or devices are available, at different times, this is transparent to the applications. A notable example of how this can be an advantage is the availability of what the authors call a generic speech modality, i.e., a modality that already tackles all aspects regarding speech interaction, e.g., speech recognition, and grammar definitions, making it simpler to use.

In light of how these multimodal architectures allow dealing with the modern interactive environments, such as smart homes, we consider that they should work as a reference context for our proposals.

2.3 Discussion

There are a number of important advantages that can come from enabling a stronger role of speech data beyond speech recognition, in smart environments, particularly when the integration of adaptability and health state monitoring are indisputable goals, such as in those scenarios aiming to provide assistance to daily life tasks while keeping an eye on the physical and mental health:

- advancing our knowledge and support to nonverbal cues in speech interaction is a paramount aspect to consider in our communication with interactive systems as it can potentially improve efficiency, naturalness, and adaptiveness;

– the integration of the inherent complexity of tackling nonverbal speech cues as part of the interaction framework, i.e., already residing in the core interaction features supported by the environment, and not as part of what each developer needs to master is paramount to ensure wider adoption;
– if the assessment of the health-related features can be integrated to profit from speech produced during the normal interactions with the home it adds to the naturalness of this process and lessens the feeling of being monitored with potential advantages to the ecological value of what is measured;
– building a long term record of speech features, i.e., measures systematically taken over time, can be important for the detection of changes that might work as biomarkers for early detection of certain physical and mental conditions [7,21,27,32];
– A decoupling among the speech signal, the extracted features, and how they can be used by third party applications opens space for a more versatile management and control regarding privacy of these data. This means, for instance, that a new application added to the smart home environment may profit from data extracted from speech, but without having access to the speech data.

All these aspects considered motivate our vision and proposal as described in the following sections.

3   Towards Enhancing Speech's Role in Smart Environments

Our overall vision is that the speech interactions with a smart environment, such as our home, can be harnessed to provide data for a wide range of services to improve both the role of speech in interaction and its value as a source for health monitoring. To ground our work, we designed a few scenarios to illustrate the overall envisioned features in the context of a smart home specifically designed to provide its users with services to assist in keeping or recovering their health, aligned with ongoing work with industry partners. This brings forward the relevance of adaptive interaction, but also the importance of considering speech for monitoring. While the overall monitoring context for this smart home also entails other modalities, such as, posture and physical activity, we keep to those scenarios harnessing speech, relevant for the work presented here.

3.1   Illustrative Scenarios

The provided scenarios illustrate two different audiences that can profit from the envisaged features: the user, at home, to obtain a more adaptive response from the system, and a caregiver or health professional, to be able to monitor for particular conditions, over time, or receive a notification about a notable event.

In a first scenario, Rosa is at home and the system is able to infer some instability and take some action to understand the situation, help Rosa handle it, and monitor the outcomes.

Scenario 1: Rosa having a different day—Rosa is a 76-year-old female who is a health smart home patient. Rosa is a well disposed, calm and active person, but she has heart and anxiety problems. On a particular day, the health smart home realizes that something unusual is going on with Rosa, through her continuous monitoring and comparison of her user context model, unusual values have been detected in her interactions since her speech rate as lower then the normal and as well as the emotion associated are classified as "sad". The conversational agent at the health smart home proceeds to interact in order to ask Rosa and understand what might be the reason for the problem. She responds by informing it that she is feeling a little anxious. The assistant then advises some diaphragmatic breathing and guides Rosa in how to proceed. After this, the system asks Rosa about how she his feeling now and detects less distress and a more positive attitude.

In a second scenario, Rita, who is Rosa's caregiver, is notified of some changes in Rosa's behavior and tries to understand what is happening, in a first instance, analysing some data about the past days.

Scenario 2: Rita follows Rosa's Day Remotely—Rita is a 38-year-old female who is the health smart home caregiver. In a special way, Rita is the caregiver responsible for Rosa, who is a patient at the health smart home. Rita, although a very attentive caregiver, can't dedicate 100% of her time to her patient. On Monday morning, Rita is notified by the system that Rosa during the weekend made use of multiple interactions with a negative sentiment associated with her speech, a high speech rate as well as an emotion associated with "anger" which are completely different values from Rosa's context model of a patient who is a well disposed, calm and active person. Rita checks that the assistant already tried to suggest some breathing exercises without any long-lasting impact. In this sense, and in order to evaluate and analyze these interactions herself, Rita searches for all the interactions made by Rosa during that weekend. The result of this query is returned to her on a dashboard containing different parameters about the queried period, including voice parameters, semantic graphs, and word clouds of most used vocabulary so that she can evaluate when and how Rosa's situation changed and what dimensions are affected. She notices that words such as "alone" and "pain", came up more frequently than usual, in the last couple of days. Rita goes out to visit Rosa.

One important aspect to note is that the overall idea is not to provide the third-parties with a complete account of the dialogues the person had, at home, but a set of aggregate data. And different people will only have access to data with relevance for their role. Access to complete sentences, for instance, may be possible, but solely for very well defined contexts, e.g., a remote consultation with a therapist. This overall principle is intended as a first rule to preserve some degree of privacy. Additionally, the system is not intended to be the last instance of diagnosis, but rather a tool that allows and facilitates the collection of additional information, in other words, the system serves only as a first line of indication for the therapist not a diagnostic tool.

3.2 Overall Requirements

In light of the proposed vision and scenarios, there are a few notable high level features that need to be considered:

- adopt a modular design, given the diversity of methods that can be relevant for integration, also enabling expansion, over time, to serve new purposes and integrate novel methods;
- obtain data from different sources of speech audio (and, eventually, written speech) in the environment;
- integrate with multimodal interaction architectures that have already been adopted to support the interaction in increasingly complex interactive environments entailing multiple services, devices, and interaction modalities;
- make the outcomes of the different methods available to a broad set of services that might not know how to deal with specific results and need a higher level (semantic) outcome;
- support different timespans for analyses: (a) as a long-term repository, to provide a baseline and as an history of parameter evolution; (b) as a source for overall characterization over smaller periods of time, e.g., daily mood or status; and (c) as a source for immediate system reaction, e.g., adapting to a particular emotional change;

These overall requirements inform our first proposal for a broader consideration of speech-related features serving adaptivity and monitoring as described in what follows.

4 Development

We start by the proposal of the overall architecture that should address the identified overall requirements. At this first stage, and as further explained ahead, we did not go into full detail regarding a complete integration with multimodal interactive frameworks, since this is not essential to demonstrate the feasibility of our proposal. After, we detail the first instantiation of this architecture and showcase some of its potential.

4.1 Proposed Architecture

Figure 1 shows the overall architecture of the proposed system, as explained in what follows.

Core Modules. The audio stream can come from a wide variety of microphones integrated in the house and can be accessed by the SPEECH PROCESSING module. This module is responsible for extracting both verbal and nonverbal (e.g., words, speech rate, fundamental frequency) data. The purpose of this module is solely the computation of different features from the speech data and their storage, and no conclusions about what the data might mean or if it requires some action are drawn, at this point.

To make sense of the data extracted by the processing module, the ANALYZER module provides features to further process and interpret the data according to particular goals. This can be done by resorting to the data provided by the processing module, for different time windows (current or past), along with data from the user context providing reference values or states. This module may enable, for instance, detecting a change in a voice property of interest or updating the user context with relevant information, such as the current mood. The analyser module can even implement more complex logic to, for instance, perform semantic analysis based on transcriptions of the speech data, with known relevance, e.g., through semantic graphs analysis, to monitor cognitive aspects [24].

Finally, the system integrates the INFORMATION AND INSIGHTS module that supports providing relevant information from what has been collected/analyzed, e.g., a dashboard exhibiting interactive visualizations of data required by the caregiver/healthcare professional to assess the patient's state. This module can provide a set of off-the-shelf solutions for visualization and features allowing the inclusion of new ones. It profits from the DATA INSPECTOR module for querying the available data.

Integration with Multimodal Interactive Framework. The architecture in Fig. 1 also depicts, delimited by a dashed line, some elements that should already be a part of the existing interaction infrastructure, in the environment, including applications and those components belonging to the multimodal interactive framework, e.g., the interaction manager and interaction modalities [3], with just speech modalities represented, for the sake of simplicity.

The ASSISTANT element represents an application, e.g., a home assistant, working in the interactive environment. It is this application that receives the interactions from the users through speech (and other modalities) and can serve a wide range of purposes, such as enabling them to control equipment in the house or ask questions about its functioning.

In a first instance, our proposal can be integrated with existing multimodal interactive frameworks, such as AM4I [3], through the user context, providing the interaction modalities and applications (such as the Assistant) with data potentially informing system behaviour and adaptability. Naturally, deeper levels of integration may be devised, over time, e.g., with analysers being able to request the assistant to initiate an interaction to obtain more speech data from the user or clarify context, e.g., to confirm if the user as a cold (which could affect the voice).

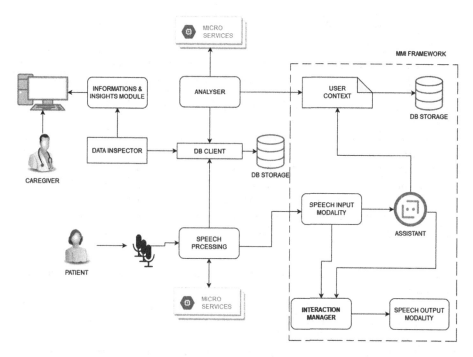

Fig. 1. Overall architecture to address the identified requirements- The modules to the right, inside the dashed area, represent the overall components of a multimodal interaction framework to illustrate the points of contact/integration with the current stage of our proposal.

It is also important to note that the Speech Input Modality already present, in the environment, as part of the framework supporting multimodal interaction, can also be an important point for integration. The diagram in Fig. 1 shows two alternatives. A first alternative is that the speech modality obtains the audio stream as before, bypassing the speech processing and analysis modules, and does not need any change. If it already had some logic to deal with context changes, it can profit from them, as explained above. This is the simplest level of integration, requiring no changes to the framework. The second alternative is that the speech input modality receives speech data that has already gone through some processing/analysis and thus provides more metadata for the speech modality, e.g., which word was emphasized. This second option is the desirable long-term integration method as it enables nonverbal speech cues to be more widely explored during interaction.

In the following sections, additional details are provided about the concrete technical aspects regarding a first implementation of the different architectural modules.

4.2   Data Management

One important aspect of the proposed architecture pertains how to deal with the speech data and all the data that is subsequently produced by the different modules. In this regard, there are some aspects that need to be considered:

- there is no speech data continuously pouring into the system, which means that the selected approach needs to be driven by data availability;
- given the modularity of the proposal, multiple methods will need to access the data in parallel;
- for particular analyser methods, only a subset of data made available by processors will be of interest from the whole range that is produced, meaning that a data source selection mechanism should enable this focus;
- some methods may need to provide results on the currently arriving data, while others may do so only at certain times, e.g., over a day, and based on past data.

Aligned with these needs, our approach adopts a producer/consumer approach based on streams using Apache Kafka[1]. This allows for the different modules to subscribe to the topics of interest and an elegant way to manage the asynchronous nature of data availability and production.

DB Storage is a non-relational and document-oriented database that uses MongoDB[2]. The database is responsible for keeping the data extracted from each speech sentence and data related of the user context. As a non-relational and document-oriented database this allow us to store variations in the documents structure and also storing documents that are halfway complete.

DB client is a module responsible to store and retrieve the data extracted and stored providing a versatile way to inspect the wide range of available data according to the needs of each analyser, e.g., some may require more than one parameter, others may work on different time windows.

Finally, the data required to build the required dashboards is supplied by a **Data Inspector** developed in Flask that queries the stored data through the DB client.

4.3   Speech Processors

The SPEECH PROCESSING module adopts a micro-services based implementation with the purpose to be used according to the needs of the system, but also, because it is possible to include or remove micro-services without affecting how the module integrates with the remaining architecture acting as a hub of micro-services. For this first implementation, we wanted to deploy processing services actuating at different levels of the speech data (acoustic and language) entailing:

- **Speech-To-Text:** This micro-service transforms the audio stream into words and also the segmentation of it, i.e., given a word, extract its duration, and the

---

[1] https://kafka.apache.org.

[2] https://www.mongodb.com/.

instant when it occurred. To perform this transcription we use the "Speech to Text" service provided by Microsoft Azure.

– **Speech Rate:** This micro-service calculates the number of words spoken per minute.
– **Speech Emotion Recognition:** This micro-service computes the probability associated with different emotions (in a set of 6) from the audio stream.
– **Sentiment Analysis:** This micro-service classifies each spoken sentence into "Positive", "Neutral" or "Negative" with a probabilistic value. To perform this classification we integrate the "Azure Text Analytics" service provided by Microsoft Azure.
– **Audio Features:** This micro-service extracts a set of audio features, such as fundamental frequency, intensity, and energy, from the audio stream integrating the OpenSMILE library.

4.4   Speech Analyzers

The ANALYSER also adopts a micro-services based implementation and is responsible for retrieving the data stored and analyse it for specific goals, e.g., if pitch changed significantly, or to compute the monthly baseline speech rate to populate the user context with a reference value. Furthermore, this module is also responsible for triggering actions, e.g., alerting the assistant and the caregiver if there are anomalous values in the interaction/monitoring. At this stage, the analyser implements three micro-services, which are:

– **Sentiment Analyser:** This micro-service compares the classification and probability of the spoken sentence with the user overall expressed sentiment in a specific time period, e.g., the past hours or week.
– **Emotion Analyser:** This micro-service monitors for emotion changes given a period of reference or the mood set in the user context.
– **Speech Rate Analyser:** This micro-service checks, using the the user context model or data from a reference time period, if there were very abrupt speech rate variations.
– **Acoustic Features Analyser:** This micro-service, at this stage, and for illustrative purposes, can understand if there were many variations in the fundamental frequency.

All the data considered by the analysers is generated by processing microservices or other analysers and selected according to the analyser's needs. Therefore, the inclusion of a new analyser micro-service may also entail the integration of novel processing features. On the other hand, some analysers may just profit from already existing data.

4.5   Assistant and User Context

The ASSISTANT and USER CONTEXT depicted in the architecture represent elements belonging to the framework dealing with multimodal interaction with which our proposal aims to integrate. Since our purpose, at this stage, was the deployment of the core features described in the previous sections, as a proof-of-concept, these two elements have received minimal intervention. The assistant inherits from our ongoing work with smart homes and allows controlling the house's lights and appliances, and provides information about water and energy consumption. Its sole purpose for the scope of this work was to provide a motive to interact with the house and, thus, generate speech data.

The USER CONTEXT is an important element, in our proposal, since it is a first path to foster integration of the work presented here with the multimodal interactive framework. By populating the user context with relevant information about the user, e.g., current mood, emotional changes, or speech rate, – through the analyser module features – the interactive services, e.g., the assistant, may be able to adapt their functioning or behavior accordingly. This integration method keeps the interactive services agnostic to all the processing and analysis that is being performed in our proposal.

4.6   Visualization Dashboard

The INFORMATION & INSIGHTS module supports providing third parties such as caregivers, health professionals or, researchers with ways of interactively exploring relevant data to inform assessing the user status, e.g., looking for any abnormal change. To this end, we required an approach that could easily allow the visualization of different types of data, over time or even, consume the data directly from streams, e.g., if a more immediate visualization is required, e.g., during remote consultation with a Speech and Language Therapist. For this purpose, different solutions were considered, such as Kibana[3], Grafana[4] and the development of dashboards from scratch. While all provided the overall features required, a dashboard developed from scratch that provides much more adapted visualization and versatile, was the selected approach.

To demonstrate the envisaged functionality and usefulness, we developed a minimal dashboard that illustrates how a healthcare professional/language pathologist might have access to relevant data concerning the patient's monitoring.

Figure 2 illustrates a simple dashboard built using ReactJS[5] showing different information concerning the suprasegmental characteristics of the speech resulting from reading a small text collected from the fable "The North Wind and the Sun" which is phonetically balanced [18]. It includes data on parameters such as the speech rate, the fundamental frequency contour (intonation), or the intensity trace. For a Speech and Language Pathologist, this type of information can be used to, e.g., characterize the speech of an individual through the comparison with normative/baseline data, or to assess the effectiveness of an intervention process. For instance, if an abrupt and sustained decrease is observed in the

---

[3] https://www.elastic.co/pt/kibana/.

[4] https://grafana.com/.

[5] https://reactjs.org/.

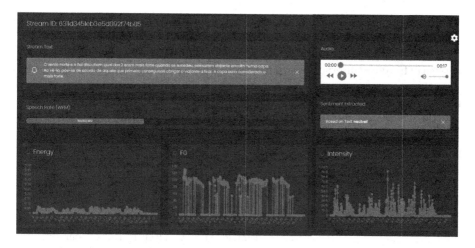

Fig. 2. Dashboard showing different information concerning the suprasegmental characteristics collected from a user reading the fable "The North Wind and the Sun" such as: speech rate, energy, fundamental frequency and, intensity.

fundamental frequency plot, it may mean the emergence of laryngeal pathology. In addition, if a marked decrease in speech rate is verified, it can also be linked to different communication pathologies or even mood disorders, for example.

While these parameters can be collected from routine interactions with the system, asking the user to read a small text, e.g., to learn it to tell a grandchild – a challenge that can be presented by the assistant –, is also an important aspect that can be explored. In this regard, the literature may provide a strong background to support the speech and language pathologist's assessment from that specific set of data and the person will not need to leave home to have a first checkup or follow-up.

5   Conclusions and Future Work

In light of the importance of speech in our daily life and its growth as a form of interaction with machines, the work presented here argues that the different dimensions provided by speech may play a greater role to inform adaptivity and eHealth approaches. In this regard, we reflect on the overall requirements to address this vision and propose a first iteration of an architecture that should serve this purpose along with a first instantiation, as a proof-of-concept.

Currently, this first iteration of our proposal is integrated in a smart home lab designed to test solutions for monitoring and supporting users with their daily living and health, at different levels (e.g., motor activity, posture, and our proposal for speech). While already enabling the collection of baseline data, and informing on mood changes, this scenario will provide us with a richer context for testing integration and further advance system features, particularly regarding, at this point, the consideration of nonverbal features extracted from the acoustic speech signal.

In the work presented here, we have implemented the different modules independently from the interaction architecture as a proof-of-concept of our proposal. Nevertheless, and as we argued, these features should progressively become an integral part of a multimodal interactive framework, e.g., The AM4I [3], to maximize their potential and the next stage of the work will progressively address that aspect. In this regard, a stronger integration between the speech input modality and the speech processing module is a step to follow. This will enable a greater integration of nonverbal cues as part of interaction in a more immediate fashion.

References

1. Abbaschian, B.J., Sierra-Sosa, D., Elmaghraby, A.: Deep learning techniques for speech emotion recognition, from databases to models. Sensors **21**(4), 1249 (2021)
2. Abdullah, H., Warren, K., Bindschaedler, V., Papernot, N., Traynor, P.: SoK: the faults in our ASRs: an overview of attacks against automatic speech recognition and speaker identification systems. In: 2021 IEEE Symposium on Security and Privacy (SP), pp. 730–747. IEEE (2021)
3. Almeida, N., Teixeira, A., Silva, S., Ketsmur, M.: The AM4I architecture and framework for multimodal interaction and its application to smart environments. Sensors **19**(11), 2587 (2019)
4. Bertini, F., Allevi, D., Lutero, G., Calzà, L., Montesi, D.: An automatic Alzheimer's disease classifier based on spontaneous spoken English. Comput. Speech Lang. **72**, 101298 (2022)
5. Bozkurt, E., Yemez, Y., Erzin, E.: Affective synthesis and animation of arm gestures from speech prosody. Speech Commun. **119**, 1–11 (2020)
6. Calvaresi, D., Cesarini, D., Sernani, P., Marinoni, M., Dragoni, A.F., Sturm, A.: Exploring the ambient assisted living domain: a systematic review. J. Ambient. Intell. Humaniz. Comput. **8**(2), 239–257 (2017)
7. Chojnowska, S., Ptaszyńska-Sarosiek, I., Kępka, A., Knaś, M., Waszkiewicz, N.: Salivary biomarkers of stress, anxiety and depression. J. Clin. Med. **10**(3), 517 (2021)
8. Dahl, D.A.: The W3C multimodal architecture and interfaces standard. J. Multimodal User Interfaces **7**(3), 171–182 (2013)
9. Dunbar, R., Robledo, J.P., Tamarit, I., Cross, I., Smith, E.: Nonverbal auditory cues allow relationship quality to be inferred during conversations. J. Nonverbal Behav. **46**(1), 1–18 (2022)
10. Eyben, F., Wöllmer, M., Schuller, B.: OpenEAR-introducing the Munich open-source emotion and affect recognition toolkit. In: 2009 3rd International Conference on Affective Computing and Intelligent Interaction and Workshops, pp. 1–6. IEEE (2009)
11. Eyben, F., Wöllmer, M., Schuller, B.: OpenSMILE: the Munich versatile and fast open-source audio feature extractor. In: Proceedings of the 18th ACM International Conference on Multimedia, pp. 1459–1462 (2010)
12. Farrús, M., Codina-Filbà, J., Escudero, J.: Acoustic and prosodic information for home monitoring of bipolar disorder. Health Inform. J. **27**(1), 1460458220972755 (2021)

13. Fu, J., et al.: Sch-net: a deep learning architecture for automatic detection of schizophrenia. Biomed. Eng. Online **20**(1), 1–21 (2021)
14. Garain, A., Singh, P.K., Sarkar, R.: FuzzyGCP: a deep learning architecture for automatic spoken language identification from speech signals. Expert Syst. Appl. **168**, 114416 (2021)
15. Guidi, A., et al.: Voice quality in patients suffering from bipolar disease. In: 2015 37th Annual International Conference of the IEEE Engineering in Medicine and Biology Society (EMBC), pp. 6106–6109. IEEE (2015)
16. Hampsey, E., et al.: Protocol for rhapsody: a longitudinal observational study examining the feasibility of speech phenotyping for remote assessment of neurodegenerative and psychiatric disorders. BMJ Open **12**(6), e061193 (2022)
17. Hoste, L., Dumas, B., Signer, B.: Mudra: a unified multimodal interaction framework. In: Proceedings of the 13th International Conference on Multimodal Interfaces, pp. 97–104 (2011)
18. Jesus, L.M., Valente, A.R.S., Hall, A.: Is the Portuguese version of the passage 'The North Wind and the Sun' phonetically balanced? J. Int. Phon. Assoc. **45**(1), 1–11 (2015)
19. Karam, Z.N., et al.: Ecologically valid long-term mood monitoring of individuals with bipolar disorder using speech. In: 2014 IEEE International Conference on Acoustics, Speech and Signal Processing (ICASSP), pp. 4858–4862. IEEE (2014)
20. Kwasny, D., Hemmerling, D.: Gender and age estimation methods based on speech using deep neural networks. Sensors **21**(14), 4785 (2021)
21. Laguarta, J., Subirana, B.: Longitudinal speech biomarkers for automated Alzheimer's detection. Front. Comput. Sci. **3**, 624694 (2021)
22. Lenain, R., Weston, J., Shivkumar, A., Fristed, E.: Surfboard: audio feature extraction for modern machine learning. arXiv preprint arXiv:2005.08848 (2020)
23. Marques, G.: Ambient assisted living and internet of things. In: Harnessing the Internet of Everything (IoE) for Accelerated Innovation Opportunities, pp. 100–115 (2019)
24. Mota, N.B., et al.: Speech graphs provide a quantitative measure of thought disorder in psychosis. PLoS ONE **7**(4), e34928 (2012)
25. Ramanarayanan, V., Lammert, A.C., Rowe, H.P., Quatieri, T.F., Green, J.R.: Speech as a biomarker: opportunities, interpretability, and challenges. Perspect. ASHA Spec. Interest Groups **7**(1), 276–283 (2022)
26. Sanden, C., Befus, C.R., Zhang, J.Z.: Camel: a lightweight framework for content-based audio and music analysis. In: Proceedings of the 5th Audio Mostly Conference: A Conference on Interaction with Sound, pp. 1–4 (2010)
27. Schwoebel, J.W., et al.: A longitudinal normative dataset and protocol for speech and language biomarker research. medRxiv (2021)
28. Sun, H., De Florio, V., Gui, N., Blondia, C.: Promises and challenges of ambient assisted living systems. In: 2009 Sixth International Conference on Information Technology: New Generations, pp. 1201–1207. IEEE (2009)
29. Tanaka, H., Sakti, S., Neubig, G., Toda, T., Nakamura, S.: Linguistic and acoustic features for automatic identification of autism spectrum disorders in children's narrative. In: Proceedings of the Workshop on Computational Linguistics and Clinical Psychology: From Linguistic Signal to Clinical Reality, pp. 88–96 (2014)
30. Tumuluri, R., Kharidi, N.: Developing portable context-aware multimodal applications for connected devices using the W3C multimodal architecture. In: Dahl, D.A. (ed.) Multimodal Interaction with W3C Standards, pp. 173–211. Springer, Cham (2017). https://doi.org/10.1007/978-3-319-42816-1_9

31. Tursunov, A., Choeh, J.Y., Kwon, S.: Age and gender recognition using a convolutional neural network with a specially designed multi-attention module through speech spectrograms. Sensors **21**(17), 5892 (2021)
32. Usman, M., Gunjan, V.K., Wajid, M., Zubair, M., et al.: Speech as a biomarker for Covid-19 detection using machine learning. Comput. Intell. Neurosci. **2022** (2022)
33. Vacher, M., et al.: Evaluation of a context-aware voice interface for ambient assisted living: qualitative user study vs. quantitative system evaluation. ACM Trans. Accessible Comput. (TACCESS) **7**(2), 1–36 (2015)
34. Vacher, M., Fleury, A., Portet, F., Serignat, J.F., Noury, N.: Complete sound and speech recognition system for health smart homes: application to the recognition of activities of daily living (2010)
35. Weiner, L., Doignon-Camus, N., Bertschy, G., Giersch, A.: Thought and language disturbance in bipolar disorder quantified via process-oriented verbal fluency measures. Sci. Rep. **9**(1), 1–10 (2019)

Integrated Design Method and Usability Outcomes of a Mobile Application for Psychological Well-Being During Pregnancy

Paolo Perego$^{(\boxtimes)}$ and Maria Terraroli

Design Department, Politecnico di Milano, via Candiani 72, 20158 Milan, Italy
paolo.perego@polimi.it
http://www.tedh.polimi.it

Abstract. The last decade has seen a radical change in the use of technologies. Mobile computing is the main technology of this decade. More and more often we are dealing with portable tools, and portable devices; medical instrumentation such as portable and connected electrocardiographs, pulse-oximeters... is widespread, especially due to COVID-19 pandemic situation in the last two years. However, mental healthcare is a critical domain which however is often unexplored, especially in terms of human factors and ergonomics. Few studies analyze the ergonomics factor and usability of mobile applications in the mental health field. This paper reports a study on the creation of a digital system with a tailor-made application for monitoring the mental health of pregnant women. The paper proposes a methodological analysis carried out with future moms and different stakeholders, to identify the most suitable solution for the psycho-physical needs of mothers and at the same time those of the various actors during pregnancy (dads, psychologists, psychiatrists). The work shows the ergonomic effectiveness of an app for the collection of the Edinburgh Scale (EPDS), designed with the users, both from the point of view of usability and the data collected. The result shows good adherence in terms of the App's active users and EPDS data gathering, a decrease in the evaluation of the EPDS scale, and therefore a reduced severity of depressive symptoms using a combination of app and home interventions by psychologists.

Keywords: Mobile application design and ergonomics · User-centered design · Mobile application for mental health · Usability

1 Introduction

Mental health has become a global issue for public health service [1] and especially during and after COVID-19 pandemic [2]. Perinatal Depression (PND) affects up to 15% of women during pregnancy and 10% within 1 year after giving birth [3, 4]. These percentages are higher in women living in poor socio-economic

A. Cunha et al. (Eds.): MobiHealth 2022, LNICST 484, pp. 287–303, 2023.
https://doi.org/10.1007/978-3-031-32029-3_25

conditions or belonging to minority ethnic groups [5], in first-time adolescents [6], and in the female population of non-Western countries [7].

Local studies underline the amplitude of perinatal mental disorders despite the lack of national population-based studies. In fact, it must be taken into account that suicide and homicide have been identified as one of the main causes of maternal and newborn death within the first year after birth. Since 2017, the Italian public primary care service offers free psychological interventions dedicated to pregnancy and puerperium assistance, but yet half of those who were known to be prone to depression and suicide during the postpartum period had not been referred to this Family Care Centers.

Italy has about 60.3 million inhabitants and more than 430,000 live births per year [8]. If we take into consideration the Lombardy region about 80,000 births occur in a year: it is realistic to think that about 9,000 women suffer from perinatal depression and that only a minority of these are diagnosed today and receive treatment (about 9%).

If treated, the prognosis of perinatal depression results basically favorable; if left untreated, however, it has a significant risk of becoming chronic. About one-third of women are still suffering from depression one year after giving birth and the risk of subsequent depressive recurrences or independent from new pregnancies is high and equal to 40% [3,4]. Currently, the attention of health services is directed almost exclusively to the physical health of the woman, while the interest in her mental health is less systematic and structured. Today, many pregnant women and new mothers do not receive a correct diagnosis of the perinatal mental disorder and just as many, recognized as clinically affected by depression, do not benefit from adequate therapeutic care. Furthermore, their family members, including the child, are not routinely offered appropriate help by the local health and social health services responsible for safeguarding maternal, child and family health. These problems are mainly related to a lack of information. The information, under the dual profile of information to the woman on perinatal psychic disorders and collection of information on the mental health of pregnant and puerperium women, represents a critical element to intercept situations with emotional disorders in the perinatal period. On the one hand, women often do not have easy access to scientific information, expressed in a popular form, on perinatal emotional disorders; on the other hand, active and population screening activities, i.e. the systematic collection of information on women's mental health status through assessment tools, the Edinburgh Postnatal Depression Scale (EPDS) [9] and Whooley's question [10] are not structured in many areas at both regional and national level. Even today, even in the case of an active offer, screening is entrusted to paper tools and is carried out "forcibly" on the occasion of either the birth or the pediatric check of the newborn, not optimal moments for this activity both for the woman and for the operators.

The Thinking Healthy Programme (THP) [11], which is endorsed by WHO (World Health Organization), is an evidence-based intervention for perinatal depression. With the aim to ease the workload of healthcare operators, and to keep the rate of use by mothers-to-be/mothers high, this work shows the ergonomic effectiveness of an application for the collection of Edinburgh Perinatal Depression Scale, designed with the users for the users.

This work comes from the goals to encourage the screening activity, simplify it through the use of technological tools, and improve the information of the woman through the possibility of connecting to other informative tools.

2   Perinatal Depression - Baby Blues

Pregnancy and becoming a mother can be described as a wonderful experience in a woman's life. But the sudden changes in physiology and endocrine status, in addition to other social circumstances and predispositions, can also produce undesirable or even pathological effects in all human domains: physical, physiological, and psychological. Among psychological disorders, perinatal depression is one of the most important for incidence and prevalence.

Perinatal depression (PD) is a mood disorder that can affect women during pregnancy and puerperium [12]. PD is considered a medical disease and can affect any mother-regardless of age, race, income, culture, or education.

Mothers with perinatal depression experience feelings of extreme sadness, anxiety, and fatigue that may make it difficult for them to carry out daily tasks, including caring for themselves or others. The word "perinatal" refers to the time before and after the birth of a child. Perinatal depression includes depression that begins during pregnancy (called prenatal depression) and depression that begins after the baby is born (called postpartum depression).

Many women have baby blues in the days after childbirth. It is characterized by having mood swings or feeling sad, anxious, or overwhelmed, having crying spells, and accompanied by a loss of appetite or sleeping troubles. This situation rapidly evolves and baby blues disappear in the first 2 weeks after having a baby. So, the two conditions must not be confused.

There are several screening tools that have been developed to diagnose PD. Those specific to detect maternal depression in the peripartum or postpartum period include the Edinburgh Postpartum Depression Scale (EPDS) [9], the Postpartum Depression Screening Scale (PDSS), and the Pregnancy Risk Questionnaire (PRQ). Another very short test is represented by the Whooley Questions for depression screening, a 2 items questionnaire that also demonstrated its reliability [10]. Despite the severe consequences that PD has on both the mother and the child, due to tests still in paper format and with only occasional meetings with nurses and caregivers, up to 50% of these cases are undiagnosed.

The situation has only worsened in this specific moment of COVID-19 pandemic. The worsening occurs on two fronts: the lockdown measures emphasized the isolation from family and friends of some women and mothers, while security measures are anticipated to decrease the opportunities to meet operators, reducing to the strictly essential and therefore decreasing access to psychological or pharmacological diagnosis and treatment [13]. A Canadian study of the Program for Pregnancy and Postpartum Health, University of Alberta, recruited 900 women who were pregnant or within the first year after delivery to participate in an online survey. Among the questions, respondents were asked to self-report levels of depression/depressive symptoms, anxiety, and physical activity. The results showed 40.7% of respondents had survey scores indicative of depression, compared with 15% pre-pandemic, while moderate to high anxiety was identified in 72% of women versus 29% pre-pandemic [13]. An Italian cross-sectional study of 100 pregnant women showed that more than half of the respondents rated the psychological impact of the COVID-19 outbreak as severe, and about two-thirds reported higher than-normal anxiety. It's therefore important to formulate psychological interventions to improve mental health and psychological resilience during the COVID-19 pandemic [14].

For these reasons, there is a huge need for effective screening administration methods to ensure that all women with PD are identified. mHealth (Mobile Health) represents a possible exploitable solution [15]. It is defined as medical or public health practice supported by mobile devices [16], encompasses a variety of contexts: use of mobile phones to improve point of service data collection, care delivery, patient communication, use of alternative wireless devices for real-time medication monitoring, and adherence support [17].

mHealth could be an interesting solution to provide punctual and continuous monitoring to mothers and future mothers, as it is a rapid and remote "touchpoint" with healthcare professionals to communicate feelings and moods.

Recent studies indeed suggest that the potential for mHealth tools to improve access to stepped mental health care for women with either perinatal depression or anxiety is now beginning to be realized [18].

This framework led to the idea to design and develop two digital tools within a public health service, with the aim of promptly intercepting cases of PD and offering a first treatment intervention.

3   The Bluebelly System

This project, called "Bluebelly", is developed with the aim of combining active psychological treatment and addressing continuity of care during the perinatal period to realize the potential of mHealth. An increasing number of Apps and websites for pregnant women and mothers are also now used as a source of information, despite research showing that information and how it is reported is often incomplete and inaccurate. A valid source of information should be provided by healthcare professionals to women, to avoid disinformation and unwarranted fears. Therefore, the project includes three different parts:

- *the website* (www.pensarepositivo.org/), where all the most important information - approved by the Istituto Superiore di Sanità Italiano (ISS) - are collected: the perinatal period and its related facts, problems, advice; information about the app and its use; material about the project, to reach easily help if needed and how to find it not far from home.
- *the Bluebelly mobile app*, downloadable from Apple store and Google Play store for the most popular smartphones' operative systems; the app was mainly created for the administration of the EPDS Scale, but also to ease

the management and the organization of the EPDS paper questionnaires. Moreover, the app eases finding information, help, and to follow the pregnancy. The app is designed to be used by as many people as possible, so it can be enjoyed in Italian and English.

- *the Bluebelly web-app*, accessible only to medical operators, allows to check the results of collected EPDS and automatically generates a warning in case of values outside the norms. Based on stringent GDPR regulations, the web app obscures most of the data so that privacy is always guaranteed. In case there is a need to intervene, the medical staff can request the telephone number with a few clicks in order to contact the mother.

In order to develop an ergonomic environment for searching information, EPDS gathering, and visualization, the User-Centered Design (UCD) approach has been implemented. User-Centered Design (UCD) is the commonly used approach to develop products and solutions by involving the human perspective (the users) in all the steps of the process [19]. Users (and stakeholders) have been involved since the first steps of project ideation; this allows the creation of a system that is fully tailor-made for users' needs. Research and design sessions for the website, web app, and mobile app were conducted by the TEDH group, from the Design Department of Politecnico di Milano, supported by psychiatrist Dr. A. Lora and psychologist Dr. S. Ciervo from ASST Lecco. The project has been divided into five main steps:

- Project Research: to identify requirements and concepts, and develop a first mockup of the website and apps.
- Focus groups with stakeholders: to test the system and find limits, difficulties, and suggestions from the direct users.
- System development: all three parts of the system were developed.
- Quantitative analysis: by means of digital tools, the developed system is tested in order to verify accessibility and usability.
- User test: the system is used to collect data from selected and limited users in order to test everything in an environment similar to the final one.

3.1   Project Research

The project research phase starts with the study of possible stakeholders. This allows clarifying which are the main users and which are the secondary or indirect ones. Main users correspond to people that use directly the system; these can be divided into two groups:

- Pregnant women and new mothers: they are the users of the mobile app and the website. Mothers would like to access the website for gathering homogeneous and certified information regarding pregnancy and the puerperium. They use the mobile application, as suggested by physicians, in order to insert EPDS ad Whooley scale based on the timing suggested by health professionals. The mobile application is also a tool that allows the women to keep in contact with their pregnancy, check the growth of the baby, and access a session where they can ask for help at the nearest center.

– Healthcare professionals: they are the users of the web app. They would like to access inserted EPDS in order to check warnings and the status of every woman. They need to access also private data such as the telephone number in order to contact the woman in case of EPDS values are out of the norm.

Secondary users are instead people that come into contact with the system, but without using it directly; an example is a "new dad" searching for information about feeding time who accesses the website. The system needs to be developed also with secondary users in mind, in order to optimize the experience. In fact, optimizing the experience avoids frustration, in a difficult period such as the one of the puerperium.

The definition of main and secondary users allows for defining the features of the system from different points of view.

3.2 Mockup and Prototype

Designing an app means bringing an idea to reality. There are four main steps in the development phase before starting coding:

1. Sketch: a low-fidelity freehand drawing of how the app should look like.
2. Wireframe: the drawing of the overall structure of the app. This allows the understanding of all the functionality; e.g. what happens when a button has been clicked.
3. Mockup: a medium-fidelity visual representation of how the app will look. It gives the user an impression of the final product.
4. Prototype: a high-fidelity representation of the UI and functionality. It focuses on interactions and shows also how the app will work.

As described above, the mockup is a detailed outline of the appearance of a mobile app. The difference between an app mockup and a wireframe is that the first one is more detailed and contains an almost defined design system with colors, layout, images, and typos... There are many advantages to creating an app design mockup. The first one is that it gives you an opportunity to make revisions to the final appearance app without spending time coding. Another benefit of creating a mockup is that it allows you to explain precisely what you want from stakeholders. This is essential to rally your team in the early stages of the app development process. A mockup is the best way to give everyone a clear vision of what the final app will look like and how it will function.

By means of all these steps, designers can understand the usability of the app and validate it by means of Heuristics [20]. In the project, different mockups have been created via FIGMA software. We decided to build different mockups in order to test different Design Systems, layouts, and also features with all the stakeholders. During the project, two mobile app mockups and one for the website have been created.

These mockups have been used in the focus group in order to gather information regarding usability, but also aesthetics, and interaction Fig. 1 shows the two main screens in the app: the dashboard and the question screen. The mockup implements also two different ways for login: a standard layout and a conversational layout which is a simulated chat to interact with the users. Focus Groups and user tests have been run in order to understand also the capability of conversational layout and clarify if they generate a more comfortable feeling for the users.

3.3 Focus Groups

Three different focus groups were organized to test the first prototype of the website and the app. Most of the stakeholders (expectant mothers, women who had recently given birth, and healthcare workers) were involved in the focus groups, in order to extract opinions and feelings from every possible future user.

We collected information from a total of 19 expectant mothers and women who had recently given birth; 17 healthcare workers (midwives, psychologists, and psychiatrists). In every focus group, a team of moderators composed of 1 engineer, 1 designer, and 1 psychologist was present. All the participants filled out a survey to investigate the relation they have with technologies; this allowed us to verify the level of digital literacy, in order to better understand the suggestions and errors reported during the focus group.

The result of the survey shows that the group participants are used to smartphones, mainly because most of the group use social networks and app daily (84%). There isn't a significant difference in this data between the population of healthcare workers and the mothers.

Pregnant women are users that are more familiar with apps (75%), and they are almost entirely in an age between 26 and 35 years old.

The opinions regarding the website and app helped define the best structure and form of the content. Other received suggestions are about the website on the clarity of the text, the structure of the content, how to make it more readable, and what information could be the most wanted. For the app, by means of FIGMA mockup, login and EPDS administration have been tested.

3.4 User Tests

All the advice acquired during focus groups and questionnaires has been used to redefine information, components, interactions, and UI inside the website and the mobile application. This allows the creation of a new mockup to test internally mainly with psychologists and designers. The new mockups have then been used for creating prototypes with most of the interactions, making it possible to test them with real users. The tests have been accomplished in two different steps:

– on real users via direct observation (ghosting); the designer's team observes the user's behavior while using the website and the app and tries to get information from the latter's expressions and speeches. At the end of the test, an interview is also made.

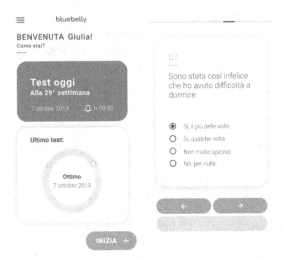

Fig. 1. Example of the main screen and question screen developed for the mockup

- with software tools. Two different software have been used: maze.co [21] allows the remote testing of prototypes and rapidly collects user insights across teams and creates better user experiences; visualeye.design [22] and VAS 3m [23], two software for visual attention detection which simulate eye-tracking studies by means of machine learning algorithm with 93% accuracy.

Two main task have been analyzed by maze.co:

- first-time sign-in;
- EPDS administration.

The first task has been analyzed in order to understand which solution between test sign-in and conversational sign-in fits better for this particular app. EPDS administration has been tested to measure the average time taken to fill the EPDS questionnaire and the two Whooley's questions. This average time depends on the question's text length but also on the interaction for the answer selection. Maze.co allows to automatically collect information regarding the interaction with app screens (number of clicks, the position of the clicks, miss-clicks, correctness of the path, time for the screen...), but gives also the possibility to implement ad-hoc questions for gathering other data. For both tasks, we add two ten-level Likert scale questions:

1. First-time sign-in task:
   - Taking into account that the required data are the bare minimum, how easy do you think creating an account is?
   - Do you think that the conversational mode can make it easier to interact with the app, especially during first use?

2. EPDS administration task:
   - Taking into account that the text and the questions shown are standard and cannot be changed, how easy do you think it is to insert the test?
   - How long do you feel about the test administration?

These questions give the possibility to clarify some doubts that arose mainly during the implementation of the mobile application.

VAS software like 3M VAS and VisualEye allows to speed up the test times on visual attention that usually involves the use of an eye tracker, and therefore requires a lot of time and subjects. These software have the capability to simulate an eye tracker thanks to thousand of data used for training the algorithm. The software are able to compute visual attention maps (a color map that indicates where the user focuses most - e.g. Fig. 2), and a clarity index that gets information from the app screen and computes how much it is clear to understand, or if there are too many information, colors, text... Figure 5 shows an example of clarity analysis done on two different versions of the dashboard screen.

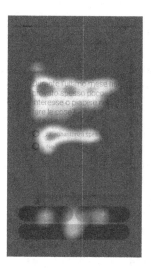

Fig. 2. An example of a visual attention map generated on an app screen.

4   Results

In this chapter, the results of the analysis, both with users and software, are reported. Focus groups and questionnaires gave the possibility to collect different information about the website and the mobile app. The need for implementing the web app for generating alerts and displaying data came after the focus groups; however, being an app for healthcare professionals only, it was developed with them to their specifications and for this reason, it was not analyzed in the focus groups. Focus group participants pointed out that the website has excellent and useful content, but is too long and dispersive. The mothers stressed the importance of a simple structure to consult, and the need to insert a search option. Furthermore, it was requested not only the inclusion information related to mental health problems but also information regarding pregnancy in general (breastfeeding, visits ...).

The website is the core of the project, being the collection of the most relevant information and notions; for this reason, thanks to the advice of the users, we restructured the website. As one enters the website, a pop-up about COVID-19 appears. There is a dedicated page about maternity, and perinatal periods related to the pandemic situation. All the organized sections refer to the website of Istituto Superiore Sanità [24]. The menu is divided into three main sections: Becoming a parent; Emotional well-being; Get support.

In the first section, all the main topics of the perinatal journey are described, together with all the findings that could create anxiety or insecurities in the parents.

In the second section, a description of conditions, symptoms, and feelings that should be monitored or, on the other hand, are exactly normal, are described in detail.

The third section is dedicated to the description of the various supports women and families can count on, and centers where one can find healthcare professionals, contacts, and main information.

The app was mainly created to administer the EPDS questionnaire to women. In order to be used by as many people as possible, the app was developed in both Italian and English. The fundamental idea is to install the app during the first meeting with a healthcare professional; then the app asks women to insert recursively the EPDS questionnaire. This method is the gold standard that should be implemented in hospitals, but - for reasons of timing and logistics - it is almost never carried out correctly. Usually, the EPDS questionnaire is given only once, a couple of days after the baby is born. It is rarely given during pregnancy or during the first year. This means that many cases of perinatal depression go undiagnosed. Using the mobile app can solve this problem. In fact, gynecologists or midwives are in charge to present and inform women about the app. They will explain how the app works and for whom the results are intended. The app is used to fill the EPDS at least 5 times in 10 months, and the scheduled timing of each questionnaire is automatically set in relation to the peak of risks for depression symptoms in the perinatal period. Figure 4 shows the entire system service blueprint. As described above, at the first visit the gynecologist or midwives introduce the system to the pregnant woman and give her a one-time code to enable the app; she can access the website to gather information and access the link for downloading and installing the application on an iOS or Android smartphone. At the first access, the app requires a login. The login phase is carried on by means of a conversational agent that follows the woman in all the steps. The one-time code is mandatory to create an account; this was a very important aspect discussed with the medical stakeholders; limiting access to the system only to users who have received the code allows to avoid system congestion and gives operators the possibility to correctly view the collected EPDSs. The EPDSs are automatically labeled with three different colors:

- green, if less than 9 and different from 0;
- yellow, if between 9 and 11;
- red, if more than 11 or the answer to the last question is different from the fourth.

Depending on the history of the woman and the value of the EPDS, the healthcare professional can then call her to ascertain the state of her mental health. The web app allows the physicians to access the woman's personal data in order to contact her and shows the answers to the last questionnaire inserted. The standard schedule for the EPDSs is related to the expected delivery date; the first EPDS is inserted when the app is installed; then a new questionnaire is requested thirty days before delivery, ten days after delivery, and then every three months until the tenth month. The time schedule for the EPDSs is automatically changed based on the previous EPDS inserted. Figure 3 shows the modified schedule based on the previous EPDS result. All the data are recorded on the cloud (by means of Firebase cloud service) in an anonymized form. Only when it is necessary to contact the user, personal data are correlated by code and shown to health care personnel. The system in this way is GDPR compliant and has been verified by the data protection officer of the Politecnico di Milano.

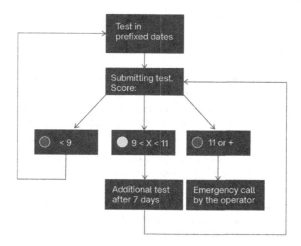

Fig. 3. EPDS schedule related to the score.

The left image in Fig. 1 shows the final dashboard. In the bottom part of the image, there is a circle that represents the feedback on the evaluation of the last EPDS inserted. Previous research [25] mentions the importance of feedback in this kind of app to promote and ensure the engagement of the users, but there is a need to explore more factors that influence it and the effect they could create in the users. During focus groups and conversations with midwives and psychologists, they were worried about the feelings or the implications that "score feedback" shown at the end of the questionnaire could arise.

In particular, a numeric score would not have an immediate meaning if not properly communicated, and could impoverish the perception of the test. Users could try to focus on beating the previous score, or they could lose the reliability in completing the answers [25]. The same effect, or worse, would be created if given "good or bad" feedback. Those results could be interpreted as a judgment on the person, or on her doing.

Everyone in the focus group agreed on the awareness that a user has during the test, implying that the feedback would be only a confirmation of what the user feels. Nonetheless, the feedback most likely could not be a surprise, everyone agreed on being extremely careful with the response after the test. The main idea of this feedback is to offer a hint, a constructive approach to keep the users engaged: in this way they know the results are controlled and checked by their professionals, and they know that there is always someone available to help or simply to listen. If the EPDS has an intermediate score (between 9 and 11), the users are informed that they will have to complete soon (in a few days) a new questionnaire; if it is over 11, the users are informed that they will have to complete a new questionnaire the day after and they will be reached out in the next days by a caregiver. If the results are under 9, the users receive a simple message which informs them that the next date for the EPDS follows the standard scheduling.

5 Discussion

As described in the previous chapter, all the parts of the system have been tested both with user tests and quantitative tests. The quantitative tests were executed with maze.co on 5 Italian users and 25 international users (women aged between 22 and 35). Maze.co allows the collection of data via screens, Likert scale-based questions, and final notes from the users.

For the first-use sign-in analysis, we found out that all the users succeeded in creating the account, with an average time of 4 min and 37 s for the entire procedure.

The most complicated part seems the estimated date of delivery selection and notification time; this was underlined by the timing for each screen and from the number of misclicks on the calendar and on the clock. It seems that the input method is not easy to use, despite being the standard for Android calendars and alarm clocks. The use of a conversational login interface was appreciated with 89% of positive responses; the user feels more familiar with and easy to use this method, as also underlined in the focus groups.

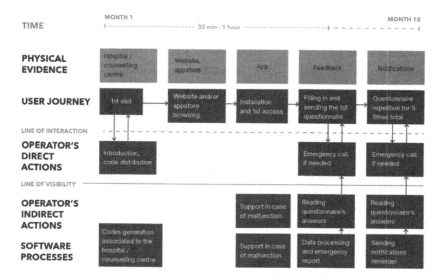

Fig. 4. Service blueprint for the entire system. The blueprint shows all the steps for using all three components of the system.

The selection of the notification time is considered very useful by all 30 users who responded to the test (Likert score average greater than 8).

The second task analyzed was the EPDS administration. The app provides two ways to start the test: by clicking on the fab button with the plus or by clicking on the card with the reminder for the next test. The success rate also for this task was 100%; all users were able to complete the insertion of the test, although some of them did not immediately understand which button to press to start EPDS (some misclick on the first screen).

From the analysis of the taps/clicks, it appears that the app is very usable; each screen has only a few interactions, which are suggested by a different contrast of colors and shadows. This allows users to better identify the possible buttons on which they can interact by reducing misclicks to a minimum. The presence of the "back" button and the possibility to go back to modify the data entered at login, facilitates the correction of any errors.

The administration of the EPDS questionnaire does not foresee a temporary interruption and resume, because this could affect the results. For this reason, to satisfy the requests of women to be able to stop the compilation, a back button has been added that allows users to return to the dashboard. This proved to be very useful because often the new mothers have to stop everything they are doing to meet the needs of their newborns.

During the analysis, we evaluated the Screen Usability Score (SCUS). The score, reported by maze.co, reflects how easy it is for a user to perform a given task (mission) with the prototype. A high usability score indicates the design will be easy to use and intuitive. This score goes from 0 to 100 and usability points are lost when a user:

- clicks on another hotspot than the expected one. This means the user got off the expected path(s), which is a live product results in frustration or a lost user;
- gives up on a task. This is a clear indication something isn't right and should be checked;
- misclicks. It's common that in a prototype not every area is clickable, but a misclick in a live product would take the user to an "incorrect" page which leads to the first point;
- spends too much time on a screen.

For every percent of users dropping off or giving up, 1 usability point is lost.

Not every misclick is an indication of a wrong action so for every percent of a misclick, 0.5 usability points are lost.

Time on screen is expressed in average duration and the lost point are:

- From 0 to 15 s: no usability points lost
- From 15 to 45 s: 1 usability point lost every 2 s
- From 45 s and on: 10 usability points lost

These timing values are optimized based on the length of the questions to be read. Here is the SCUS formula:

$$SCUS = MAX(0, 100 - (DOR * dW) - (MCR * mW) - (MIN(10, MAX(0, \frac{AVGD - 5}{2})))))$$

Which has these variables:

- SCUS for Screen Usability Score;
- DOR for drop-off and bounce rate;
- dW for DOR weight; The dW equals 1 point for every drop-off/bounce;
- MCR for misclick rate;
- mW for MCR weight; The mW equals 0.5 points for every misclick;
- AVGD for Average Duration in seconds.

The main task (EPDS administration) gets a SCUS total usability score of 84: a very good starting point for a new application. The value 84 mainly depends on the misclick on the main page, the only page where there is more information. This is underlined also by means of the VAS analysis. Examples of VAS results are reported in Fig. 2 and Fig. 5. Figure 2 shows the visual attention (red is a hot point, blue is a cold one) on-screen elements for a single EPDS question. The color map shows great attention to the question and answers, less on the navigation button below, and no attention to the status on the top. This underlines that the screen is well-defined because the question gets most of the attention without distraction. The top bar is an Instagram-based stories bar that underlines the completeness of the number of answers filled in. The top bar starts to get visual attention after the user filled some questions when the users need to know how much time he needs to complete the questionnaire.

Figure 5 shows the clear difference between two different versions of the dashboard on the main screen. The image on the left uses fewer colors and elements than the right image. The analysis of the two screens underlines a loss of clarity of 7 points in the screen with more elements and colors.

The notification process to request the insertion of a new EPDS is a very delicate part of the system: it is very important that, when a notification appears, the user chooses to open it. During focus groups, pregnant women and new mothers underlined the importance of not to over-stress themselves with many notifications. For this reason, the system is programmed in order to send the notification once a day, at the pre-selected time, and repeat the notification the day after only if the woman does not insert the EPDS. The sentence used for the notification is very important in order to convince the user of the importance of inserting the test, without pressing too hard, so as not to inadvertently change the result. The sentence is a way to create confidence and reassure that the test won't take too much time but only a few minutes. During the focus groups, we tested different sentences and feedback with real users in order to understand which one could fit better in this use case. The notification needs to be personal, informal, and inviting; here is the final result: "(Name of the user), how are you? It's time to fill in the test, it will take only 3 min."

Answering the requirements of women, opening the main menu of the app, the user could see an icon with the mom's belly, and on the side her name with the reminder of what month she (and her baby) are in and the selected name of the baby. In fact, customizing the application allows for creating a greater involvement with the user, in order to have her more willing to continue the path and to insert the EPDS when required.

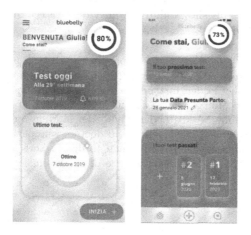

Fig. 5. Clarity difference between two UI versions

The system described in the previous chapter has been tested before by a small number of caregivers (ten psychologists and midwives from ASST Lecco - Italy). After this first bench test, the system move to production and was tested with real users in the restricted area of ASST Lecco, before being released to all health organizations taking part in the project.

6   Conclusion

Preliminary tests carried out on the developed system first only with health personnel, and subsequently with some volunteer mothers have given excellent results. The pre-tests have in fact made it possible to optimize both the UI part of the application and the structure of the site in order to make them more usable and complete.

The app is now used daily for the administration of EPDS in the Lecco area. During use, a new need has emerged: being able to insert the way in which the baby came into the world (natural birth, cesarean...), as it is often related to perinatal depression. Given the optimized structure of the application, it was possible to easily add it as an application update to the store, without invalidating the data already collected.

The app continuously collects usage times and any errors and crashes generated. This allows for checking both the stability of the entire system and how it is used by new users.

The web app proved to be stable and clear for healthcare personnel, as it was developed in a minimal way as a list of inserted EPDSs. Healthcare personnel only access the EPDS in their area and are able to immediately check, through the color code, which user needs an intervention. Thanks to the user-centered approach, based on the involvement of stakeholders from the initial stages, the system is still stable and usable after 6 months of use. The number of errors found is minimal (and largely depends on the use of old Android versions that struggle to support the app). As for the timing of use, the SCUS index remains stable at around 80. This shows high usability despite the different form factors of the supported devices.

Acknowledgments. This work has been part of the BLUES project funded by the Ministry of Health, provided by Lombardy Region, and which involved, in addition to Lecco Hospital as project leader, further nine Lombard health institutes (Ats Brianza, Asst di Vimercate and Monza, Papa Giovani XXIII hospital and Asst Bergamo Est, Niguarda hospital in Milan, Asst Rhodense and Asst in Mantova). The authors would like to thank all the moms, psychologists, and doctors who participated in the focus groups for their willingness and patience, and to dr. A. Lora and dr. S. Ciervo for supervising the research. A big thanks also to dr. R. Sironi for the help during the focus groups.

References

1. GBDC Network: Global Burden of Disease Study 2016 (GBD 2016) Causes of Death and Nonfatal Causes Mapped to ICD Codes. Institute for Health Metrics and Evaluation (IHME) (2015)
2. Layton, H., Owais, S., Savoy, C.D., Van Lieshout, R.J.: Depression, anxiety, and mother-infant bonding in women seeking treatment for postpartum depression before and during the COVID-19 pandemic. J. Clin. Psychiatry **82** (2021)
3. Breese McCoy, S.J.: Postpartum depression: an essential overview for the practitioner. South. Med. J. **104**, 128–132 (2011)

4. Grussu, P., Lega, I., Quatraro, R.M., Donati, S.: Perinatal mental health around the world: priorities for research and service development in Italy. BJPsych Int. **17**, 8–10 (2020)
5. Yonkers, K.A., et al.: Onset and persistence of postpartum depression in an inner-city maternal health clinic system. Am. J. Psychiatry **158**(11), 1856–1863 (2001)
6. Lanz, R.G., Bert, S.C., Jacobs, B.K.: Depression among a sample of first-time adolescent and adult mothers. J. Child Adolesc Psychiatr. Nurs. **22**(4), 194–202 (2009)
7. Rahman, A., et al.: Interventions for common perinatal mental disorders in women in low- and middle-income countries: a systematic review and meta-analysis. Bull World Health Organ. **91**, 593–601 (2013)
8. ISTAT: Demography in figures. http://demo.istat.it/. Accessed 06 June 2022
9. Cox, J.L., Holden, J.M., Sagovsky, R.: Detection of postnatal depression: development of the 10-item Edinburgh post-natal depression scale. Br. J. Psychiatry **150**, 782–786 (1987)
10. National Collaborating Centre for Mental Health: Antenatal and postnatal mental health: the NICE guideline on clinical management and service guidance. British Psychological Society (2007)
11. World Health Organization: Thinking healthy: a manual for psychosocial management of perinatal depression, WHO generic field-trial version 1.0 (2015)
12. Alhusen, J.L., Alvarez, C.: Perinatal depression. Nurse Pract. **41**(5), 50–55 (2016)
13. Davenport, M.H., Meyer, S., Meah, V.L., Strynadka, M.C., Khurana, R.: Moms are not OK: COVID-19 and maternal mental health. Front. Glob. Women's Health **1** (2020)
14. Saccone, G., et al.: Psychological impact of COVID-19 in pregnant women. Am. J. Obstet. Gynecol. **222**(2), 293–295 (2020)
15. Olla, P., Shimskey, C.: mHealth taxonomy: a literature survey of mobile health applications. Heal. Technol. **4**(4), 299–308 (2015). https://doi.org/10.1007/s12553-014-0093-8
16. Van Heerden, A., Tomlinson, M., Swartz, L.: Point of care in your pocket: a research agenda for the field of m-health. Bull. World Health Organ. **90**(5), 393–394 (2012)
17. Tomlinson, M., Rotheram-Borus, M.J., Swartz, L., Tsai, A.C.: Scaling up mHealth: where is the evidence? PLoS Med. **10**(2) (2013)
18. Hussain-Shamsy, N., Shah, A., Vigod, S.N., Zaheer, J., Seto, E.: Mobile health for perinatal depression and anxiety: scoping review. J. Med. Internet Res. **22**(4) (2020)
19. LUMA Institute: Innovating for People Handbook of Human-Centered Design Methods (2012)
20. Machado Neto, O., Pimentel, M.D.G.: Heuristics for the assessment of interfaces of mobile devices. In: Proceedings of the 19th Brazilian Symposium on Multimedia and the Web, pp. 93–96 (2013)
21. Maze.co. https://maze.co/. Accessed 06 June 2022
22. VisaulEye. https://www.visualeyes.design/. Accessed 03 Mar 2022
23. VAS 3M. https://vas.3m.com/. Accessed 10 June 2022
24. Istituto Superiore di Sanità: Epicentro - L'epidemiologia per la sanità pubblica. https://www.epicentro.iss.it/. Accessed 10 June 2022
25. Doherty, K., et al.: A mobile app for the self-report of psychological well-being during pregnancy (BrightSelf): qualitative design study. JMIR Mental Health **5**(4) (2018)

Investigating the Perception of the Elderly Population About Comfort, Safety and Security When Using Active Modes of Transport

Soraia Felício[1]([⊠]), Joana Hora[1], Marta Campos Ferreira[1,2], Diogo Abrantes[3], Fábio Luna[1], Jorge Silva[4], Miguel Coimbra[2,3], and Teresa Galvão[1,2]

[1] Faculty of Engineering of the University of Porto,
Rua Dr. Roberto Frias, s/n, 4200-465 Porto, Portugal
up201900015@up.pt
[2] INESC TEC - Institute for Systems and Computer Engineering,
Technology and Science, R. Dr. Roberto Frias s/n, Porto 4200-465, Portugal
[3] Faculty of Sciences of the University of Porto,
Rua do Campo Alegre, s/n, 4169-007 Porto, Portugal
[4] Bosch Security Systems, R. Pardala, Zona Ind. de Ovar,
Estrada Nacional 109 Aptd. 653, Aveiro, Portugal

Abstract. Promoting active modes of transport, such as walking and cycling, has a positive impact on environmental sustainability and the health and well-being of citizens. This study explores the elderly population's perception of comfort, safety and security when using active modes of transport. It begins with a systematic review of the literature considering research works that relate to active travel, the elderly population, and random forest. Then a questionnaire was applied to 653 participants and the results were analyzed. This analysis consisted of using statistics to evaluate the socio-demographic profile, the preferences regarding the use of active modes of this population, and the importance given to each dimension: comfort, safety, distance, and time, comparing these indicators through the Wilcoxon Rank Sum test and the Random Forest algorithm. The results showed that people over 56 years old walk as much as younger people. Furthermore, the importance given by this group of people to indicators referring to active modes is related to safety and security, distance, time, and comfort. The statistical results of the Wilcoxon Rank Sum test indicate the most important indicators: Adequate Travel Distance & Time and Existence of Commercial Areas by age group [0–55], and Absence of Allergenics and Existence of Green Areas by age group [56+]. Finally, the Random Forest algorithm provides the relative importance for both age groups, [0–55] and [56+], where the indicators that stand out in the [56+] age group, which is the focus of our study, are air quality, adequate travel distance & time, adequate crowd density, adequate thermal sensation, absence of allergenic, good street illumination level, adequate traffic volume, and adequate noise level.

Keywords: Active modes · Comfort · Safety · Security · Descriptive statistic · Wilcoxon Rank Sum test · Random Forest · Erdely

© ICST Institute for Computer Sciences, Social Informatics and Telecommunications Engineering 2023
Published by Springer Nature Switzerland AG 2023. All Rights Reserved
A. Cunha et al. (Eds.): MobiHealth 2022, LNICST 484, pp. 304–321, 2023.
https://doi.org/10.1007/978-3-031-32029-3_26

1   Introduction

The improvement of urban mobility is a concern regarding the growth of cities. There is an incentive to use less polluting means of transport, such as active modes, which include cycling and walking, for the sustainable development of cities.

Several studies show that safety, security, and comfort are decisive factors in the choice of mode of transport [3,18] and [13]. With the lack of perception of safety, security, and comfort among the main issues that deter people from bicycling [16], and walking [4]. The importance of these perceptions is even more pressing in the case of more vulnerable populations, such as the elderly [9].

The goal of this study is to evaluate the users' preferences related to comfort, safety, and security in urban mobility for users above 56 years old that use active modes.

The research questions of this work are described below.

1. What indicators related to the perception of comfort, safety, and security are more important for people above 56 years old?
2. What is the relative importance attributed to the indicators on the use of active modes by the age group over 56 years old?

The methodology followed in this work includes the following three steps: 1) systematic review of the literature related to the use of active modes by the elderly population; pre-processing of collected data from a questionnaire applied over a period of one year to understand the perception of comfort, safety and security related to active travel and a socio-demographic analysis; 2) statistical analysis to understand the differences among a set of attributes related to active travel applied to different ages; 3) descriptive statistics for an overview of all responses related to the importance given to each indicator, Wilcoxon Rank Sum test analysis to find out which indicators related to the perception of comfort, safety and security are more important for people above 56 years old, and the relative importance given to each indicator by this age group using the Random Forest algorithm.

This study uses the dataset obtained through an online questionnaire to understand the importance of comfort, safety, and security of people who use active modes of transport in urban areas. The dataset includes the responses from 653 participants. However, we used a sample of this questionnaire with participants above 56 years old, i.e., 18.07% of the population studied.

Several statistical analyzes were carried out to deepen the understanding of the data collected through the questionnaire. Sociodemographic data was evaluated using descriptive statistics, also the Wilcoxon Rank Sum tests were performed and the Random Forest algorithm was used to assess the relative importance attributed to each indicator within a group of people over 56 years of age.

2   Literature Review

This section includes a systematic review of the literature that was conducted to identify other research studies related to this work. This review follows the extensive review conducted in [3], but with a focus on the elderly population.

The literature search was conducted on the Scopus database, using the following queries: *TITLE-ABS-KEY ("active modes" AND "elderly")*; *TITLE-ABS-KEY ("active modes" AND "elderly" AND "random forest")*; and *TITLE-ABS-KEY ("active modes" AND "random forest")*. The research carried out resulted in 22 documents, some of which are not concerning this work. Thus, we highlight the most relevant ones that are presented below, which bring a comprehensive view of active modes, almost all related to the elderly. Most of the articles disregarded dealt with issues restricted to the medical field. There is an article that deals with security and presents a solution related to the infrastructure of the streets. In addition, there are two articles that are more than 10 years old, so they were also disregarded. Therefore, of the total of 22 articles, 13 articles were disregarded and 9 articles were included in this study. The second search query did not return any documents. The third search query resulted in 4 documents.

In this paper, only the two most relevant articles on transportation mean to use the Random Forest algorithm because of its relation to our study, which involves active modes in urban areas.

The authors [10] investigated walking behavior for discretionary and mandatory trips at different distances and ages. They achieved some results that reveal that people under the age of 14 are more likely to choose to walk on mandatory trips over 2400 m, those aged 25–44 years old or over 65 are less likely to choose to walk on mandatory trips with distances of 2000–2400 m and 800–1200 m, respectively. These findings are almost different on discretionary trips. Compared to other age groups, people aged 15–24 years are less likely to choose to walk on discretionary trips with 800–1200 m. In addition, in distances covered from 1200 m to 1600 m, the elderly are more likely to opt for walking compared to other age groups.

Another study [14] aimed to investigate and compare factors that affect the choice of active modes of transport by the elderly in the pre-and post-COVID-19 outbreak and evaluated changes in their active mobility behavior. The results indicate that in the post-outbreak the average duration of walking per week decreased from 59 to 29 min; while the share of this transport mode increased from 40% to 65%. Also, the proportion of bicycles and the average duration of cycling per week increased from 9% to 18% and from 9 to 15 min, respectively. In addition, travel frequency, bicycle ownership, quality of walking and cycling routes, safety at intersections, neighborhood security, vegetation, traffic calming, CBD accommodation, and accessibility of public transport have positive effects on the choice of active modes of transport by elderly; while trip distance and vehicle ownership affect negatively. The results reveal that older people have resorted to cycling on most of their long journeys during the pandemic because it is not subject to traffic restrictions.

Examples of contributions using active travel are the works of [1,5] and [19] that explored the physical activity related to the transport activity. These studies can encourage public health and transport policies so that people reach daily recommendations of physical activity using active modes. The authors [5] and [19] directly surveyed the elderly population.

Following the same bias, the works of [11] and [17] are exploratory research. The first work explored studies published up to December 2019 on the relationship between active commuting and depression among adults and older adults, suggesting that active commuting can be used as physical activity to protect against depression. The second work explores 20 articles researching studies on bicycle safety that include a description of how cycling exposure was measured, and what exposure units were used, such as distance, time, trips. Retrospective studies indicated a higher incidence of accidents for men compared to women and a higher risk of injury for cyclists aged 50 years and over. There was a lack of data for cyclists under the age of 18. The risk of bicycle accidents increased when riding in the dark. Wearing visible clothing or a helmet, or having more cycling experience did not reduce the risk of being involved in an accident. Better awareness of cyclist drivers and more interaction between car drivers and cyclists and well-maintained bicycle-specific infrastructure should improve bicycle safety.

Another contribution concerning the well-being of the elderly population is the study [12] that evaluates the fundamental linkages between subjective well-being or happiness and transport mobility-travel behavior of the elderly population, based on data from the Supplement on Disability and Use of Time for 2009, which specifically targeted senior couples with an average age of 68, using the scores to a set of satisfaction questions about life, health, memory, finances, and marriage, latent class clusters are estimated, which leads to four distinct clusters of respondents that depend on the degree of happiness in each of the satisfaction questions. The results show that respondents who engage in active modes (walking-bicycling) at the home, socialize, and enjoy better mobility also report higher levels of subjective well-being leading to a better quality of life. Additionally, the model outcomes also show that illness and pain are related to lower well-being and that quality of life in older age is correlated to mobility.

On the other hand, with a focus on the sustainable environment, the study of [8] was motivated by the promotion of low-carbon and active modes of transportation, due to the impacts of negative health and environment by the predominance of automobile dependency on North America. This study explores the potential for e-bikes to support independent mobility and active aging among the older adult population in Canada's auto-dependent context, according to a conceptual framework for older adult mobility.

They used qualitative methods to gather perceptual and experiential data from 17 community stakeholders and 37 older adults in the Region of Waterloo, Ontario. The findings highlight the importance of cycling life histories, social connection, and physical limitations to adopting cycling later in life. Specific individual and structural factors were discussed in relation to e-bike adoption including facilitators such as increased convenience, reduced physical exertion, reduced reliance on a vehicle, and fun. Barriers included cycling infrastructure and road safety, regulation, and stigmatization barriers. E-bikes as a more convenient and supportive mode of transit for older adults are discussed alongside the importance of e-bikes as a replacement for traditional bicycles in a subset of this population.

The authors [6] define the Random Forest technique as a supervised learning algorithm. The "forest" it builds is an ensemble of independent decision trees aimed to assess the importance of the variables and those that most contributed to the model's prediction. However, the technique loses the precision of the interpretation, as it is not possible to analyze all the generated trees, but rather a set of important variables based on them. In the end, it results in a graph of important variables showing, within all the trees analyzed, which variables stood out the most. It is in this graph of importance that we are interested in our study.

The studies of [6] and [15] use the Random Forest algorithm regarding the active modes (walking and bike). The first study aims to examine how volume traffic and speed limits affect walking trips in a medium-sized Brazilian city, São Carlos city in São Paulo state, Brazil. The second study addresses people's willingness to go shopping by bike or kick-scooter and to transport lightweight goods in cities with low maturity for cycling and scooting applied in the two largest cities of Brazil (São Paulo and Rio de Janeiro) and Portugal (Lisbon and Porto). These researches contribute to understanding mobility behavior changes and identifying barriers that affect the use of active modes and also present some policy recommendations to encourage the use of these means of transport as more sustainable.

3   Methodology

The research methodology adopted in this study is shown in Fig. 1.

This study uses the data obtained from an online questionnaire. A process of data cleansing was performed on the responses obtained with the questionnaire to ensure that the dataset used in the study is complete and consistent.

The dataset was then used to perform a socio-demographic characterization of respondents. The socio-demographic characterization included an overview of the following features: gender, age group, educational level, nationality, and country of residence.

The descriptive statistics display the travel habits of respondents regarding two active modes of transport (walking and bicycle) for seven age groups. The descriptive statistics also portray the importance given by respondents to a set of thirteen indicators considering two main age groups: under 55 and over 56 years old.

A non-parametric statistical test comparing two paired groups, the Wilcoxon Rank Sum test, showed the most important indicators for both age groups ([0–55] and [56+]).

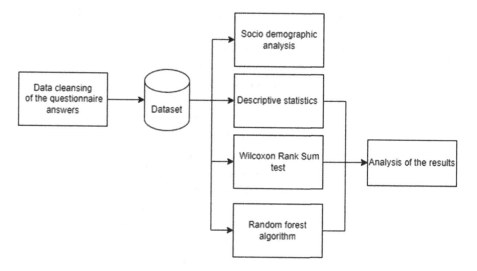

Fig. 1. Overview of the methodology adopted in this study.

Next, the random forest algorithm was applied to the dataset for the same purpose as the previous test, ranking the importance of the thirteen indicators. The random forest analysis considered the same age groups as the previous analyses for the same indicators (i.e., under 55 and over 56). For each age group, the random forest algorithm returned the relative importance of the thirteen indicators (thus ranking the indicators from most important to least important).

The analysis of results aimed to extract the main findings from the previous steps, namely regarding the identification of the perceived importance of each indicator by each age group related to the research questions.

4   Data

The data set used in this study was gathered from an online survey, conducted between August 2021 and August 2022. The questionnaire included a set of questions to provide the socio-demographic context of respondents. These include age range, nationality, country of residence, gender, educational level, employment situation, and the number of children.

The questionnaire continued by asking respondents to rate the importance they attribute to a set of thirteen indicators considering their personal experience when using active modes of transport. To classify the importance of each indicator, the respondents used a Likert scale, where 1 referred to not important and 5 to very important. Table 1 shows the set of indicators organized in the following dimensions: Distance & Time, Comfort, and Safety & Security. The identification of this set of indicators and dimensions follows the work published in [2], which evolved with further studies and literature review.

Table 1. Indicators used in the questionnaire organized by dimension.

Dimension	Indicators
Distance & time	Adequate Travel Distance & Time
Comfort	Absence of Allergenics
	Air Quality
	Adequate Thermal Sensation
	Adequate Noise Level
	Adequate Crowd Density
	Existence of Commercial Areas
	Existence of Green Areas
Safety & security	Adequate Speed Limit of the Street
	Adequate Street Visual Appearence
	Adequate Surveillance Level
	Adequate Traffic Volume
	Good Street Illumination Level

The questionnaire had a total of 660 responses, of which 7 responses were discarded due to missing values and inconsistency. Therefore, a total of 653 responses were considered in this study.

Regarding gender, 51.91% of respondents identified as female, 47.93% as male, and 0.15% as other. Moreover, 55.59% of the respondents had no children and 44.41% of the respondents had children.

Table 2. Number and proportion of respondents by age group.

Age Group	No.	%	Age Group	No.	%
[0−17]	32	4.90	[0−55]	535	81.93
[18−25]	140	21.44			
[26−35]	106	16.23			
[36−45]	136	20.83			
[46−55]	121	18.53			
[56−65]	78	11.94	[56+]	118	18.07
[66+]	40	6.13			

Table 2 shows the number and proportion of responses for each age group. Accordingly, 4.90% of respondents had less than 18 years old, 21.44% had between 18 and 25 years old, 16.23% had between 26 and 35 years old, 20.83% had between 36 and 45 years old, 18.53% had between 46 and 55 years old, 11.94% had between 56 and 65 years old, and 6.13% had more than 65 years old.

Moreover, in order to investigate the perception of the elderly when using active modes of transport, we performed statistical analyses comparing the following two main age groups: the age group [0–55] included respondents up to 55 years old, and the age group [56+] included respondents over 56 years old (both obtained by aggregating the corresponding data). The number and proportion of respondents in these two categories is also displayed in Table 2.

Table 3. Number and proportion of respondents by the degree of education.

Education	[0–55]		[56+]		Total	
	No.	%	No.	%	No.	%
1st cycle of basic education (4th year)	0	0.00	2	0.31	2	0.31
2nd cycle of basic education (6th year)	5	0.77	0	0.00	5	0.77
3rd cycle of basic education (9th year)	24	3.68	1	0.15	25	3.83
Secondary education (12th year)	92	14.09	11	1.68	103	15.77
Lic./bachelor's degree	188	28.79	46	7.04	234	35.83
Master's degree	142	21.75	23	3.52	165	25.27
Doctorate degree	73	11.18	29	4.44	102	15.62
Other	11	1.68	6	0.92	17	2.60

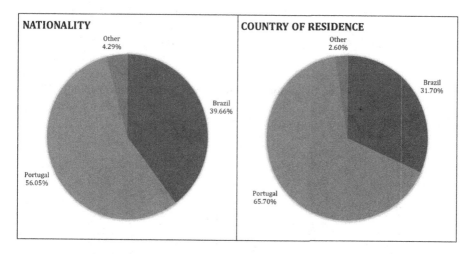

Fig. 2. Number and proportion of responses regarding nationality (left) and country of residence (right).

Table 3 shows the number and proportion of respondents with each education level for the age group [0–55] in columns 2 and 3, for the age group [56+] in columns 4 and 5, and for the total of respondents in columns 6 and 7. The number of respondents with 2nd cycle of basic education or less was almost residual, around 1%. Respondents with at least the 3rd cycle of basic education accounted for 3.83%, while respondents with at least the 12th year of education accounted for 15.77%. Furthermore, 35.83% of respondents had at least a bachelor's degree, 25.27% a master's degree, and 15.62% a doctorate degree.

Figure 2 shows the number and proportion of respondents regarding their nationality and country of residence. Accordingly, 56.05% of respondents had Portuguese nationality, 39.66% had Brazilian nationality and 4.29% had other nationalities. Regarding country of residence, 65.70% of respondents lived in Portugal, 31.70% in Brazil, and 2.60% in other countries.

5   Results and Discussion

5.1   Descriptive Statistics

Figure 3 shows the proportion of people who walked more than 2 km per day in each age group. Similar proportions were obtained for the age groups [0–17], [18–25], [56–65], and [66+], with 43.75%, 45.71%, 46.15%, and 45.00%, respectively. The proportion of respondents walking at least 2 km per day in age groups [26–35], [36–45], and [46–55] was lower than in the other age groups, with 30.19%, 28.68% and 34.71%, respectively.

Figure 4 shows, for each age group, the proportion of respondents who cycle more than 2 km per day. The age groups with the highest proportion of respondents were [36–45] and [46–55], with 28.68% e 36.36% respectively. Older age groups showed lower proportions: the age group [56–65] had a proportion of 17.95%, and the age group [66+] had a proportion of 7.50%. The remaining age groups showed the following proportions: age group [0–17] with 25.00%, age group [18–25] with 13.57%, and age group [26–35] with 11.32%.

The proportion of respondents who cycle at least 2km per day (Fig. 4) was lower than the proportion of respondents who walk at least 2 km per day (Fig. 3) for age groups [0–17], [18–25], [26–35], [56–65], and [66+]. While for age groups [36–45] and [46–55], this comparison returned similar values.

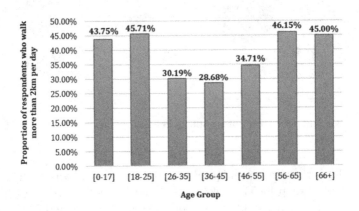

Fig. 3. Proportion of respondents in each age group who walk more than 2 km per day.

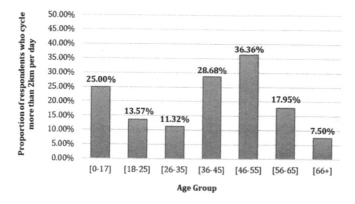

Fig. 4. Proportion of respondents in each age group who cycle more than 2 km per day.

Figure 5 and Fig. 6 show, for age groups [0–55] and [56+] respectively, the number of respondents who rated each indicator in each level of the Likert scale (varying from 1 not important to 5 very important). These figures allow us to visualize the distribution of responses obtained.

Considering only the very important answers in the descriptive statistics for the [0–55] group, the set of people evaluated gives more importance to good street illumination of the street, adequate surveillance level, adequate traffic volume, adequate travel distance & time, air quality, adequate speed limit on the street, existence of green areas, adequate noise level, adequate street visual appearance, adequate crowd density, adequate thermal sensation, absence allergenic, existence of commercial areas, in this order. Next, applying the same analysis to the [56+] group, the set of people evaluated gives more importance to good street illumination of the street, adequate traffic volume, existence of green areas, surveillance level, air quality, adequate speed limit of the street, distance & time, adequate street visual appearance, adequate noise level, adequate thermal sensation, absence of allergenic, adequate crowd density, existence of commercial areas indicators, in this order.

However, this analysis does not consider all the answers on a scale between 1 (not important) and 5 (very important).

Therefore, the Wilcoxon Rank Sum test and the Random Forest algorithm described in the following sections solve this problem, because these analyses consider all responses to establish an importance ranking.

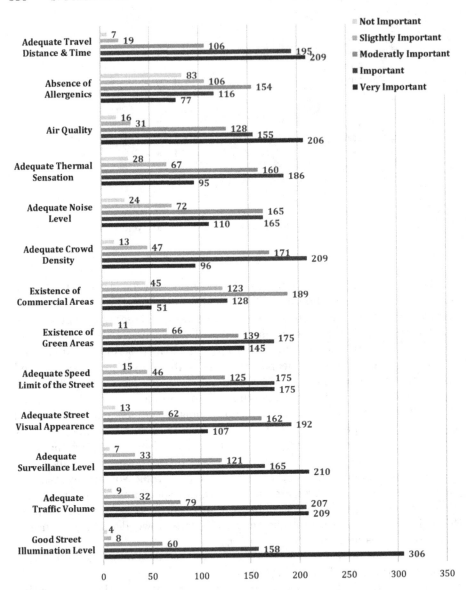

Fig. 5. Number of respondents in age group [0–55] who rated each indicator in each level of the Likert scale.

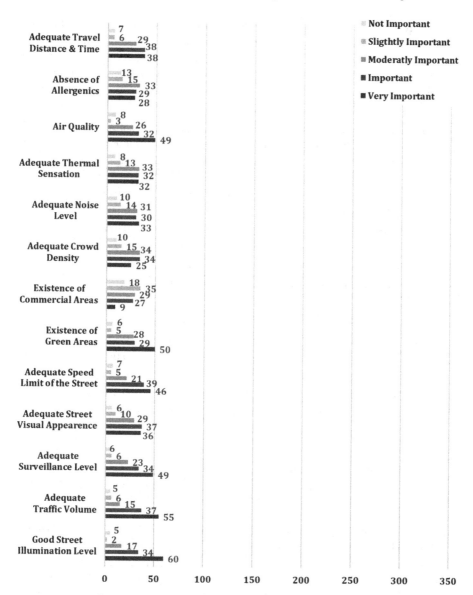

Fig. 6. Number of respondents in age group [56+] who rated each indicator in each level of the Likert scale.

5.2 Wilcoxon Rank Sum Test for Independent Samples

In this section, we compare whether the importance attributed to each indicator is different in age groups [0–55] and [56+], considering a statistical significance of 5%. To this end, we performed the Wilcoxon Rank Sum test for independent samples. This statistical test is adequate to compare two populations whose samples are independent (i.e., they are not paired), from ordinal data. The null hypothesis H0 is that the two population locations are the same, and the alternative hypothesis H1 is that the location of population A is different from the location of population B (two-tail test) [7, p. 584]. The results are summarized in Table 4.

Table 4. Comparing the importance given by age groups [0–55] and [56+] to each indicator using the Wilcoxon Rank Sum test for independent samples.

Indicator	W statistic	p-value
Adequate Travel Distance & Time	35655	0.020
Absence of Allergenics	26256	0.003
Air Quality	30854	0.687
Adequate Thermal Sensation	29692	0.295
Adequate Noise Level	30475	0.543
Adequate Crowd Density	34006	0.168
Existence of Commercial Areas	35446	0.030
Existence of Green Areas	26824	0.008
Adequate Speed Limit of the Street	29062	0.158
Adequate Street Visual Appearance	28454	0.080
Adequate Surveillance Level	31283	0.873
Adequate Traffic Volume	29822	0.316
Good Street Illumination Level	34306	0.098

The results showed that there was evidence at the 5% significance level to establish that the two age groups attribute different importance to the following indicators: *Adequate Travel Distance & Time, Absence of Allergenics, Existence of Commercial Areas,* and *Existence of Green Areas.* These are the cases where we can reject the null hypothesis of equal medians comparing the two age groups.

Also with a statistical significance of 5%, we investigated the age group attributing more importance to each one of these four indicators, using the single-tailed results of the same statistic test. The results showed that: i) indicators *Adequate Travel Distance & Time* and *Existence of Commercial Areas* were given more importance by age group [0–55], with p-values of 0.010 and 0.015, respectively; ii) indicators *Absence of Allergenics* and *Existence of Green Areas* were given more importance by age group [56+], with p-values of 0.002 and 0.004 respectively.

5.3   Random Forest

The Random Forest method works by assuming that each feature is a root node of a decision tree, and the set of features forms the forest. In our case, each feature is an indicator, the algorithm calculates the relative importance of each feature as a function of the answer given by the survey participants returning a vector with this importance as graphics shown in the figures below.

The application of the Random Forest algorithm to the age group [0–55] highlighted the relative importance given by people to indicators: adequate thermal sensation, absence of allergenic, adequate crowd density, an adequate speed limit of the street, adequate traffic volume, adequate noise level, adequate street visual appearance, existence of commercial areas, adequate travel distance & time, adequate surveillance level, air quality, existence of green areas, and good street illumination in this order, as shown in Fig. 7. In this analysis, there were no indicators with zero relative importance.

Furthermore, the algorithm returned a relative importance of the different indicators for the age group [56+] in the following descending order: air quality, adequate travel distance & time, adequate crowd density, adequate thermal sensation, absence of allergenic, good street illumination level, adequate travel volume, and adequate noise level. These results are shown in Fig. 8.

Additionally, in the analysis for the age group [56+], the following indicators returned zero relative importance: existence of commercial areas, existence of green areas, adequate speed limit of the street, adequate street visual appearance, and adequate surveillance level.

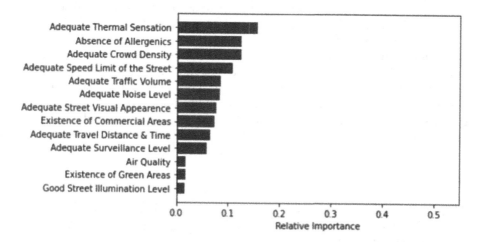

Fig. 7. Relative importance for the different indicators obtained with the Random Forest algorithm in age group [0–55].

It is noted that within the age group [56+], the descriptive statistics presented an emphasis important on the safety & security dimensions considering only the answers "very important", but this analysis is incomplete by difficult to compare using a scale of importance to each indicator. On the other hand, the results of the Random Forest algorithm showed a relative importance ranking

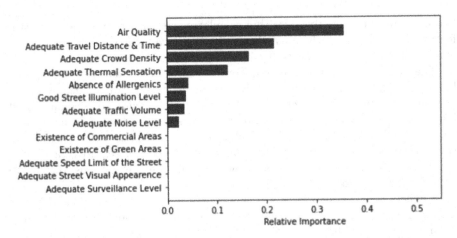

Fig. 8. Relative importance for the different indicators obtained with the Random Forest algorithm in age group [56+].

easier to compare that includes the indicators of the comfort dimension as air quality, adequate crowd density, adequate thermal sensation, absence of allergenic, and adequate noise level, while the safety & security dimension stand out good street illumination level and adequate traffic volume, besides of distance & time dimension. Therefore, these analyzes revealed that in this [56+] group the comfort dimensions stand out.

In this study, the indicators that stand out in both analyzes can be deepened in future works, as well as those that were not so satisfactory. In addition, the context in which these groups of people are included as their residences must be considered, as the environment in which they live influences these results. For example, there are cities or countries where the safety & security dimension is more important, while others where comfort is more important.

6   Conclusion and Future Work

There is a growing encouragement to use active modes of transport such as cycling and walking, as a way to promote sustainability, as well as increased health and well-being for all ages.

Our contribution is to bring more analyses within this group of people above 56 years old to know their preferences regarding the active modes and the importance given to each indicator of comfort and safety & security dimensions because the literature review showed that there are few works that treat this subject to this set of people.

In this study, we analyzed the responses to an online questionnaire conducted between August 2021 and August 2022 to understand the preferences in active modes of different age groups. Respondents were asked a set of socio-demographic questions (i.e., age range, nationality, country of residence, gender, educational level, employment situation, and the number of children), and to rate the importance they attributed to a set of thirteen indicators.

The set of indicators was organized into three dimensions: i) the *Distance & Time* dimension (including Adequate Travel Distance & Time); ii) the *Comfort* dimension (including Absence of Allergenics, Air quality, Adequate Thermal Sensation, Adequate Noise Level, Adequate Crowd Density, Existence of Commercial Areas, and Existence of Green Areas); iii) the *Safety & Security* dimension (including Adequate Speed Limit of the Street, Adequate Street Visual Appearance, Adequate Surveillance Level, Adequate Traffic Volume, and Good Street Illumination Level).

The two main age groups considered for this analysis were: [0–55] including all respondents 55 years old or less, and [56+] encompassing all respondents 56 years old or more.

We applied descriptive statistics to the questionnaire responses to provide a sociodemographic characterization of the respondents, as well as show an overview of the responses for each indicator.

To address the first research question (i.e., What indicators related to the perception of comfort, safety, and security are more important for people above 56 years old?) we applied the Wilcoxon Rank Sum test for independent samples, considering the comparison of the two age groups under analysis. The results showed that: i) the indicators *Adequate Travel Distance & Time* and *Existence of Commercial Areas* were perceived as having more importance for the [0–55] age group than the [56+] age group; ii) the indicators *Absence of Allergenics* and *Existence of Green Areas* were perceived as having more importance for the [56+] age group than the [0–55] age group.

To address the second research question (i.e., What is the relative importance attributed to the indicators on the use of active modes by the age group over 56 years old?) we applied the random forest algorithm to the answers in each age group and compared the results obtained. The results of the Random Forest algorithm for the age group [56+] returned the following relative importance of the indicators (sorted from most important to least important): 1) air quality, 2) adequate travel distance & time, 3) adequate crowd density, 4) adequate thermal sensation, 5) absence of allergenic, 6) good street illumination level, 7) adequate traffic volume, and 8) adequate noise level.

Our suggestion for future work is more studies using active modes for people above 56 years old investigating more the indicators that stand out in this work to encourage more people the use active modes and public politics directed toward the improvement of infrastructure and get along with other means of transport promoting cities more sustainable.

Additionally, future work could include studying the differences in the importance of these indicators with respect to the country of residence.

Acknowledgements. This paper is a result of the project Safe Cities - Inovação para Construir Cidades Seguras, with the reference POCI-01-0247-FEDER-041435, cofunded by the European Regional Development Fund (ERDF), through the Operational Programme for Competitiveness and Internationalization (COMPETE 2020), under the PORTUGAL 2020 Partnership Agreement.

References

1. Bista, S., Debache, I., Chaix, B.: Physical activity and sedentary behaviour related to transport activity assessed with multiple body-worn accelerometers: the RECORD MultiSensor study. Public Health **189**, 144–152 (2020). https://doi.org/10.1016/j.puhe.2020.10.009
2. Felicio, S., et al.: Characterizing soft modes' traveling in urban areas though indicators and simulated scenarios (2021)
3. Ferreira, M., et al.: Identifying the determinants and understanding their effect on the perception of safety, security, and comfort by pedestrians and cyclists: a systematic review. Transp. Res. Part F: Traffic Psychol. Behav. **91**, 136–163 (2022). https://doi.org/10.1016/j.trf.2022.10.004
4. Ferrer, S., Ruiz, T., Mars, L.: A qualitative study on the role of the built environment for short walking trips. Transp. Res. Part F: Traffic Psychol. Behav. **33**, 141–160 (2015). https://doi.org/10.1016/j.trf.2015.07.014
5. Hatamzadeh, Y., Hosseinzadeh, A.: Toward a deeper understanding of elderly walking for transport: an analysis across genders in a case study of Iran. J. Transp. Health **19**, 100949 (2020). https://doi.org/10.1016/j.jth.2020.100949
6. de Jesus, M.C.R., da Silva, A.N.R.: Barrier effect in a medium-sized Brazilian city: an exploratory analysis using decision trees and random forests. Sustainability **14**(10), 6309 (2022). https://doi.org/10.3390/su14106309
7. Keller, G., Warrack, B., Bartel, H.: Statistics for Management and Economics: A Systematic Approach. Business Statistics. Wadsworth Publishing Company (1988). https://books.google.pt/books?id=YBdZAAAAYAAJ
8. Leger, S.J., Dean, J.L., Edge, S., Casello, J.M.: "If i had a regular bicycle, i wouldn't be out riding anymore": perspectives on the potential of e-bikes to support active living and independent mobility among older adults in Waterloo, Canada. Transp. Res. Part A: Policy Pract. **123**, 240–254 (2019). https://doi.org/10.1016/j.tra.2018.10.009
9. Lord, S., Cloutier, M.S., Christoforou, Z., Garnier, B.: Crossing road intersections in old age-with or without risks? Perceptions of risk and crossing behaviours among the elderly. Transp. Res. Part F Traffic Psychol. Behav. **55** (2018). https://doi.org/10.1016/j.trf.2018.03.005
10. Macioszek, E., Karami, A., Farzin, I., Abbasi, M., Mamdoohi, A.R., Piccioni, C.: The effect of distance intervals on walking likelihood in different trip purposes. Sustainability **14**(6), 3406 (2022). https://doi.org/10.3390/su14063406
11. Marques, A., Peralta, M., Henriques-Neto, D., Frasquilho, D., Gouveira, É.R., Gomez-Baya, D.: Active commuting and depression symptoms in adults: a systematic review. Int. J. Environ. Res. Public Health **17**(3), 1041 (2020). https://doi.org/10.3390/ijerph17031041
12. Ravulaparthy, S., Yoon, S.Y., Goulias, K.G.: Linking elderly transport mobility and subjective well-being. Transp. Res. Rec.: J. Transp. Res. Board **2382**(1), 28–36 (2013). https://doi.org/10.3141/2382-04

13. Schneider, R.: Theory of routine mode choice decisions: an operational framework to increase sustainable transportation. Transp. Policy **25**, 128–137 (2013). https://doi.org/10.1016/j.tranpol.2012.10.007

14. Shaer, A., Haghshenas, H.: The impacts of COVID-19 on older adults' active transportation mode usage in Isfahan, Iran. J. Transp. Health **23**, 101244 (2021). https://doi.org/10.1016/j.jth.2021.101244

15. Silveira-Santos, T., Vassallo, J.M., Torres, E.: Using machine learning models to predict the willingness to carry lightweight goods by bike and kick-scooter. Transp. Res. Interdisc. Perspect. **13**, 100568 (2022). https://doi.org/10.1016/j.trip.2022.100568

16. Thigpen, C., Driller, B., Handy, S.: Using a stages of change approach to explore opportunities for increasing bicycle commuting. Transp. Res. Part D: Transp. Environ. **39**, 44–55 (2015). https://doi.org/10.1016/j.trd.2015.05.005

17. Vanparijs, J., Panis, L.I., Meeusen, R., de Geus, B.: Exposure measurement in bicycle safety analysis: a review of the literature. Accid. Anal. Prevent. **84**, 9–19 (2015). https://doi.org/10.1016/j.aap.2015.08.007

18. Wardman, M., Tight, M., Page, M.: Factors influencing the propensity to cycle to work. Transp. Res. Part A: Policy Pract. **41**, 339–350 (2007). https://doi.org/10.1016/j.tra.2006.09.011

19. Winters, M., Voss, C., Ashe, M.C., Gutteridge, K., McKay, H., Sims-Gould, J.: Where do they go and how do they get there? Older adults' travel behaviour in a highly walkable environment. Soc. Sci. Med. **133**, 304–312 (2015). https://doi.org/10.1016/j.socscimed.2014.07.006

Machine Learning for Drug Efficiency Prediction

Hafida Tiaiba[1]([⊠]), Lyazid Sabri[1,2], Abdelghani Chibani[2], and Okba Kazar[3,4]

[1] Maths and Informatics Faculty, Mohamed El Bachir El Ibrahimi University, Bordj Bou
Arreridj, Algeria
{hafida.tiaiba,lyazid.sabri}@univ-bba.dz

[2] LISSI-The Laboratory of Images, Signals and Intelligent Systems, University Paris-Est
Vitry-sur-Seine, Île-de-France, France
{sabri,chibani}@lissi.fr

[3] LINFI Laboratory, Computer Sciences Department, University of Biskra, Biskra, Algeria
o.kazar@univ-biskra.dz

[4] Department of Information Systems and Security, College of Information Technology, United
Arab Emirates University, Al Ain, United Arab Emirates
o.kazar@uaeu.ac.ae

Abstract. Health-related social media data, particularly patients' opinions about drugs, have recently provided knowledge for research on the adverse reactions, allergies that a patient experiences and drug efficacy and safety. We develop an effective method for analyzing medicines' efficiency and conditions-specific prescription from patient reviews provided by Drug Review Dataset (drug.com). Our approach relies on the Natural Language Processing (NLP) principle and a word embedding vectorization method to preserve semantics. For this purpose, we conducted experiments using various sampling techniques, precisely random sampling and balanced random sampling. Furthermore, we applied several statistical models: Logistic Regression, Decision Tree, Random Forests, K-Nearest Neighbors (KNN) and Neural Network models (simple perceptron, multilayer perceptron and convolutional neural network). We varied the size of training and test data sets to study the effect of the sampling techniques on model efficiency. Compared to other models, the results show that the proposed models in this paper: KNN, Embedding-100, and CNN-Maxpooling outclass models proposed by several researchers. Indeed, Embedding-100 has achieved better training accuracy and test accuracy. Moreover, during our study, we concluded that different factors influence the effectiveness of the models, mainly the text preprocessing method, sampling techniques in terms of size and type, text vectorization method and machine learning models.

Keywords: Machine Learning · Text Classification · Word Embedding · Health · Predict Drug Efficiency · Natural Language Processing

A. Cunha et al. (Eds.): MobiHealth 2022, LNICST 484, pp. 322–337, 2023.
https://doi.org/10.1007/978-3-031-32029-3_27

1 Introduction

The prescription of a drug is crucial; an initial step in the circuit in the personalization of diagnosis and treatment helps therapeutic education and promotes more effective precision medicine. The effectiveness of a cure is closely linked to the positive results obtained by minimizing the adverse effects. Nevertheless, the efficacy of a drug relies on an important criterion, namely, whether a patient strictly adheres to the dosing schedule dosage. Treatment may work well in clinical trials but may not produce the same results in the real world due to side effects. That is why patients stop taking this drug without a doctor's advice. Implementing new technologies for patient well-being depends on many factors, such as personal experience, patient practices and expert opinion. One can also ask whether patients' reviews (i.e., feedback) on medicine can help evaluate drugs. The High Authority of Health (HAS) [1] answers this question for Health. HAS assesses health technologies from a clinical and medico-economic point of view. HAS has been integrating patients into the drug evaluation process for several years (November 2016). The result is clear, the HAS advocates collaboration between health actors and patients.

Among the HAS surveys, a pharmaceutical association observed that patients resorted to cutting a pill at the level of a groove for lack of drugs and inadequate doses. However, it is not possible to regularly break a tablet; therefore, getting the required dose becomes difficult. Thus, everyone's participation (e.g., patients and pharmacists) in audits and/or assessments made available to doctors is an asset for the patient's well-being. Analyzing side effects and the effectiveness of drugs based on opinions and feedback from patients is our approach's objective. The results will aid the medical staff in better preventing and providing care. The proposed approach relies on the following mechanisms and techniques:

1. Investigate the impact of dataset sampling on model performance.
2. Analyze the effect of preprocessing method on model accuracy.
3. Apply the word embedding principle for reasoning with the textual semantic in formation.
4. The use of data mining models, statistical models, and neural network models to compare the two types of models and select the best model.

Natural Language Processing (NLP) is a field of Computer Science and Artificial Intelligence. NLP is either a rule-based or statistical-based technique. In addition, NLP and machine learning can analyze large volumes of data written in natural language [2]. We proceeded to textual classification to extract knowledge from patients' narrative opinions on drugs for a specific disease. This approach aims to find a better textual classification model based on NLP. It automatically assigns an opinion on whether or not the drug used for a specific disease is effective. The results should provide healthcare partners, pharmacists, physicians, and managers with valuable drug information.

A class assignment relies on the drug's designation, the type of disease, and the patient's opinion. We have opted for two strategies to prepare the data: The first preserves the semantics of the texts (i.e., does not modify the content of the reviews written in natural language). The second strategy relies on the lemmatization principle. Moreover, instead of representing each word using a numeric vector using the one-hot representation, we have described each document in unstructured (narrative) text format using a numeric vector. To increase the performance of our approach, we used the word embedding representation, in which similar words have an identical encoding, using the Embedding layer of Keras [2]. Finally, we used data mining algorithms for data analysis.

Previous works on analyzing patient reviews of medications have focused on improving learning methods. However, the document preprocessing phase (i.e., text cleaning) differs slightly from traditional methods. This phase influences the classification result and the medical textual data since the sentences-preprocessing can lead to the deletion of words and contexts and bias the meaning. In addition, a medical (clinical) record is a sequence of structured chronological elementary events (i.e., the dynamic narrative of the patient's history). Thus, lexical processing via lemmatization can alter temporal knowledge. Indeed, reporting all the past tenses to their corresponding infinitive tenses will change the meaning of a patient's medical history. The work carried out by Bemila et al. [3] and Mascio et al. [4] relied on removing stop words, special characters and punctuation, and then the authors applied lemmatization and stemming. The only difference between the two authors is that Mascio, Aurelie, et al. used SciSpacy during the lemmatization process. Unlike Bemila, Mercadier, Yves [5] did not use stemming. Gräber et al. [6], Vijayaraghavan, and Basu [7] preferred to delete the terms whose frequency is lower than a threshold in addition to the preprocessing phase. In [6], the authors used Drug.com and applied the logistic regression classifier.

In this work, we use Drug.com data sets that include 215,063 patient reviews. We compare different statistical models, namely LogisticRegression, RandonForest, DecisionTree, KNeighbors and neural network models: Embedding-100, Simple10, Embedding-32-, Embedding-32-Maxpooling and CNN-Maxpooling. We also studied the effect of sampling training and test datasets and the text-cleaning process on the effectiveness of the proposed models. Furthermore, we analyze the impact of semantic reasoning using word embedding on the performance of neural network models. Finally, we also analyze the effect of the dimension size of the vectors resulting from word embedding on the efficiency of the models. The automatic analysis of the evaluations of patient opinions made by our study makes it possible to obtain relevant information on side effects, drug interactions, and the effectiveness of drugs.

To our knowledge, the proposed model allows for determining drug efficiency using drug.com data sets is the first to achieve 0.9984 accuracies. For example, the following opinion is categorized as negative (i.e., this class indicates that the drug used has side effects): "This medicine does not work for me, each time I take it, it makes me drowsy, but I could not sleep". The following patient's opinion, "It has no side effects, I take it in combination of Bystolic 5 Mg and Fish Oil", has been labelled positive (i.e., positive opinion) and therefore allows inferring that the drug is efficient.

This paper is organized as follows: Sect. 2 presents state-of-the-art. Section 3 describes our approach to classifying large-scale drug.com data. We also detail the pseudo algorithms we developed in this section with the results. Finally, Sect. 4 concludes the paper and proposes new research directions and perspectives.

2   Related Work

Several studies have been devoted to information representing the experiences and opinions of consumers. For example, the authors Jiménez-Zafra et al. have examined how patients express their opinions in the medical forum [8]. They aim to determine the best way to exploit sentiment analysis in this area. They applied supervised learning and lexical sentiment analysis approaches to two different corpora extracted from the social web. Among the datasets most used in studies on the opinion of patients on drugs is drug.com. Most of the studies were based only on the patients' opinions for the classification of their reviews.

However, those studies ignored the drug designation and conditions. Patient reviews are characterized by a combination of informal language with specific terminology and a high degree of lexical diversity, making it more challenging to analyze. The authors in [9] proposed a text vectorization method based on Term Frequency-Inverse Document Frequency (TF-IDF) and FastText word embeddings. They used five classifiers: Support Vector Machine (SVM), Decision Tree, Random Forests, Naïve Bayes, and K-nearest neighbors. Colón-Ruiz et al. proposed a system based on word embedding, and Long short-term memory (LSTM) classifier. Their approach achieved an accuracy of 0.9046 compared to other models they studied, such as Convolutional Neural Network (CNN) and CNN combined with LSTM [10]. As for Gräber et al. studied the performance of their models on the data on a single condition [6]. Then they evaluated the models on other subsets related to the conditions. Specific conditions are selected by extracting five of the most common disorders in the Druglib.com dataset. Such as Depression, Pain, Anxiety, Contraception and Diabetes Type 2. The logistic regression model applied to drug.com achieved an accuracy of 0.9224. In [11], the authors used the principle of TF-IDF and obtained an accuracy of 0.316 achieved by the Roberta classifier with the Data Augmentation and Inference Augmentation (DAIA) method. While in [3], the authors applied the Bag of Words principle and used Naive Bayes, Random Forest, Linear Support Vector Classification (SVC), Logistic Regression and RNN-BiLSTM (Recurrent neural networks - A Bidirectional Long Short-Term Memory) algorithms. MIN, Z. used AskaPatient data sets and proposed a combined WSM-CNN-LSTM (Weakly Supervised Mechanism) model of CNN and LSTM. His model provided an accuracy of 86.72 [12].

3   Classification Approach

3.1   Theoretical Study

We recall here our approach for a better prediction of drug intake. Thus, we considered different criteria, such as the size of the samples, the semantic contribution and the study of the deep-learning and statistical models. The process of our research is as follows:

1. Relying on the binary classification to predict patient satisfaction with medication use and perceptions of side effects and efficacy.
2. Study the impact of data set sampling on model performance.
3. Analyze the effect of preprocessing method of model accuracy.
4. Apply word embedding for the semantic reasoning of texts.
5. Compare statistical models and artificial neural network models.

A Machine Learning Dataset. We chose the drug.com dataset from the UCI Machine Learning Repository [13]. It includes 215,063 samples presented in two files (training and test).

Each sample has the following fields: drug name and a drug's number, terms that describe the reason for using the drug or the patient's illness, user reviews, ratings given by the user, the date on which the drug was reviewed, and the number of users who found the review useful.

In this paper, we concatenated the two files (drug_train, drug_test), and then we reconstituted the training and test data set by randomly choosing the documents for two case studies.

For the first case, we selected 75% for training and 25% for the test. While for the second case, we used 80% for training and 20% for the test. We also carried out random and random balanced sampling. The second sampling method aims to maintain the proportion of ranking values across the training and testing sets. Our approach relies on the 'stratify' parameter of the 'train_test_split' function [14]. To evaluate the certainty of patient satisfaction, we derived two level labels for patient satisfaction. After that, we attributed positive classification "1" for a rating interval from 5 to 10 points and negative classification "0" for a rating less than five to one.

Data Preprocessing Strategies. Two strategies have been conducted; the first consists in carrying out the transformations in the sentences written in natural languages. All uppercase characters are transformed to lowercase, removing the unique character ("). Then, the spaces are deleted in the name of the drug and the conditions. The goal is to treat each as a single word (i.e., each of these data will be represented by a number). Therefore, after concatenating the drug name, condition and patient's feedback, their one-hot representations will be straightforward as long as a single number describes each word. We highlight that during the process of this first strategy, we chose to discard the stemming and lemmatization process, avoid removing punctuation marks and numbers from texts.

Removing the question's marks, dots, commas, and numbers such as '5 Mg' and '10 Mg' will change the meaning of a patient's medical history. As for a stemming process that reduces or removes a part of a word, which can completely distort the sentence's meaning, for example, the implications of the words 'suffering', 'suffered' and 'suffer' are different since the stemming result gives the same stem; hence the meaning of the sentence will be biased. At the end of this strategy's process, the obtained vocabulary size is 84,362 words, and the document's length is 2,405. While in the second strategy, we opted for the principle of lemmatization based on the Natural Language Toolkit (NLTK) library associated with the Wordnet dictionary. In this case, the vocabulary's length is 83,162 and as in the first strategy, we obtained the exact size of the longer document.

Converting text to numerical data allows describing each document by a vector instead of representing each word by a numerical vector. Since each document includes the name of the drug, the conditions, and the patient comments, and considering the numeric vectors of different sizes, we applied the padding principle to make all vectors the same length. The size of the document vectors is 2,405. Concerning the statistical classifiers, we used only one-hot; for the neural classifiers, we used One-hot and word embedding of different dimensions (32 and 100) to analyze the effect of vectorization on model performance.

A Proposed Models and Algorithms for Drug Efficiency Prediction. We opted for logistic regression, random forest, decision trees, and K-nearest neighbors among the statistical models, for this purpose we used sklearn library [15]. Concerning the random forests, we set 'n_estimators', the parameter allowing us to define the number of trees in the random forest, to 10 and the maximum depth of each tree 'max_depth' to 3. Same thing for the decision tree; we limit the maximum depth 'max_depth' to 3. For the K-nearest neighbors' models, we used the Euclidean distance and set the number of neighbors to 1.

For the neuronal models, we used the sequential model of the Keras library [16]. The latter provides a way to convert positive integer representations of words to word embedding by an embedding layer. In word embedding, words are encoded by numeric value vectors in high-dimensional space, where the similarity between words translates to proximity in vector space for semantic reasoning.

Each document that includes a drug name, condition, and patient comment is represented by One–hot. Then, relying on the embedding layer, a vector of the real numbers represents each document. Keras' embedding layer allows choosing the dimension of the vector representing the document. We treated the case of an Embedding with a size of 32 for the vectors representing the model (Embedding-32-). Also, for the Embedding-100 model, we used a representation by word embedding of dimension 100. We have proposed the artificial neural models: Embedding-100, Embedding-32-, Embedding-32-Maxpooling and CNN-Maxpooling. Embedding-100 is a simple perceptron consisting of a single neuron with an embedding layer of dimension 100. A vector of size 100 represents each word, allowing the representation of the words efficiently and densely in which similar words have similar encoding [17]. Therefore, each document will be represented by a vector of two size dimensions (2,405 and 100).

This process allowed us to apply the flatten principle to create a single vector of one dimension (240 500) to be directly used with the next fully connected layer. Simple10: is a neural network with a hidden layer consisting of 10 neurons linked to a single output neuron using One-hot representation. The Embedding-32- model has the same structure as Simple10 but with an additional Embedding layer. The latter has a dimension of 32.

We applied the Global max-pooling on the Embedding-32 model for building the Embedding-32-max-pooling model. Finally, the proposed CNN-Maxpooling model: is a convolutional neural network (CNN) composed of a one-dimensional convolution layer (Conv1D). The number of filters is 128; the kernel size is 5. We applied an embedding of size 32 and then a global max-pooling (GlobalMaxPool1D). GlobalMaxPool1D takes the maximum of each vector, which reduces the dimension of the resulting embedding matrix.

For all artificial neural models, the activation function used is Rectified Linear Unit Activation Function (ReLU) and 'sigmoid' for the output layer. Concerning the Embedding-100, we applied the sigmoid function exclusively because we have a binary classification. Furthermore, we rely on the optimization 'adam' implementation of the gradient descent function [18], and the 'binary_crossentropy' loss function suited to binary classification problems. In addition, the parameters 'metrics' is 'accuracy', representing the accuracy of the models used to evaluate the different models. Accuracy measures the labels assigned by our approach. Formally, accuracy is handled by the following formula:

$$accuracy = \frac{TP + TN}{TP + TN + FP + FN} \tag{1}$$

where, we use TP (True Positive), TN (True Negative), FP (False Positive) and FN (False Negative).

The pseudo-algorithm, 'General Pseudo Algorithm', synthesizes our approach and handles the preprocessing, sampling, vectorization, and model training, Table 1.

According to the obtained results, we chose the Embedding-100 model. The parameters of this model are:

– The sigmoid (X) activation function is: $\frac{1}{1+e^{-x}}$

Table 1. General Pseudo Algorithm.

Data1= Drug_train ∪ drug_test{union}Conversion "review" to lowercase, removing (")
Removal of drug name spaces
Removal of condition spaces
Data_drug['review'] = concatenation of (drug name, condition and review)
if (Sentiment >= 5) then Review_Sentiment=1
else Review_Sentiment=0
endif
/* Data_drug: contain review and Review_Sentiment */
Split Drug_train into sample_set = {s_75, s_75_stratify, s_75_lemmatization,
s_75_lemmatization_stratify, s_80, s_80_stratify, s_80_lemmatization,
s_80_lemmatization _stratify}
if sample in (s_75_lemmatization, s_80_lemmatization,
   s_75_lemmatization_stratify, s_80_ lemmatization_stratify))
then
        Lemmatization of review
endif
D=Data_drug['review'] /* the corpus*/
$D_i=(d_{i1},d_{i2}, \ldots ,d_{in})$ /* (n<=2405 longest document, i<=215063) */
Y= Data_drug['Review_Sentiment'] { labels}
R= One_hot(D) / $R_i= (R_{i1},R_{i2},\quad ,R_{in})$: numeric representation
P= padding(R) / $P_i=(P_{i1},P_{i2},\quad ,P_{i2405})$: make all vectors of the same size (2405) ....(a)
Set_model={ LogisticRegression, DecisionTree, KNeighbors, Embedding-100,
Simple10, Embedding-32-, Embedding-32-Maxpooling, CNN-Maxpooling }
For every sample in sample_set do
     For every model in Set_model do
              Train model
              Test model
     Endfor
Endfor
Best model = model where max (train accuracy, test accuracy)
End

Table 2. Pseudo Algorithm for generating Embeddig-100 (the best model).

Input : P ∈ R²⁴⁰⁵⁰⁰ Calculated in General Algorithm step (a) sample = s_75_stratify (75% train 25% test. case balanced random of data_drug without lemmatization) , Y= review_Sentiment
Output:Trained model
Begin
        {Train the model: 75% of dataset}
   Initialize w_0, $W_i ∈ R^{240500}$
   For each training example $(P_i, y_i) ∈ (P,Y)$
      E_i= embedding(P_i)/ E_i is matrix(2405,100)
      F_i= flatten(E_i)   / F_i =(E_{i1}, E_{i2}, , E_{i3}, , $E_{i240500}$.)/ One dimension
      yi'= sigmoid(W_{it}^T × F_i+ w_0) ……………..(b)
       /* W_{it}^Ttransposed vector of W_{it}*/
      if yi ≠ yi' then   calculate loss (yi , yi') given in (3)
        update W_{it} using dam optimizer given in formula (4)
        go to (b)
      endif
 Endfor
        {Test the model : 25% of dataset }
   Initialize w_0, $W_i ∈ R^{240500}$
   For each training example $(P_i, y_i) ∈ (P,Y)$
      E_i= embedding(P_i)/ E_i is matrix(2405,100)
      F_i= flatten(E_i)   / F_i =(E_{i1}, E_{i2}, , E_{i3}, , $E_{i240500}$.)/ One dimension
      yi'= sigmoid(W_{it}^T × F_i+ w_0) ……………..(c)
       /* W_{it}^Ttransposed vector of W_{it}*/
      if yi ≠ yi' then   calculate loss (yi , yi') given in (3)
        update W_{it} using dam optimizer given in formula (4)
        go to (c)
      endif
 Endfor
Return final weights vector
Save the model: Embedding_100_75final.h5
(to use it in Predictions)
End

- The performance of a classification model, the binary cross-entropy loss function is handled by the following formula:

$$L = -\frac{1}{output\ size} * X. \qquad (2)$$

$$X = \sum_{i=1}^{out\ put\ size} y_i.\log y'_i + (1 - y_i).\log(1 - y'_i)$$

$$L = -y.\log y' + (1 - y).\log(1 - y') \tag{3}$$

where: y' is the label computed by the model, and y is the predicted label. Adam optimiser is used as follows for updating weights [19]:

$$w_{i,t+1} = (w_{i,t} - \alpha.m_t) \tag{4}$$

where: $m_t = \beta m_{t-1} + (1 - \beta)\frac{\partial L}{\partial W_{i,t}}$

m_t: aggregate of gradients at iteration t initially $m_t = 0$,
α: learning rate,
$W_{i,t}$: weights at time t,
$W_{i,t+1}$: weights at iteration $t + 1$,
∂L: derivation of loss function,
$\partial W_{i,t}$: derivation of weights at iteration t,
β: moving average parameter,

The pseudo algorithm illustrated in Table 2 explains the sequence of steps of the Embedding_100 model approach.

To exploit our Embedding_100 model, we use the Prediction pseudo algorithm presented in Table 3 that makes predictions regarding drug reviews.

Table 3. Prediction Pseudo Algorithm.

Input   : Drug name, Condition, Patient review
Output: drug efficiency
Begin
  Enter drug name and condition
  Enter review
  Conversion patient review to lowercase
  Removal of drug name spaces
  Removal of condition spaces
  review = concatenation of (drug name, condition and review)
  r=one_hot(review)
  p=padding(r)
  Embedding_100_75final(p)
  If y=0 then 'the drug presents conflit'
      else ' the drug presents no conflit'
End

3.2 Practical Study

Example Illustrating Stages in Natural Language Processing. Consider the following sentences taken from the drug.com: The first approach transforms the text into lowercase and removes spaces in the name of the drugs and the instructions for use (i.e.,

Table 4. Text Vectorization.

Approach 1: The length of the largest document is 2,405 and the vocabulary size is 84,362
Azithromycin ChlamydiaInfection was prescribed one dose over the course of one day, took 4 pills of 250mg after a light lunch, and had nausea and mild stomach pains/upset. lying down did not alleviate the discomfort and threw up 3 hours later. called up my doctor to check if i needed to take another dose but he said my body would have absorbed the pills by then. still experiencing mild stomach pains but nausea is mostly gone now.stomach pains but nausea is mostly gone now.
One hot : [13084, 50875, 62892, 38293, 1436, 6294, 46079, 26091, 52962, 4736, 1436, 38726, 65804, 33200, 18587, 4736, 78333, 10937, 8946, 10470, 70093, 36469, 31023, 20051, 36469, 43536, 9610, 83427, 82756, 7416, 69605, 45744, 66264, 34414, 26091, 6303, 36469, 52222, 13236, 78384, 76910, 58260, 49736, 13236, 61167, 74271, 77306, 65408, 43571, 65228, 25474, 77306, 55872, 16926, 6294, 65610, 53047, 1232, 61167, 23363, 48658, 15209, 57011, 26091, 18587, 10796, 70690, 22086, 32677, 43536, 9610, 83427, 65610, 20051, 68236, 9373, 49136, 75495]
Padding : [13084 50875 62892 ...   0   0   0]
Embedding : tf.Tensor([[-0.00030909 0.04441366 -0.01012845 ... -0.01254865 -0.02349045 -0.03326954] [-0.03938956 0.0266563 -0.02233372 ... 0.02533278 0.04644166   0.01073159]... [-0.00268913 -0.03778163 -0.04249182 ... 0.04519937 -0.00611898   0.04797543] [-0.00268913 -0.03778163 -0.04249182 ...   0.04519937 -0.00611898   0.04797543]], shape=(2405, 100), dtype=float32)
Flatten: [-0.00030909 0.04441366 -0.01012845 ... -0.01254865 -0.02349045   -0.03326954 -0.03938956   0.0266563   -0.02233372 ... 0.02533278 0.04644166   ... 0.04519937 -0.00611898   0.04797543 -0.00268913 ... 0.04519937 -0.00611898   0.04797543]
Approach 2: The length of the largest document is 2,405 and the vocabulary size is 83,162
Azithromycin ChlamydiaInfection wa prescribed one dose over the course of one day, took 4 pill of 250mg after a light lunch, and had nausea and mild stomach pains/upset. lying down did not alleviate the discomfort and threw up 3 hour later. called up my doctor to check if i needed to take another dose but he said my body would have absorbed the pill by then. still experiencing mild stomach pain but nausea is mostly gone now.
One hot : [12172, 39241, 39536, 68005, 22878, 48912, 81513, 17567, 70694, 44772, 22878, 17104, 56100, 42384, 25484, 44772, 5599, 49865, 2936, 81692, 4995, 64433, 15463, 26371, 64433, 22062, 57770, 26197, 31686, 20524, 61211, 77066, 29682, 70526, 17567, 23297, 64433, 8632, 57916, 6464, 71041, 11634, 8126, 57916, 46389, 58551, 35636, 79304, 52635, 13974, 9880, 35636, 48878, 22702, 48912, 25530, 31781, 81052, 46389, 72903, 79338, 80701, 56709, 17567, 25484, 24160, 75320, 72300, 63521, 22062, 57770, 51437, 25530, 26371, 52854, 16037, 48754, 16579]
Padding : [12172 39241 39536 ...   0   0   0]
Embedding: tf.Tensor([[0.03626031 -0.00316075 0.0112661   ... -0.02691853 -0.03584041 0.00848019] [-0.01687868 -0.03148886 -0.03002917 ... -0.03701594 -0.03470857   -0.01378261]... [0.02724567 0.01433365 -0.01567432 ... -0.00919002 -0.03320863   -0.00234286] [0.02724567   0.01433365 -0.01567432 ... -0.00919002 -0.03320863   -0.00234286]], shape=(2405, 100), dtype=float32)
Flatten: [0.03626031 -0.00316075 0.0112661   ... -0.02691853 -0.03584041   0.00848019 - 0.01687868 -0.03148886 -0.03002917 ... -0.03701594 -0.03470857   -0.01378261 0.01509024

(*continued*)

Table 4. (*continued*)

-0.04584317 -0.031525   ... -0.00919002 -0.03320863   -0.00234286]

Approach 3: The length of the largest document is 1,036 and the vocabulary size is 61,318

azithromycin chlamydiainfect wa prescrib one dose cours one day took pill mg light lunch nausea mild stomach painsupset lie not allevi discomfort threw hour later call doctor check need take anoth dose said bodi would absorb pill still experienc mild stomach pain nausea mostli gone

One hot : [45626, 28111, 3375, 52534, 31538, 28868, 10091, 31538, 57765, 34662, 32504, 18006, 58030, 12401, 21328, 22967, 23849, 15936, 40673, 49312, 40475, 30382, 49223, 54143, 4428, 4676, 14683, 7214, 6879, 2871, 10144, 28868, 15097, 15031, 52534, 12338, 32504, 26673, 39566, 22967, 23849, 51801, 21328, 26871, 13077]

Padding : [45626 28111 3375 ...   0   0   0]

Embedding: tf.Tensor([[-0.03886646 -0.0198079   0.01174947 ... -0.03995751 -0.04186364 0.01677601]
[-0.04668018 -0.04458895 -0.00548612 ... -0.01382007 0.01983864 -0.03390007]...
[0.03535514 -0.04283841 -0.04564927 ... 0.031701 -0.03638158   0.0310008]
[0.03535514 -0.04283841 -0.04564927 ... 0.031701   -0.03638158   0.0310008]],
shape=(1036, 100), dtype=float32)

Flatten: [-0.03886646 -0.0198079   0.01174947 ... -0.03995751 -0.04186364   0.01677601 - 0.04668018 -0.04458895 -0.00548612 ... -0.01382007 0.01983864 -0.03390007 0.04955867 0.03802111 0.03902782 0.03535514... 0.031701 -0.03638158   0.0310008]

conditions). As for the second approach, we likewise integrate the process of lemmatization. As the majority of the state-of-the-art learning methods, we remove symbols, special characters, numbers, and punctuation in the third approach. Furthermore, we use lemmatization and stemming. The experiments highlight those two approaches' limitations that cause the general loss of vital knowledge in health care. For clarity, the words (i.e., term) emphasized with yellow are deleted in the third or second approach. Otherwise, the terms highlighted in grey color are edited (i.e., modified) within the third and second approaches. We have exploited only the first and second approaches in this study.

An example of the different types of text vectorization in different approaches is presented in Table 4 to show the impact of pre-processing on the text, in particular, the semantics of the text.

Experimental Results. We studied the models' performance according to three criteria: The classifier's impact, the sampling method, and the size of the training and test data sets.

Discussion. The first strategy shows that in the case of a random sampling of 75% for training and 25% for testing, the Embedding-100 classifier achieved better results with a training accuracy of 99.83%, Table 5. This result is similar to the Embedding-32- (99.72%), and CNN-Max-pooling (99.71%) models. Within the random sampling process, the train's accuracy increased for all models except for the decision tree model. In the case of a random sampling of 80% for training and 20% for testing, the train's accuracy value increases by 0.0026 for the KNeighbors model. The best test accuracy

Table 5. Models' accuracy in case of random sampling without lemmatization.

Model	75% train 25% test		80% train 20% test	
	Train accuracy	Test accuracy	Train accuracy	Test accuracy
LogisticRegression	0.7508	0.7512	0.7506	0.7521
RandonForest	0.7508	0.7512	0.7506	0.7521
DecisionTree	0.7525	0.7534	0.7506	0.7521
KNeighbors	0.9960	0.7928	0.9986	0.8037
Embedding-100	0.9983	0.9983	0.9983	0.9983
Simple10	0.7508	0.7512	0.7506	0.7521
Embedding-32-	0.9972	0.9011	0.9976	0.9083
Embedding-32-Maxpooling	0.9176	0.8591	0.9236	0.8703
CNN-Maxpooling	0.9971	0.9322	0.9973	0.9365

Table 6. Models' accuracy in case of balanced random sampling ('stratify' parameter) without lemmatization.

Model	75% train 25% test		80% train 20% test	
	Train accuracy	Test accuracy	Train accuracy	Test accuracy
LogisticRegression	0.7509	0.7509	0.7509	0.7509
RandonForest	0.7509	0.7509	0.7509	0.7509
DecisionTree	0.7509	0.7509	0.7509	0.7509
KNeighbors	0.9986	0.7938	0.9986	0.8032
Embedding-100	0.9984	0.9984	0.9984	0.9984
Simple10	0.7509	0.7509	0.7509	0.7509
Embedding-32-	0.9961	0.8937	0.7509	0.7509
Embedding-32-Maxpooling	0.9152	0.8638	0.9179	0.8664
CNN-Maxpooling	0.9972	0.9340	0.9970	0.9347

(0.9984) is achieved by the Embedding_100 model for the two sampling cases (75% and 80% for training and 25% and 20% for test). Indeed, the CNN-Maxpooling model obtained 0.9972 (for 75%) and 0.9970 (for 80%) in the training case and test accuracy of 0.9340 and 0.9347. Therefore, the size of the training and test data sets impacts the models' performance. We notice well from the results that we have different results for most cases by changing the number of training and test data. Table 6 describes that the KNeighbors model (0.9986) obtains the best performance in the training case. The best test accuracy (0.9984) is achieved by the Embedding_100 model for the two sampling

Table 7. Models' accuracy in case of random sampling with lemmatization.

Model	75% train 25% test		80% train 20% test	
	Train accuracy	Test accuracy	Train accuracy	Test accuracy
LogisticRegression	0.7508	0.7512	0.7481	0.7491
RandonForest	0.7508	0.7512	0.7506	0.7521
DecisionTree	0.7537	0.7541	0.7506	0.7521
KNeighbors	0.9960	0.7782	0.9986	0.8054
Embedding-100	0.9982	0.9015	0.9984	0.9104
Simple10	0.7508	0.7512	0.7506	0.7521
Embedding-32-	0.9974	0.8996	0.7506	0.7521
Embedding-32-Maxpooling	0.9093	0.8610	0.9091	0.8626
CNN-Maxpooling	0.9960	0.9271	0.9962	0.9345

Table 8. Models' accuracy in case of balanced random sampling ('stratify' parameter) with lemmatization.

Model	75% train 25% test		80% train 20% test	
	Train accuracy	Test accuracy	Train accuracy	Test accuracy
LogisticRegression	0.7509	0.7509	0.7508	0.7508
RandonForest	0.7509	0.7509	0.7509	0.7509
DecisionTree	0.7509	0.7509	0.7523	0.7521
KNeighbors	0.9986	0.7745	0.9986	0.7924
Embedding-100	0.9984	0.9031	0.9983	0.9082
Simple10	0.7509	0.7509	0.7509	0.7509
Embedding-32-	0.9972	0.8966	0.9968	0.9026
Embedding-32-Maxpooling	0.9122	0.8632	0.9181	0.8683
CNN-Maxpooling	0.9963	0.9307	0.9965	0.9385

cases (75% and 80% for training and 25% and 20% for the test). Indeed, the CNN-Maxpooling model obtained 0.9972 (for 75%) and 0.9970 (for 80%) in the training case and test accuracy of 0.9340 and 0.9347.

Table 7 shows that in the case of data lemmatization and random sampling for 75% training data sets, the best accuracy obtained is 0.9982 for Embedding-100. While in the case of training data sets of 80%, we notice that the K-Neighbors model gets a slight performance evaluated to 0.9986 (i.e., a difference of 0.0004 compared to

Table 9. The best machine learning model.

Model	Train accuracy	Test accuracy	Sampling
Embedding-100	0.9983	0.9983	75% train 25% test random sampling without lemmatization
Embedding-100	0.9984	0.9984	80% train 20% test and 75% train 25% test balanced random sampling without lemmatization
KNeighbors	0.9986	0.8054	80% train 20% test random sampling with lemmatization

Embedding-100). In Table 8, the balanced random sampling case with lemmatization K-Neighbors achieved a better training accuracy of 0.9986. However, K-Neighbors model achieves very low test accuracy compared to Embedding-100, Embedding-32-, and CNN-Maxpooling. We concluded that, on the one hand, the use of GlobalMaxpooling negatively affects the accuracy of the Simple10.

On the other hand, lemmatization also causes a decrease in performance for the models: Embedding-32-Maxpooling and CNN-Maxpooling. With an exciting reduction for the Embedding-32- model in the case of 80% training data sets with random sampling, except for the K-Neighbors model (i.e., presents the stability of these results). As for word embedding, it has increased the performance of neural network models. It is important to note that the results show the effect of word embedding for the Simple10 model for all the study cases. We propose choosing the Embedding-100 model for the case, 75%–25%, with balanced random sampling without lemmatization. Indeed, this model has a training accuracy of 0.9984 and a test accuracy of 0.9984, Table 6.

In our comparative state-of-the-art learning models, however, we retained only the models having obtained better performances, as indicated in Table 9. Comparative studies on different deep learning architectures, such as recurrent short-term memory neural networks (LSTM) and convolutional neural networks (CNN), have been conducted by Colón-Ruiz and Segura-Bedmar [10]. This study highlighted the importance and performance of the combination of Bert and Word2vec representation-based models. All the techniques studied proceed by deleting numerical expressions.

Furthermore, Bemila et al. [3] tested several classifiers on bags of words, such as Naive Bayes, logistic regression and RNN-BiLSTM. The best accuracy score is 0.83906, obtained using an RNN-BiLSTM classifier. Additionally, Na and Wai [20] proposed a rule-based linguistic approach. Their method takes a purely linguistic approach to calculating the sentiment orientation of a clause from prior sentiment scores assigned to words, taking into account grammatical relationships and semantic annotation of words in the text. Their approach achieved an accuracy of 0.69.

Table 10 highlights that our approach overcame the logistic regression model proposed by F. Gräber et al. [6], whose precision was 0.9224. The proposed text preprocessing method relies on word embedding, which keeps the text's semantics. Based on our study's research, the models: KNeighbors, Embedding-100, Embedding-32- and CNN-Maxpooling proposed by our study achieved the best accuracy of all analysis and classification models for drug.com dataset.

Table 10. Comparison with previous studies.

Study	Year	Method	Accuracy
Mercadier, Yves [5]	2021	XLNet [a]	0.3678
S. Vijayaraghavan et D.Basu [7]	2020	ANN [b]	0.887309
Na, Jin-Cheon, and Wai Yan Min Kyaing [20]	2015	Linguistic Approach	0.69
Gräber, Felix, et al. [6]	2018	Régression logistique	0.9224
Bemila, et al. [3]	2020	RNN-BiLSTM	0.83906
Y. Mercadier et al. [11]	2020	Roberta avec DAIA	0.316
C. Colón-Ruiz and I. Segura-Bedmar [10]	2020	LSTM	0.9046
M.E BASIRI et al. [21]	2020	3W3DT-NB	0.8836
Our approach	2022	Embedding-100	0.9984

[a] A Generalized Autoregressive Pretraining for Language Understanding (XLNet).
[b] Artificial Neural Network.

4 Conclusion and Future Work

In this work, we propose the Embedding-100 model to predict the drug's effectiveness and efficiency. We rely on natural language processing. As a new approach, we tackle a crucial challenge: the medical semantics to analyze and extract knowledge from medical text. The proposed model is the result of an extensive study. The latter shows that the accuracy of the models depends on their architecture and type.

Furthermore, those models are influenced by the text preprocessing method and sampling type. Experiments indicate that the accuracy (Training accuracy is 0.9984, and the test accuracy is 0.9984) of our model is better than others handled by the totality of the state-of-the-art learning model. Embedding-100 combines artificial neural network, one hot encoder and word embedding. In the future, our work can be extended to analyzing drug effectiveness for other types of data sets, especially medical records. In addition, medical text preprocessing remains a critical research area.

References

1. Haute Autorité de Santé. https://www.has-sante.fr/. Accessed 01 Aug 2022
2. Campesato, O.: Artificial intelligence, machine learning, and deep learning. Mercury Learning and Information (2020)
3. Bemila, T., Kadam, I., Sidana, A., et al.: An approach to sentimental analysis of drug reviews using RNN-BiLSTM model. In: Proceedings of the 3rd International Conference on Advances in Science & Technology (ICAST) (2020)
4. Mascio, A., Kraljevic, Z., Bean, D., et al.: Comparative analysis of text classification approaches in electronic health records. arXiv preprint arXiv:2005.06624 (2020)
5. Mercadier, Y.: Classification automatique de textes par réseaux de neurones profonds: application au domaine de la santé. Diss. Université Montpellier (2020)

6. Graber, F., Kallumadi, S., Malberg, H., et al.: Aspect-based sentiment analysis of drug reviews applying cross-domain and cross-data learning. In: Proceedings of the 2018 International Conference on Digital Health, pp. 121–125 (2018)
7. Vijayaraghavan, S., Basu, D.: Sentiment analysis in drug reviews using supervised machine learning algorithms. arXiv preprint arXiv:2003.11643 (2020)
8. Jiménez-Zafra, S.M., Martín-Valdivia, M.T., et al.: How do we talk about doctors and drugs? Sentiment analysis in forums expressing opinions for medical domain. Artif. Intell. Med. **93**, 50–57 (2018)
9. Yadav, A., Vishwakarma, D.K.: A weighted text representation framework for sentiment analysis of medical drug reviews. In: 2020 IEEE Sixth International Conference on Multimedia Big Data (BigMM), pp. 326–332. IEEE (2020)
10. Colón-Ruiz, C., Segura-Bedmar, I.: Comparing deep learning architectures for sentiment analysis on drug reviews. J. Biomed. Inform. **110**, 103539 (2020)
11. Mercadier, Y., Azé, J., Bringay, S.: Divide to better classify. In: Michalowski, M., Moskovitch, R. (eds.) AIME 2020. LNCS (LNAI), vol. 12299, pp. 89–99. Springer, Cham (2020). https://doi.org/10.1007/978-3-030-59137-3_9
12. Min, Z.: Drugs reviews sentiment analysis using weakly supervised model. In: 2019 IEEE International Conference on Artificial Intelligence and Computer Applications (ICAICA), pp. 332–336. IEEE (2019)
13. UCI Machine Learning Repository: Drug Review Dataset. https://archive.ics.uci.edu/ml/datasets/Drug+Review+Dataset+%28Drugs.com%29. Accessed 26 Aug 2022
14. Split Your Dataset With scikit-learn's train_test_split() Real Python. https://realpython.com/train-test-split-python-data/. Accessed 14 Apr 2022
15. Userguide: contents scikit learn. https://scikitlearn.org/stable/user_guide.html. Accessed 10 June 2022
16. Le modèle séquentiel TensorFlow Core. https://www.tensorflow.org/guide/keras/sequential_model. Accessed 12 May 2022
17. Géron, A.: Hands-On Machine Learning with Scikit-Learn, Keras, and TensorFlow: Concepts, Tools, and Techniques to Build Intelligent Systems. O'Reilly Media Inc., USA (2019)
18. Kingma, D.P., Jimmy, L.B.: Adam: A method for stochastic optimization. arXiv preprint arXiv:1412.6980 (2014)
19. Intuition d'Adam Optimizer – StackLima. https://stacklima.com/intuition-d-adam-optimizer/. Accessed 14 Apr 2022
20. Na, J.C., Kyaing, W.Y.M.: Sentiment analysis of user-generated content on drug review websites. J. Inf. Sci. Theory Pract. **3**(1), 6–23 (2015)
21. Basiri, M.E., Abdar, M., Cifci, M.A., et al.: A novel method for sentiment classification of drug reviews using fusion of deep and machine learning techniques. Knowl.-Based Syst. **198**, 105949 (2020)

Remote Secured Monitoring Application for Respiratory Ventilator Implementations

Sérgio Branco[1]([✉])(iD), Ertugrul Dogruluk[1](iD), Pedro Mestre[1,2,4](iD),
Carlos Ferreira[1](iD), Rui Cordeiro[1](iD), Rui Teixeira[1](iD), João Valente[1](iD),
Bruno Gaspar[3](iD), and Jorge Cabral[1,4](iD)

[1] CEiiA Centro de Engenharia e Desenvolvimento de Produto, 4450-017 Matosinhos, Portugal
{antonio.branco,ertugrul.dogruluk,pedro.mestre,
carlos.ferreira,rui.cordeiro,rui.pteixeira,joao.valente,
jorge.cabral}@ceiia.com
[2] Universtity of Trás-os-Montes e Alto Douro, Vila Real, Portugal
[3] NOS Comunicações, 1600-404 Lisboa, Portugal
bruno.gaspar@nos.pt
[4] ALGORITMI Research Centre/LASI, University of Minho, 4800-058 Guimarães, Portugal
https://www.ceiia.com, https://www.utad.pt, https://www.nos.pt/,
https://algoritmi.uminho.pt

Abstract. Internet of Things (IoT) applications have recently significantly increased, especially in health-related services. This movement also brings security issues to the applications, especially for those where the life of patients can be put in risk. This work presents the implementation of an application with remote monitoring for real respiratory ventilator implementation scenarios. To provide secure communications for the devices and applications, a custom protocol (Blackwing) was used. This protocol provides integrity and confidentiality to the application and also has as an objective to be lightweight and micro-service oriented. Lastly, communications from the ventilators are integrated using an architecture for IoT based on a mediator that allows the integration with devices that use other communication protocols.

Keywords: IoT · Remote health IoT application · Respiratory Ventilator · IoT Mediator

A. Cunha et al. (Eds.): MobiHealth 2022, LNICST 484, pp. 338–346, 2023.
https://doi.org/10.1007/978-3-031-32029-3_28

1 Introduction

Recently, the interaction between devices and the Internet has increased significantly. The Internet of Things (IoT) technologies attempt to answer these needs by providing various communication designs, methodologies, network technologies, and others. IoT applications can also answer to health-related services such as patient health tracking, medication supply management, hospital/billing records, remote patient health monitoring, etc. [3].

Therefore an area of research that has increasingly been the target of the research community. In fact, in the literature, we can find several health service-related IoT solutions and their applications. For instance, wearable health sensors and intelligent medicine packages (iMedBox and iMedPack) application are proposed by [9]. The work [5] proposed and deployed a health IoT application (IoTM) monitoring cardiopulmonary functions. Authors of [7] proposed a solution to optimize the management of medicines for patients or elderly users. In [2], it is described the mobile health architecture for the IoT technologies and discussed connectivity, low-power-based devices, and wearable health applications to monitor ECG, blood sugar level, etc. The work [6] developed an IoT architecture for remotely monitoring service with the support of efficient software engines such as rapid summarization for effective prognosis (RASPRO) and criticality measure index (CMI), which are deployed at edge IoT services. This remote monitoring tool is deployed in a hospital to be an alternative clinical device for remote monitoring. Last but not least, in [1], it used a user-centered design (UCD) to analyze the users' requirements and intention of usage for the m-health approaches.

In this work, it is proposed a solution, based on IoT technologies, to monitor respiratory ventilators in a medical environment. These ventilators are connected using a custom protocol that is being tested for this type of applications. This protocol is named Blackwing. It is based on standard encryption algorithms, and uses a two phase communication (as we can find in other protocols): in the first phase asymmetric encryption is used to exchange encryption and authentication information, and in the second phase, a symmetric key is used to cipher the information.

To aggregate the information from the ventilators an architecture based on a Mediator is used. This Mediator architecture will allow the integration of other medical devices that can be using other protocols. Also, data from the ventilators are made available for remote access to the medical staff.

This work is organized as follows: Introduction, the current section, summarizes the related works within the motivation of the IoT healthcare services and presents the motivations and objectives for deployment of a secure remote respiratory ventilator application. Section 2 summarizes the literature review on IoT healthcare services architectures and the implementation of remote monitoring tools/applications. Section 3 introduces the main contribution of this paper by presenting the developed work and the results related to the monitoring application and the used security protocol. Finally, Sect. 4 concludes this work's findings.

2   Health Applications in the Internet of the Things

Within increasing to Machine-to-Machine communication and devices is leading
to IoT applications to be increased significantly. For instance, healthcare-related
IoT applications cover several implementations such as intelligent health patient
monitoring, vehicular emerging services tracing, healthcare, structural health,
hospital patient records, etc. The health-related applications have the capability
or requires to enable real-time or remote patient monitoring [8].

All health-related applications require service, performance, reliability, and
integrity to maintain available services, access patient information and health-
related platforms or applications.

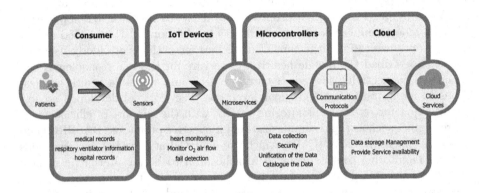

Fig. 1. Health IoT structure

Figure 1 illustrates the health IoT system architecture. The system starts by
receiving patient or health data (respiratory ventilator, hospital/patient records,
emergency service tracing, etc.) through IoT devices (sensors). Then, micro-
services granted lightweight protocols to bring health IoT services independent
of other complex architectures. Finally, using communication protocols (HTTP,
NB-IoT, and others), the health IoT data or services are secured and maintained
by cloud providers. Additionally, some cloud providers can support service availability (*e.g.* Kubernetes) to maintain the services up and running.

2.1   Design a Mobile Secured Respiratory Monitoring Architecture

The recent movement of IoT architectures brings smart and easy accessibility to
applications. These services can be to tracking the emergency services, monitoring the patient health records, alarming depending on the patient situation, etc.
Because these IoT services are crucial and must be reliable, security and other
related services matter.

In this work, we have created a secured application to monitor real respiratory
ventilator devices remotely. The application supports a user-friendly interface to
analyze patient data. A protocol also secures this architecture for the application
at the application layer, which will be explained next.

3   Remote Respiratory Ventilator Application

Other works propose several monitoring applications for IoT implementations. However, secure remote application on the specific m-health IoT implementation is a lack in the literature.

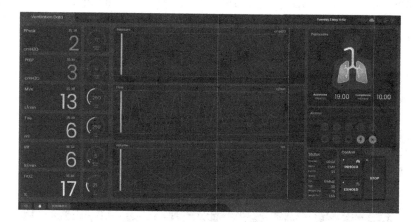

Fig. 2. Health IoT structure

A remote monitoring service or application is required in hospitals or other related services. In this work, the application was created to monitor and analyze the patient parameters in real-time. This health IoT application analyzes respiratory ventilator devices using Internet Protocol.

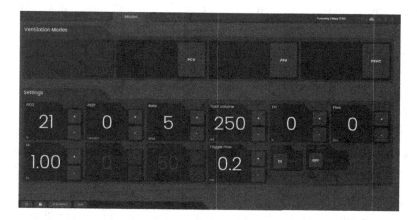

Fig. 3. Defining the parameters for the respiratory ventilator machine

Figure 2 illustrates the application dashboard interface. The application mainly illustrates the following main parameters: - Pressure, Flow, Volume,

PPeak, PEEP, MVe, TVe, and RR from the respiratory ventilator device, which is called Atena.

Figures 3 and 4 illustrate the inserting of the auxiliary parameters for the device (respiratory ventilator). These parameters include the ventilation modes/settings, Alarms, and Patient details (sex, age, weight, and height). The PSV backup settings include 1;E, Rate, Positive end expiratory pressure (PEEP), and inspiratory pressure (Plnsp). Under the setting also ventilator setting includes parameters the Insp/Exp hold, O_2, and Flow calibrations.

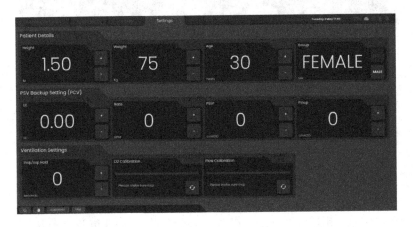

Fig. 4. Defining the parameters for the respiratory ventilator machine

In device modes, the Fraction of inspired oxygen (F_iO_2), PEEP, Rate, Tidal Volume, transpulmonary pressure (TP_i), Flow, inspiratory time: expiratory time (I: E), Pinssp, Slope, Trigger Flow, and other settings for the ventilator.

Figure 5 illustrates the secured application on the remote device. This application is synchronized with the Atena respiratory device in real-time. The application also supports remotely setting the patients' data. The remote application was tested to meet the requirement to be accessed remotely through the Internet.

3.1 Securing the Monitoring Application

This work considers all IoT-related services critical and must be secured to maintain the services' integrity. To do so, we have used a specific security protocol at the application layer to maintain the application service integrity. This security tool is called Blackwing and uses encryption between endpoints. Blackwing protocol uses both asymmetric and symmetric encryption to secure data transmission. In the initial phase, RSA is used to cipher the initial communication parameters and to cipher an AES key negotiated between the client and the server. In all other transactions, communications are encrypted using that key [4].

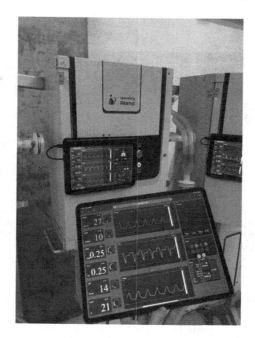

Fig. 5. Application with the Atena Respiratory Ventilator

Blackwing works based on a micro-service architecture. When a client sends information to the server, it specifies which micro-service will handle that request. In this work setup, the Blackwing tool is used to secure the data between Atena (respiratory ventilator device) and Application device micro-services.

The remote secured application we developed supports monitoring/managing multiple devices in this work. Figure 6 illustrates the real-time application dashboard for the five ventilator devices. Each ventilator device can be managed remotely by setting the parameters of the patient, device, and others.

Figure 7 illustrates the application performance with a network analyzing tool on real Atena ventilator devices. We deployed five respiratory ventilator devices in this experiment, as presented previously. The results are obtained for Packets/sec. for the application dashboard. As expected during the application dashboard, the traffic is increasing, and 150 packets/s are obtained from five ventilators.

3.2   Integration with an IoT Mediator

Using devices from different IoT manufacturers and applications can be challenging when integrating devices and applications. Distinctive IoT health brands, databases, communication protocols, and others can be problematic in communicating with other health IoT architectures. For example, various data sets, patient billing, ventilator records, tracing patient information, etc., can increase the complexity of health-related IoT architectures.

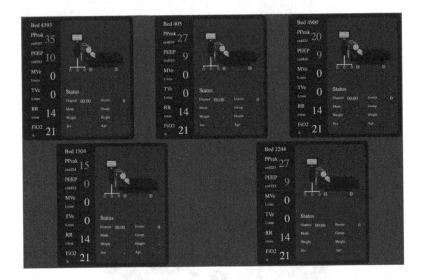

Fig. 6. Multiple Atena Respiratory Ventilators in the Application

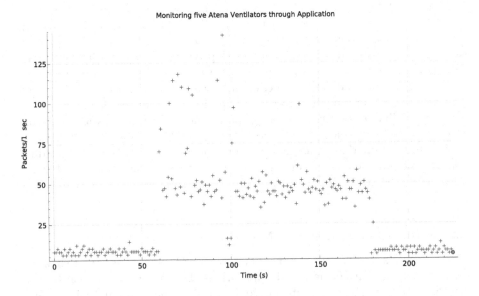

Fig. 7. Application with the Atena Respiratory Ventilator

The IoT mediator (another definition is "platform") overcomes the challenges identified above. IoT platform makes the IoT architecture(s) understandable and easy to manage between IoT architectures. In addition to the respiratory ventilator application, this work also proposes an adaption to the IoT mediator.

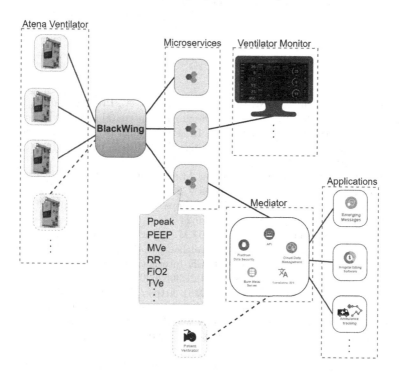

Fig. 8. Atena Respiratory Ventilator adaption the Mediator

Figure 8 illustrates the proposal of health IoT device adaption to the IoT Mediator, as also stated for future works. In this mediator adaption architecture, the Ventilator devices use the Blackwing security protocol to get managed microservices (e.g., Ventilator parameters) and then use through the Mediator, which answers the applications and other ventilator brands.

4   Conclusions and Future Works

This work presented a remote secured monitoring application for a real respiratory device called Atena. Preliminary findings with traffic analyzing tools for a remote monitoring application edge side. Additionally, a security protocol was adapted to keep the application and device integrity for the edge consumers and server.

Lastly, to maintain services availability and integrity of the monitoring application, an IoT mediator integration is modeled, and this work is stated as a future work.

Acknowledgements. Project "(Link4S)ustainability - A new generation connectivity system for creation and integration of networks of objects for new sustainability paradigms [POCI-01-0247-FEDER-046122 | LISBOA-01-0247-FEDER-046122]" is financed by the Operational Competitiveness and Internationalization Programmes COMPETE 2020 and LISBOA 2020, under the PORTUGAL 2020 Partnership Agreement, and through the European Structural and Investment Funds in the FEDER component.

References

1. Afrizal, S.H., Hidayanto, A.N., Hakiem, N., Sartono, A., Priyambodo, S., Eryando, T.: Design of mHealth application for integrating antenatal care service in primary health care: a user-centered approach. In: Proceedings of 2019 4th International Conference on Informatics and Computing, ICIC 2019 2, 0–5 (2019). https://doi.org/10.1109/ICIC47613.2019.8985911

2. Almotiri, S.H., Khan, M.A., Alghamdi, M.A.: Mobile health (m-Health) system in the context of IoT. In: Proceedings - 2016 4th International Conference on Future Internet of Things and Cloud Workshops, W-FiCloud 2016, pp. 39–42 (2016). https://doi.org/10.1109/W-FiCloud.2016.24

3. Bhuiyan, M.N., Rahman, M.M., Billah, M.M., Saha, D.: Internet of Things (IoT): a review of its enabling technologies in healthcare applications, standards protocols, security, and market opportunities. IEEE Internet Things J. 8(13), 10474–10498 (2021). https://doi.org/10.1109/JIOT.2021.3062630

4. Branco, S.: Blackwing Specifications (2018). https://blackwing.readthedocs.io

5. Liu, J., Miao, F., Yin, L., Pang, Z., Li, Y.: A noncontact ballistocardiography-based IoMT system for cardiopulmonary health monitoring of discharged COVID-19 patients. IEEE Internet Things J. 8(21), 15807–15817 (2021). https://doi.org/10.1109/JIOT.2021.3063549

6. Pathinarupothi, R.K., Durga, P., Rangan, E.S.: IoT-based smart edge for global health: remote monitoring with severity detection and alerts transmission. IEEE Internet Things J. 6(2), 2449–2462 (2019). https://doi.org/10.1109/JIOT.2018.2870068, https://ieeexplore.ieee.org/document/8464257/

7. Pinto, A., Correia, A., Alves, R., Matos, P., Ascensão, J., Camelo, D.: eHealthCare - A Medication Monitoring Approach for the Elderly People. In: Gao, X., Jamalipour, A., Guo, L. (eds.) MobiHealth 2021. LNICST, vol. 440, pp. 221–234. Springer, Cham (2022). https://doi.org/10.1007/978-3-031-06368-8_15, https://link.springer.com/10.1007/978-3-031-06368-815

8. Stoyanova, M., Nikoloudakis, Y., Panagiotakis, S., Pallis, E., Markakis, E.K.: A survey on the internet of things (IoT) forensics: challenges, approaches, and open issues. IEEE Commun. Surv. Tutorials 22(2), 1191–1221 (2020). https://doi.org/10.1109/COMST.2019.2962586

9. Yang, G., et al.: A fealth-IoT platform based on the integration of intelligent packaging, unobtrusive bio-sensor, and intelligent medicine box. IEEE Trans. Industr. Inf. 10(4), 2180–2191 (2014). https://doi.org/10.1109/TII.2014.2307795

Understanding User Trust in Different Recommenders and Smartphone Applications

Siva Simhadri and Sudip Vhaduri[✉]

Purdue University, West Lafayette, IN 47907, USA
{ssimhadr,svhaduri}@purdue.edu

Abstract. In recent times, we are witnessing rapid growth in smartphone applications due to various types of services ranging from bank transactions to health and well-being monitoring, that these apps are providing. However, most often these apps suffer from low user trust and that directly impacts the utility and adherence to the apps. Thereby, it is crucial to understand the user trust in different types of apps and recommenders to improve the utility and adherence of the apps. In this work, we perform a detailed investigation of user trust in four major types of apps, including health apps, payment apps, news apps, and gaming apps, and four major groups of recommenders, i.e., friends, family members, external recommenders (healthcare providers, news channels, or advertisements), and no recommender. From our detailed analysis of a study with 60 smartphone users with different backgrounds, we find a higher trust in health apps and payment apps when recommended by healthcare providers or physicians, and friends or family members. In general, we do not find any significant differences among users with different backgrounds. Thereby, we recommend considering specific groups of recommenders and their recommended features while developing relevant apps to achieve higher utility and adherence.

Keywords: Smartphone app · Recommenders · User trust

1 Introduction

1.1 Motivation

Due to the rise of sensing power and computing capability of smartphones and advancement in mobile networks [8], major app stores, including Google Play, Apple App Store, and Amazon Appstore, are flooded with more than 3.48 million apps [5] providing various services, including discovering places of interest [35,41,43,46,47], security and user authentication [11–13,20,29,31,38–40, 44,45], assessing respiratory diseases and their stages [14,26,28,49,50], assessing

© ICST Institute for Computer Sciences, Social Informatics and Telecommunications Engineering 2023
Published by Springer Nature Switzerland AG 2023. All Rights Reserved
A. Cunha et al. (Eds.): MobiHealth 2022, LNICST 484, pp. 347–361, 2023.
https://doi.org/10.1007/978-3-031-32029-3_29

health and wellbeing [10, 22, 27, 33, 34, 36, 37, 42, 48], and call behavior assessment [15, 18, 30, 32]. The global market for smartphone applications is expected to grow by 11.5% compound annual growth rate (CAGR) from 2020 to 2027 [6]. With the increase of smartphone apps, we are experiencing an increased number of downloads, i.e., a 7% rise in 2021 compared to 2020 [4]. Among various types of app that people download and use, mobile health (mHealth) apps, news apps, gaming apps, and payment apps are found to be the most common types [1].

The global market for mobile health (mHealth) apps is predicted to increase at a CAGR of 11.8% from 2022 to 2030 [2]. This rapid increase in the adoption of mHealth apps is due to the various benefits, including real-time and remote patient monitoring, diagnosis, and treatment based on physicians' recommendations, that the mHealth apps provide to the users [3]. During the COVID-19 global pandemic, around 900 million new mobile payment apps were added to the App stores (in 2020), most of which are primarily targeted to help users make online payments [7]. However, a user's decision to use an app from a set of apps could affect the user's trust in people who are recommending the app. Thereby, knowing users' trust in different recommenders can help the app designer and developer involve the specific group of recommenders to develop apps with a higher utility and adherence.

1.2 Related Work

Since the compliance of smartphone apps drop over time, researchers have been actively trying to find factors that affect a user's trust in apps in order to improve the compliance and utility of the apps. Along this line, a group of researchers has investigated the popularity of different categories of mobile applications using *monthly active users* (MAUs) [23]. They have analyzed important features of mobile apps and their association with global market share and growth rate. Another group of researchers has tried to determine the variables that lead to shorter *application life cycles* (ALCs) of an app [25]. Researchers have found several factors, including telecommunication infrastructure, smartphone hardware specifications, application user interfaces, data privacy, security, trends, and ads that affect a user's choice to install and continue specific smartphone apps. Additionally, some researchers have found attractiveness, value, ease-of-use, trust, social support, diffusiveness, and user reviews are some key elements that influence users' decisions to download and utilize apps from the vast choices accessible in the app stores [9, 16, 19].

To better understand different factors and their impact on app compliance, several focused studies have been conducted with specific categories of apps, such as news apps, gaming apps, health apps, social networking apps, payment apps, and many other apps [17, 21, 24, 51–53]. While some researchers investigated the major user concerns in using a social networking app [51], some found perceived performance risk, perceived financial risk, and perceived privacy risk have strong negative effects on perceived value and acceptance of payment apps [52]. Similarly, some researchers have found user experience and functionality of a health app as the main factors affecting a user's decision to continue using an app [24].

Additionally, some researchers have found the popularity of the apps and the security preferences of the users as key features to affect a user's decision to continue an app [53]. However, none of these works thoroughly investigated user trust in different types of recommender groups, such as family members, friends, and physicians, and their association with various types of apps based on users' backgrounds.

1.3 Contribution

The main contribution of this work is to understand user trust in different types of smartphone applications and recommenders. Also, we investigate whether there is any significant difference in trust among different group of app users. While we find a high level of user trust in health apps and payment apps compared to other types of apps when the apps are recommended by healthcare providers, friends, or family members, we do not find any statistically significant difference among different groups of users based on educational background, age, app development experience, and gender. Therefore, our findings are generalized to the entire population, and we recommend bringing the respective group of recommenders into the design process of different types of smartphone apps, including health and payment apps. Thereby, the apps can be developed based on various features that the recommenders think to better serve the respective users. This way the apps will have a higher chance of serving the targeted user population.

Organization: First, we present our human study data collection approach, followed by our methods to analyze the collected data in the "Approach" section (Sect. 2). Next, in "Analysis" section (Sect. 3), we present our detailed analysis using graphical and statistical techniques to determine user-trust in different recommenders and smartphone apps and to determine statistical significance of different factors, such as app development experience, age, education level, gender, and marital status. In the end, we present the conclusions in the "Conclusions" section (Sect. 4) and the limitations and future work in the "Limitations and Future Work" section (Sect. 5).

2 Approach

First, we present our human study data collection approach, followed by our methods to analyze the collected data and determine user-trust towards different types of smartphone applications and recommendation groups.

2.1 Human Study Data Collection

To understand the significance of recommender groups on a users' trust towards different types of apps, we conduct a study that is approved by the institutional review board (IRB#: IRB-2022-156). To reach out to different smartphone user

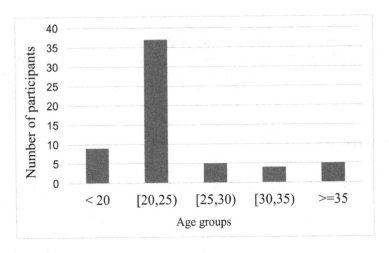

Fig. 1. Bar graphs presenting subject distribution based on age

groups, we post our flyers to various online groups in different social media platforms, such as Twitter and Facebook, in addition to posting on university advertisement boards. The flyer contains a QR code to a Google Form survey that we use to collect data. Participants can reach to the survey from the QR code posted on the flyer and participants can submit their responses anonymously without providing any email id, phone number, or person identifiable information (PPI). Additionally, participation in the survey was completely voluntary and participants could withdraw from the study any time they want while taking the survey. In the "Participant Demographics" section (Sect. 2.1), we present the demographic details of our study subjects. During the study, we use Google Form surveys to anonymously collect various demographic information about subjects, including gender and age, with some additional questions to inquire about subjects' marital status, educational background, and smartphone app development experience. To understand a users' trust towards different recommender groups and smartphone applications, we ask additional questions as discussed in the "Survey" section (Sect. 2.1).

Participant Demographics We were able to get replies from 60 anonymous participants throughout the experiment. There are 60 participants, and 65.9% of them are men. The total subject pool is divided into five age groups: 20, [20, 25], [25, 30], [30, 35], and ≥35. Figure 1 shows that the dominant age range is [20, 25] years, where 62% of the participants are found.

Since a subject's marital status may affect that subject's trust in various recommender groups, including family, we additionally collected the participants' marital status during the study. We discovered that 51 of the total 60 participants are single. We display the subjects' educational backgrounds in Fig. 2. We discover that 36.4% participants have completed their undergrad (termed as

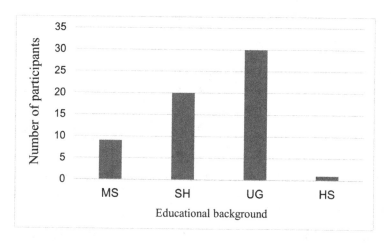

Fig. 2. Bar graphs presenting subject distribution based on educational background

UG in the figure), 43.2% have completed their senior high school, 18.2% have earned a master's degree, and the other participants have completed high school (termed as HS in the figure).

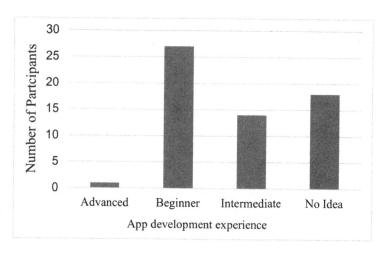

Fig. 3. Bar graphs presenting subject distribution based on app development experience

Additionally, we ask the subjects to report their smartphone app development experience (Fig. 3). Only 2.3% of the subjects had advanced experience, and 25% of the participants have no prior understanding of app development.

Table 1. Different types of smartphone apps

Types of Apps	Acronyms
Health App	H
Gaming App	G
News App	N
Payment App	P

Survey. During the study, we investigate user-trust across four major types of smartphone applications as presented in Table 1. And, participants respond to the following four questions:

1. How frequently do you install a Health app recommended by the following groups?
2. How frequently do you install an online Payment app recommended by the following groups?
3. How frequently do you install a News app (app that provides all the latest news) recommended by the following groups?
4. How frequently do you install a Gaming app recommended by the following groups?

For each app type (i.e., one of the above four questions), subjects rate their trust in different apps when they are recommended by the following four major groups:

– Friends
– Family Members
– External Recommenders (i.e., physicians or healthcare providers (H apps), news channels (N apps), or advertisements (P and G apps)
– No Recommendation

Where the "external recommender" is a term we introduced while analyzing and presenting our findings, but during the study we present them as showed inside the parenthesis based on the app type. Additionally, the "no recommendation" refers to cases where the users do not have any recommender group. Participants rate the recommender groups on a scale of 1 to 5 for each of the four app types mentioned above. A rating of 1 means a recommender group is trusted the least, and 5 means the highest level of trust.

2.2 Methods

In this work, we consider a two-step approach to analyze our data. We first utilize a visualization-based approach using stacked-bars to find user-trust variations across different types of smartphone applications and recommender groups. Next, we use statistical tests, such as the $z-test$ and χ^2-test, to determine the

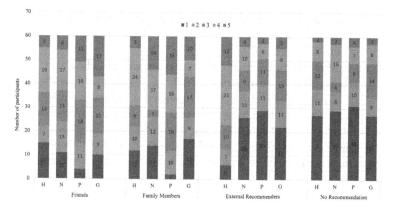

Fig. 4. User-trust rating across different types of smartphone apps and recommender groups, where 1 and 5 mean the lowest and highest level of trust

statistical significance of different features, such as educational background, age, app development experience, marital status, and gender, on user-trust across different types of apps and recommender groups.

3 Analysis

While interpreting a user's trust, i.e., willingness to use an app based on a specific recommender group, we group ratings 1 and 2 into "least likely" (i.e., low trust) category. Similarly, we group ratings 4 and 5 to "highly likely" (i.e., high trust) category. In Fig. 4, we use stacked bars to present users' rating across different types of recommenders and smartphone apps.

We first analyze **friends** as a recommender group and try to determine user-trust across different types of apps when they are recommended by friends. In the figure, we find that 80% more people (i.e., $(27 - 15)/15 * 100\%$) rate high trust ("highly likely" versus. "least likely" categories) in the case of payment apps (P-bar in the figure). However, in the case of gaming apps (G-bar) and health apps (H-bar), only 36% and 9% more people rate high trust in friends' recommendations. On the other hand, more people rate less trust in friends recommendations about news apps (N-bar). Therefore, we conclude that people consider friends' recommendations with a high level of trust when choosing payment apps.

Next, we consider **family members** as a recommender group. In the figure, we observe that the number of people who mention high trust in choosing a payment app (P-bar) based on a family member's recommendation is 2.67 times (i.e., 32 versus 12) higher than the number of people who mention low trust. Similarly, compared to the number of people who mention high trust in a family member's recommendation while choosing news apps (N-bar) and health apps (H-bar) is 1.19 times (i.e., 31 versus 26) and 1.32 times (i.e., 29 versus 22) higher than the number of people who mention low trust. On the other hand, more people mention low trust in a family member's recommendation when choosing a gaming app (G-bar). Hence, we conclude that more people are highly likely to use a payment app when recommended by their family members, compared to any other recommender group.

Next, we analyze users trust in different types of app when they are recommended by **external recommenders**, such as healthcare providers or physicians, news channels, or advertisements. In the case of health apps (H-bar), the number of people who mention high trust is 2.85 times (i.e., 37 versus 13) higher than the number of people who mention low trust. Compared to health apps, more people mention low trust in the other three types of apps when referred by external recommenders, such as news channels (P-bar) or advertisements (N-bar and G-bar). Hence, we conclude that people are more likely to use a health app when it is recommended by a health expert, such as a physician or a healthcare provider.

Finally, we consider the **no recommendation** category. In Fig. 4, we observe that in general more people rated low trust while selecting all types of apps without any recommendation. Around 1.94–3.8 times people are likely to rate low trust compared to rating high trusts. Hence, we conclude that people need some guidance either from family/friends or external recommenders while selecting smartphone apps.

As we have found people mention high trust in payment (P) apps when they are recommended by **friends** and **family members**, and high trust in health (H) apps, when they are recommended by health experts, such as healthcare providers or physicians, therefore, we will next investigate significance of different features, such as marital status, educational background, gender, app development experience, and age in choosing a health (H) app (Sect. 3.1) or payment (P) app (Sect. 3.2) with high trust (4 or 5 ratings). Throughout this manuscript, p_i and $\hat{p}_i$ are used to indicate population and sample proportions of the ith group.

3.1   Factors Affecting User-Trust in Health Apps

In this section, we analyze the statistical significance of various parameters, such as user trust, educational attainment, gender, app development experience, age, and marital status, when selecting a health app.

Significance of Gender. The percentage of men and women who have high trust in health applications that are suggested by healthcare professionals or doctors is compared using the $z-test$ to see if there is a statistically significant discrepancy between both, i.e., null hypothesis, $H_0 : p_1 = p_2$, where $\hat{p}_1 = \frac{16}{24}$ and $\hat{p}_2 = \frac{21}{36}$ are the fractions of male and female who provide a high rating when conveying their trust in health (H) apps recommended by physicians or healthcare providers. With $z = .6$ and $p = .533$, we are unable to reject the null hypothesis at the .05 level of significance. Thus, we draw the conclusion that trust in health (H) apps suggested by doctors or other healthcare professionals is not comparable for males and females.

Significance of Age. We conduct the χ^2 proportion test with the null hypothesis that "when it comes to user-trust in health apps recommended by healthcare providers or physicians, there is no statistically significant discrepancy among the fractions of individuals from different age groups" (i.e., $H_0 : p_1 = p_2 = p_3 = p_4 = p_5$, where $\hat{p}_1 = \frac{5}{9}$, $\hat{p}_2 = \frac{25}{37}$, $\hat{p}_3 = \frac{3}{5}$, $\hat{p}_4 = \frac{1}{4}$, and $\hat{p}_5 = \frac{3}{5}$ are the fractions of subjects from different age groups that provide a high rating in health app when recommended by physician or healthcare providers). At .05 level of significance, we cannot reject the null hypothesis with $\chi^2(4) = .8602$ and $p = .93$. Therefore, we draw the conclusion that user trust in health (H) apps suggested by doctors or other healthcare professionals does not significantly differ among the five age groups.

Significance of Educational Background. From our analysis, we dropped the subject who "passed high school" (Fig. 2) and does not have high trust in the health (H) apps when recommended by healthcare providers or physicians. We take into account the remaining three categories of people: those who completed senior high school, graduated, and obtained a master's degree. We use the χ^2 proportion test with the null hypothesis that "there is no statistically significant distinction among the fractions of individuals from different education backgrounds, in terms of user-trust in health apps when recommended by physicians or healthcare providers" to examine the significance among different groups. (i.e., $H_0 : p_1 = p_2 = p_3$, where $\hat{p}_1 = \frac{3}{9}$, $\hat{p}_2 = \frac{11}{20}$, and $\hat{p}_3 = \frac{23}{30}$ are the fractions of subjects from the three groups that provide a high rating in health app when recommended by physician or healthcare providers. With $\chi^2(2) = 1.5786$ and $p = .454$, we are unable to reject the null hypothesis at the .05 level of significance. Thus, we draw the conclusion that there is no discernible difference in user-trust in health (H) apps suggested by doctors or other healthcare professionals across the three groups of people.

Significance of App Development Experience. When recommended by healthcare professionals or doctors, one participant with "advanced" app development expertise (Fig. 3) did not place a high level of trust in the health (H) apps. The "advanced" app development expertise and that participant are thus excluded from this research. The remaining three categories of people—those with no experience, intermediate experience, and no experience—are taken into consideration.

With the χ^2 proportion test and the null hypothesis "there is no significant discrepancy among the fractions of individuals from different groups, in terms of user-trust in health apps when recommended by physicians or healthcare providers", we examine the significance among groups of people based on app development experience (i.e., $H_0 : p_1 = p_2 = p_3$, where $\hat{p}_1 = \frac{18}{27}$, $\hat{p}_2 = \frac{11}{14}$, and $\hat{p}_3 = \frac{8}{18}$ are the fractions of subjects from the three groups that provide a high rating in health app when recommended by physician or healthcare providers. With $\chi^2(2) = 1.0179$ and $p = .601$, we are unable to reject the null hypothesis at the .05 significance level. Thus, we draw the conclusion that there is no discernible difference in user-trust in health (H) apps suggested by doctors or other healthcare professionals across groups with different app development experiences.

Significance of Marital Status. The proportion of single and married people who have high trust in health applications that are suggested by healthcare professionals or physicians is compared using the $z - test$ to see if there is a statistically significant discrepancy, i.e., null hypothesis, $H_0 : p_1 = p_2$, where $\hat{p}_1 = \frac{2}{9}$ and $\hat{p}_2 = \frac{35}{51}$ are the fractions of married and unmarried who provide a high rating when conveying their trust in health apps (H) recommended by physicians or healthcare providers. With $z = 2.6$ and $p = .0091$, we reject the null hypothesis at the .05 level of significance. Thus, we draw the conclusion that, when advised by doctors or other healthcare professionals, health (H) applications are more trusted by unmarried people than by married people.

3.2   Factors Affecting User-Trust in Payment Apps

In this section, we evaluate the statistical importance of several variables, such as gender, age, educational attainment, expertise in app development, and marital status on user trust when selecting a payment app.

Significance of Gender. We utilize the $z - test$ to see if there is a statistically significant discrepancy between the percentage of males and females who have high trust in payment (P) apps that are recommended by family or friends, i.e., null hypothesis, $H_0 : p_1 = p_2$, where p_1 and p_2 are the fractions of male and female who provide a high rating when conveying their trust in payment apps recommended by family members or friends. In the case of family members, we find $\hat{p}_1 = \frac{15}{24}$ and $\hat{p}_2 = \frac{17}{36}$ with $z = 1.2$ and $p = .2385$. Therefore, we are unable to rule out the null hypothesis at the .05 level of significance. Similarly, in the case of friends, we are unable to rule out the null hypothesis with $z = 1.2$ and $p = .2217$. Therefore, we draw the conclusion that males and females do not have a comparable level of trust in payment (P) apps that have been suggested by family or friends.

Significance of Age. With the "there is no statistically significant variation among the fractions of people from different age groups, in terms of user-trust in payment applications when recommended by family members or friends" null hypothesis, we utilize the χ^2 proportion test to examine the significance among the different age groups (i.e., $H_0 : p_1 = p_2 = p_3 = p_4 = p_5$, where p_1, p_2, p_3, p_4, and p_5 are the fractions of subjects from the five age groups that provide a high rating in payment apps when recommended by family members or friends. In the case of family members, we find $\hat{p}_1 = \frac{6}{9}$, $\hat{p}_2 = \frac{17}{37}$, $\hat{p}_3 = \frac{4}{5}$, $\hat{p}_4 = \frac{3}{4}$, and $\hat{p}_5 = \frac{2}{5}$ with $\chi^2(4) = 1.1300$ and $p = .889$. Therefore, we are unable to rule out the null hypothesis at the .05 level of significance. Similarly, in the case of friends, we are unable to rule out the null hypothesis with z = 1.558 and p = .816. Therefore, we draw the conclusion that there is no discernible difference in terms of user-trust in payment (P) apps suggested by family or friends across the five age groups.

Significance of Educational Background. When recommended by family members, we dropped one subject, who "passed high school" (Fig. 2) and did not report a high level of trust in the payment (P) apps. We take into account the remaining three categories of people: those who completed senior high school, graduated, and obtained a master's degree. We use the χ^2 proportion test with the null hypothesis that "there is no significant distinction among the fractions of people from different educational backgrounds, in terms of user-trust in payment apps when recommended by family members or friends" to examine the significance among different groups (i.e., $H_0 : p_1 = p_2 = p_3$, where p_1, p_2, and p_3, are the fractions of people from the three groups that provide a high rating in payment apps when recommended by family members or friends. In the case of family members, we find $\hat{p}_1 = \frac{4}{9}$, $\hat{p}_2 = \frac{8}{20}$, $\hat{p}_3 = \frac{19}{30}$ with $\chi^2(2) = .9125$ and $p = .634$. Therefore, we are unable to rule out the null hypothesis at the .05 level of significance. Similarly, when considering friends, with $z = 3.9142$ and $p = .141$, we cannot reject the null hypothesis. Therefore, we draw the conclusion that there is no discernible difference in terms of user-trust in payment (P) apps suggested by family or friends across the three groups.

Significance of App Development Experience. In the case of recommendations from family or friends, we drop one subject with "advanced" app development experience (Fig. 3) that did not report high trust in the payment (P) apps. The remaining three categories of people-those with no experience, intermediate experience, and no experience - are taken into consideration. We use the χ^2 test with the null hypothesis "there is no statistically significant distinction among the fractions of individuals from different educational backgrounds, in terms of user-trust in payment apps when recommended by family members or friends" (i.e., $H_0 : p_1 = p_2 = p_3$, where p_1, p_2, and p_3 are the fractions of participants from the three groups that provide a high rating in payment apps when recommended by family members or friends. In the case of family members, we find $\hat{p}_1 = \frac{18}{27}$, $\hat{p}_2 = \frac{7}{14}$, and $\hat{p}_3 = \frac{7}{18}$ with $\chi^2(2) = 1.05524$ and $p = .59$. Therefore, we are unable to rule out the null hypothesis at the .05 level of significance. Similarly, in the case of friends, we are unable to rule out the null hypothesis with z = .6364 and p = .727. Therefore, we draw the conclusion that there is no discernible difference in terms of user-trust in payment (P) apps suggested by family or friends across the three groups of people.

Significance of Marital Status. To verify if there is a statistically significant difference in the fraction of married and unmarried people who reported high trust in payment apps that are suggested by family or friends, we perform a

$z - test$, i.e., null hypothesis, $H_0 : p_1 = p_2$, where p_1 and p_2 are the fractions of unmarried and married who provide a high rating when conveying their trust in payment (P) apps recommended by their family members or friends. In the case of family members, we find $\hat{p}_1 = \frac{5}{9}$ and $\hat{p}_2 = \frac{27}{51}$ with $z = .1$ and $p = .8854$. Therefore, we are unable to rule out the null hypothesis at the .05 level of significance. Similarly in the case of friends, where $z = .8$ and $p = .4363$, we cannot reject the null hypothesis. Thus, we draw the conclusion that there is no discernible difference between married and unmarried people in terms of user-trust in payment (P) apps that are suggested by family or friends.

4 Conclusions

To the best of our knowledge, this is the first work that conducts a thorough investigation of user trust in different types of smartphone applications and recommenders using graphical and statistical approaches. Among the four types of apps investigated in this work, we find that users have a high trust in health apps when they are recommended by healthcare providers or physicians. Similarly, we find that users have a high trust in payment apps when they are recommended by friends or family members. These groups of recommenders probably have a better understanding of the features that a specific app should have. Therefore, it will important to bring these specific groups of recommenders and their recommendations to gain higher user trust and higher app utility and adherence. Additionally, we do not observe any significant difference in user trust due to background variations, except the marital status while choosing health apps. Therefore, our findings are generic across users with different backgrounds.

5 Limitations and Future Work

This work has some limitations, which we plan to address in the future. First, the dataset used in this work is relatively small, i.e., consists of 60 smartphone users. However, we perform proportion analysis to determine the significance of user backgrounds. Therefore, findings from this work show some guidelines for future app developments. Also, some of the categories, e.g., high school in the educational background and advanced app developer, have low user count; therefore, we are not able to investigate their significance. Finally, to develop an app with high utility and adherence, it is important to understand various user concerns, including privacy and security, confidentiality, difficulty in-app usage, among many others as well as a user's choice to configure an app and its features in addition to user trust in different types of recommenders. In the future, we will further investigate user concerns and their choices to configure apps.

References

1. What are the different types of mobile apps? https://blog.duckma.com/en/types-of-mobile-apps/. Accessed March

2. Compound annual growth rate (CAGR). https://bit.ly/3jHm8OT. Accessed March 2022
3. Medical apps: Improving healthcare on a global scale. https://bit.ly/3KPSRgO. Accessed March 2022
4. Mobile app download statistics & usage statistics (2022). https://bit.ly/37nVaJF. Accessed March 2022
5. Mobile app marketing insights: How consumers really find and use your apps. https://bit.ly/3JNxRGv. Accessed March 2022
6. Mobile application market size, share & trends analysis. https://bit.ly/3vlV7pR. Accessed March 2022
7. Mobile apps have a short half life; use falls sharply after first six months. https://bit.ly/3JOnIJv. Accessed March 2022
8. Al Amin, M.T., Barua, S., Vhaduri, S., Rahman, A.: Load aware broadcast in mobile ad hoc networks. In: IEEE International Conference on Communications (ICC) (2009)
9. Chang, T.R., Kaasinen, E., Kaipainen, K.: What influences users' decisions to take apps into use? A framework for evaluating persuasive and engaging design in mobile apps for well-being. In: Proceedings of the 11th International Conference on Mobile and Ubiquitous Multimedia, pp. 1–10 (2012)
10. Chen, C.Y., Vhaduri, S., Poellabauer, C.: Estimating sleep duration from temporal factors, daily activities, and smartphone use. In: IEEE Computer Society Computers, Software, and Applications Conference (COMPSAC) (2020)
11. Cheung, W., Vhaduri, S.: Context-dependent implicit authentication for wearable device users. In: IEEE International Symposium on Personal, Indoor, and Mobile Radio Communications (PIMRC) (2020)
12. Cheung, W., Vhaduri, S.: Continuous authentication of wearable device users from heart rate, gait, and breathing data. In: IEEE RAS & EMBS International Conference on Biomedical Robotics and Biomechatronics (BioRob) (2020)
13. Dibbo, S.V., Cheung, W., Vhaduri, S.: On-Phone CNN Model-based Implicit Authentication to Secure IoT Wearables. In: Nayyar, A., Paul, A., Tanwar, S. (eds.) The Fifth International Conference on Safety and Security with IoT. EAI/Springer Innovations in Communication and Computing, pp. 19-34. Springer, Cham (2021). https://doi.org/10.1007/978-3-030-94285-4_2
14. Dibbo, S.V., Kim, Y., Vhaduri, S.: Effect of noise on generic cough models. In: IEEE International Conference on Wearable and Implantable Body Sensor Networks (BSN) (2021)
15. Dibbo, S.V., Kim, Y., Vhaduri, S., Poellabauer, C.: Visualizing college students' geo-temporal context-varying significant phone call patterns. In: 2021 IEEE 9th International Conference on Healthcare Informatics (ICHI), pp. 381–385. IEEE (2021)
16. Fu, B., Lin, J., Li, L., Faloutsos, C., Hong, J., Sadeh, N.: Why people hate your app: making sense of user feedback in a mobile app store. In: Proceedings of the 19th ACM SIGKDD International Conference on Knowledge Discovery and Data Mining, pp. 1276–1284 (2013)
17. Humbani, M., Wiese, M.: An integrated framework for the adoption and continuance intention to use mobile payment apps. Int. J. Bank Mark. **37**, 646–664 (2019)
18. Kim, Y., Vhaduri, S., Poellabauer, C.: Understanding college students' phone call behaviors towards a sustainable mobile health and wellbeing solution. In: International Conference on Systems Engineering (2020)

19. Liccardi, I., Pato, J., Weitzner, D.J.: Improving user choice through better mobile apps transparency and permissions analysis. J. Priv. Confidentiality **5**(2), 1–55 (2014)

20. Muratyan, A., Cheung, W., Dibbo, S.V., Vhaduri, S.: Opportunistic multi-modal user authentication for health-tracking IoT wearables. In: Nayyar, A., Paul, A., Tanwar, S. (eds.) The Fifth International Conference on Safety and Security with IoT. EAI/Springer Innovations in Communication and Computing. Springer, Cham (2021). https://doi.org/10.1007/978-3-030-94285-4_1

21. Natarajan, T., Balasubramanian, S.A., Kasilingam, D.L.: Understanding the intention to use mobile shopping applications and its influence on price sensitivity. J. Retail. Consum. Serv. **37**, 8–22 (2017)

22. Sharmin, M., et al.: Visualization of time-series sensor data to inform the design of just-in-time adaptive stress interventions. In: Proceedings of the 2015 ACM International Joint Conference on Pervasive and Ubiquitous Computing, pp. 505–516 (2015)

23. Tao, K., Edmunds, P., et al.: Mobile apps and global markets. Theor. Econ. Lett. **8**(08), 1510 (2018)

24. Vaghefi, I., Tulu, B., et al.: The continued use of mobile health apps: insights from a longitudinal study. JMIR Mhealth Uhealth **7**(8), e12983 (2019)

25. Vagrani, A., Kumar, N., Ilavarasan, P.V.: Decline in mobile application life cycle. Procedia Comput. Sci. **122**, 957–964 (2017)

26. Vhaduri, S.: Nocturnal cough and snore detection using smartphones in presence of multiple background-noises. In: ACM SIGCAS Conference on Computing and Sustainable Societies (COMPASS) (2020)

27. Vhaduri, S., Ali, A., Sharmin, M., Hovsepian, K., Kumar, S.: Estimating drivers' stress from GPS traces. In: International Conference on Automotive User Interfaces and Interactive Vehicular Applications (AutomotiveUI) (2014)

28. Vhaduri, S., Brunschwiler, T.: Towards automatic cough and snore detection. In: IEEE International Conference on Healthcare Informatics (ICHI) (2019)

29. Vhaduri, S., Dibbo, S.V., Chen, C.Y.: Predicting a user's demographic identity from leaked samples of health-tracking wearables and understanding associated risks. In: 2022 IEEE 10th International Conference on Healthcare Informatics (ICHI). IEEE (2022)

30. Vhaduri, S., Dibbo, S.V., Chen, C.Y., Poellabauer, C.: Predicting next call duration: a future direction to promote mental health in the age of lockdown. In: IEEE Computer Society Computers, Software, and Applications Conference (COMPSAC) (2021)

31. Vhaduri, S., Dibbo, S.V., Cheung, W.: HIAuth: a hierarchical implicit authentication system for IoT wearables using multiple biometrics. IEEE Access **9**, 116395–116406 (2021)

32. Vhaduri, S., Dibbo, S.V., Kim, Y.: Deriving college students' phone call patterns to improve student life. IEEE Access **9**, 96453–96465 (2021)

33. Vhaduri, S., Munch, A., Poellabauer, C.: Assessing health trends of college students using smartphones. In: IEEE Healthcare Innovation Point-of-Care Technologies Conference (HI-POCT) (2016)

34. Vhaduri, S., Poellabauer, C.: Design and implementation of a remotely configurable and manageable well-being study. In: Leon-Garcia, A., et al. (eds.) SmartCity 360 2015–2016. LNICST, vol. 166, pp. 179–191. Springer, Cham (2016). https://doi.org/10.1007/978-3-319-33681-7_15

35. Vhaduri, S., Poellabauer, C.: Cooperative discovery of personal places from location traces. In: International Conference on Computer Communication and Networks (ICCCN) (2016)
36. Vhaduri, S., Poellabauer, C.: Human factors in the design of longitudinal smartphone-based wellness surveys. In: IEEE International Conference on Healthcare Informatics (ICHI) (2016)
37. Vhaduri, S., Poellabauer, C.: Design factors of longitudinal smartphone-based health surveys. J. Healthc. Inform. Res. 1(1), 52–91 (2017)
38. Vhaduri, S., Poellabauer, C.: Towards reliable wearable-user identification. In: 2017 IEEE International Conference on Healthcare Informatics (ICHI) (2017)
39. Vhaduri, S., Poellabauer, C.: Wearable device user authentication using physiological and behavioral metrics. In: IEEE International Symposium on Personal, Indoor, and Mobile Radio Communications (PIMRC) (2017)
40. Vhaduri, S., Poellabauer, C.: Biometric-based wearable user authentication during sedentary and non-sedentary periods. International Workshop on Security and Privacy for the Internet-of-Things (IoTSec) (2018)
41. Vhaduri, S., Poellabauer, C.: Hierarchical cooperative discovery of personal places from location traces. IEEE Trans. Mob. Comput. 17(8), 1865–1878 (2018)
42. Vhaduri, S., Poellabauer, C.: Impact of different pre-sleep phone use patterns on sleep quality. In: IEEE International Conference on Wearable and Implantable Body Sensor Networks (BSN) (2018)
43. Vhaduri, S., Poellabauer, C.: Opportunistic discovery of personal places using smartphone and fitness tracker data. In: IEEE International Conference on Healthcare Informatics (ICHI) (2018)
44. Vhaduri, S., Poellabauer, C.: Multi-modal biometric-based implicit authentication of wearable device users. IEEE Trans. Inf. Forensics Secur. 14(12), 3116–3125 (2019)
45. Vhaduri, S., Poellabauer, C.: Summary: multi-modal biometric-based implicit authentication of wearable device users. arXiv preprint arXiv:1907.06563 (2019)
46. Vhaduri, S., Poellabauer, C.: Opportunistic discovery of personal places using multi-source sensor data. IEEE Trans. Big Data 7(2), 383–396 (2021)
47. Vhaduri, S., Poellabauer, C., Striegel, A., Lizardo, O., Hachen, D.: Discovering places of interest using sensor data from smartphones and wearables. In: IEEE Ubiquitous Intelligence & Computing (UIC) (2017)
48. Vhaduri, S., Prioleau, T.: Adherence to personal health devices: a case study in diabetes management. In: EAI International Conference on Pervasive Computing Technologies for Healthcare (PervasiveHealth) (2020)
49. Vhaduri, S., Simhadri, S.: Understanding user concerns and choice of app architectures in designing audio-based mHealth apps. Smart Health J. 26, 100341 (2022)
50. Vhaduri, S., Van Kessel, T., Ko, B., Wood, D., Wang, S., Brunschwiler, T.: Nocturnal cough and snore detection in noisy environments using smartphone-microphones. In: IEEE International Conference on Healthcare Informatics (ICHI) (2019)
51. Williams, G., Mahmoud, A.: Modeling user concerns in the app store: a case study on the rise and fall of Yik Yak. In: 2018 IEEE 26th International Requirements Engineering Conference (RE), pp. 64–75. IEEE (2018)
52. Yang, Y., Liu, Y., Li, H., Yu, B.: Understanding perceived risks in mobile payment acceptance. Industr. Manage. Data Syst. 115, 253–269 (2015)
53. Zhu, H., Xiong, H., Ge, Y., Chen, E.: Mobile app recommendations with security and privacy awareness. In: Proceedings of the 20th ACM SIGKDD International Conference on Knowledge Discovery and Data Mining, pp. 951–960 (2014)

Using Wearable Devices to Mitigate Bias in Patient Reported Outcomes for Aging Populations

John Michael Templeton[1]([⊠])[ID], Christian Poellabauer[1][ID], and Sandra Schneider[2][ID]

[1] Florida International University, Miami, FL 33199, USA
{jtemplet,cpoellab}@fiu.edu
[2] Saint Mary's College, Notre Dame, IN 46556, USA
sschneider@saintmarys.edu

Abstract. Wearable devices are increasingly used in health monitoring due to the provision of objective and longitudinal measures of physiological functions. The purpose of this work was to assess variability of perceived functionality for autonomic function, sleep, and physical activity, compared to objective physiological measures collected via device sensors. Further, this work assessed disparities between healthy aging populations and those with confirmed neurodegenerative conditions (e.g., Parkinson's Disease (PD)). 30 participants ($n = 20$ PD; $n = 10$ control) wore a smart tracker to collect objective features for autonomic function, sleep, and activity. Further, all participants completed daily questionnaires to depict perceived physiologic functionality. While previous studies note the importance of patient reported outcomes (PROs), these may be subject to variability. PROs of the control group were higher than sensor-based values across all functions; where sleep and heart rate yielded statistical significance ($p = 0.002$; $p = 0.012$; respectively). Conversely, PROs of populations with PD were significantly lower for sleep quality, heart rate, and activity ($p = 0.018$; $p = 0.009$; $p = 0.007$; respectively) compared to sensor-based values. Finally, significant differences ($p << 0.01$) were present for all functions between groups. Although PROs are commonly used to monitor health, digital health systems should be used to increase reliability and accuracy via the collection of objective sensor-based measures.

Keywords: Digital Biomarkers · Neurocognitive Assessment · Wearable Devices · Parkinson's Disease

1 Introduction

Given the pervasiveness of digital technology in everyday life, mobile and wearable devices provide clinicians (e.g., epidemiologists, neurologists, physicians,

A. Cunha et al. (Eds.): MobiHealth 2022, LNICST 484, pp. 362–374, 2023.
https://doi.org/10.1007/978-3-031-32029-3_30

and other healthcare personnel) the opportunity to collect, analyze, and interpret new and complex sensor-based health datasets [1,2]. These devices and their capabilities yield an expansive assortment of objective symptom-specific information (e.g., digital outcome measures) acquired via mobile device sensors (e.g., wearable accelerometers, gyroscopes, and optical sensors) [3–5]. The provision of this objective data is imperative to aid in the mitigation of individual subjective bias and allow for the accurate evaluation of neurocognitive functionalities (e.g., motor function, autonomic function, and sleep) necessary in patient monitoring, disease diagnosis, and subsequent rehabilitation [6].

Currently, the monitoring of a patient's thoughts and opinions with respect to short-term changes commonly come from patient reported outcomes (PROs) [7]. These PROS are also commonly used as a measure for improved disease management, as the individual is able to recognize and interpret their condition, symptoms, and triggers [8]. However, as individuals age, their perceived neurocognitive functionalities (e.g., motor, sleep, and autonomic functions) may become reliant on changes in their cognition, the memory of past experiences, and/or sensory experiences in the body [7–9]. Further, as these individuals age, there is a noted susceptibility increase for various neurodegenerative conditions (e.g., Parkinson's Disease (PD), Alzheimer's Disease, and dementia [10–13]) that may affect changes in the way individuals perceive their neurocognitive functionalities. This concept is expressed using the stereotype embodiment theory, which suggests that beliefs surrounding culture leads to self-definitions that may influence perceived functioning and health (e.g., such that if you are deemed 'healthy' you embody the perceived notion that you are comprehensively healthy, and vice versa) [14,15].

The objective of this work was to assess the variability of perceived functionality for autonomic function, sleep, and activity levels, for aging populations, in comparison to objective physiological measures collected using wearable device sensors. Further, this work was extended to assess disparities between healthy aging populations and individuals with confirmed neurodegenerative diseases (e.g., individuals with PD).

2   Related Work

Although PROs are regularly used for monitoring a patient's thoughts and opinions with respect to short-term changes, there are no well-defined criteria on what these PROs actually entail, in the perception of the individual [7,8,16]. Exploratory analyses have shown that high physical activity PROs is associated with a minimized progression of symptoms for individuals with neurodegenerative conditions [17] and rate of perceived exertion was found to increase with heart rate (HR) and maximal oxygen consumption during exercise (VO2) among older adults [18]. However, other review studies have provided mixed results between traditional objective markers and PROs [9].

Therefore the aim of digital health technology (e.g., wearable devices) is to increase both the accuracy and reliability of PROs by combining it with objective measures, thus yielding higher diagnostic and prognostic values while also reducing individual variability and/or bias [19–22]. With the use of wearable devices, the collection of vital health related data can occur both opportunistically and longitudinally via the implementation of inherent device sensors [23,24]. These wearable devices allow for an objective evaluation of neurocognitive functions (e.g., sleep and autonomic function) that are imperative to the monitoring of aging populations, especially those with neurodegenerative conditions [6]. Digital features from these devices relate to health-related monitoring (e.g., for the assessment of autonomic functions [25]), in tandem with the utilization of on-device accelerometers and gyroscopes (e.g., to aid in the assessment of physical activity and sleep) [26]. Although previous works have utilized wearable technology for the increased reliability of patient reported outcomes of healthy aging populations (e.g., for sleep and physical activity [27,28]) further work across comprehensively representative populations is necessary to capture objective disease-related symptoms and inform big data applications [29].

3   Methodology

This pilot study included thirty individuals between the ages of 50 and 85. The population was split into two groups, (a) those with a clinical diagnosis of PD ($n = 20$) and (b) age-matched healthy controls ($n = 10$). In this pilot, slightly less than half were male ($n = 13$ or 43.33%) with nine being from the PD population, and four being from the age-matched control population. Participants of the PD group were recruited for an IRB-approved study via advertisements, referrals by physicians and clinicians, and organized therapeutic programs. Age-matched health control populations were also recruited via advertisement from groups including spouses/caregivers of the clinically affected population in addition to preceding research work in this setting. In the Western world, early-to-mid 60s is the mean onset age for clinical diagnosis of PD [30]; therefore, recruitment for this study was limited to persons who are 50 years or older from the aforementioned groups.

3.1   Wearable Device Monitoring

The wearable device chosen for this study was the Fitbit Charge 5 fitness tracker. This consumer activity tracker was chosen as several reviews examined the validity and inter-reliability of Fitbit activity trackers in both the laboratory setting and free-living environments, while demonstrating the high accuracy of physical activity measures including steps, distance traveled, and energy expenditure [31–33]. All participants were instructed to wear the device for a total of 4 weeks. Participants wore this wearable device on their non-dominant hand continuously for the duration of this study (e.g., only taking the watch off to charge). Individuals were instructed to charge the device daily when they were sedentary/inactive, but not sleeping (e.g., as the collection of sleep data was imperative to the outcomes of this work).

Data from the device accelerometer and optical sensors were used for the collection of physical activity, sleep, heart rate, and breathing features. While the Fitbit software development kit (SDK) allows for the programming of these devices to access raw sensor measurements, the devices themselves use this data to compute a number of physiological parameters such as sleep quality, step count, calorie burn, metabolic rate, activity levels, that were used to calculate the normalized score of each functionality (e.g., sleep, breathing, heart rate, and physical activity).

3.2 Patient Reported Outcomes

Each participant was given a commonly administered questionnaire for aging populations. Questions included information regarding general health information, medical diagnoses, and respective disease stage, as well as any related symptoms (e.g., an individual's feeling in general, energy levels, activity levels, pain, sleep quality, medication schedule, etc.) as depicted in Tables 1 and 2. In addition, the PDQ-39 (e.g., a fixed questionnaire regarding the quality of life for individuals with PD) was administered to gain an understanding of mobility, activities of daily living (ADLs), emotional well-being, social support, cognition, communication, bodily discomfort, and their perceived stigma of PD [34]. Questionnaires depicted in Tables 1 and 2 were administered to accompany and confirm diagnoses provided by medical practitioners. Further, all participants were administered a daily questionnaire to assess autonomic functions, sleep, and physical activity as listed in Table 3. This questionnaire used the Borg Rating Scale to assess the rate of perceived exertion [9], Likert Scales for the rating of all other functions, and additional questions regarding perceived factors that may have affected functional quality. All daily questionnaires were scheduled (e.g., participants were alerted using push notifications for the completion of mobile-based daily questionnaires) for participants to maintain compliance. All participants completed the daily questionnaire at the end of each day (e.g., before bed) such that all responses were related to the previous 24 h.

3.3 Feature Normalization

The standardization of wearable device collected feature values and patient reported outcomes is necessary as part of this work as many of the collected features differ distinctly (e.g., as they come from standardized questionnaires/tools with varying ranges and units). This normalization utilized Z-scores as depicted in Eq. 1; such that Z results from x (i.e., individual scores), μ (i.e., the mean of the population) and σ (i.e., the population standard deviation).

$$Z = \frac{(x - \mu)}{\sigma} \tag{1}$$

Z-scores are measured as standard deviations with relation to the mean. These Z-scores can be either + or −, where a positive Z-score indicates a value greater than the mean, a negative Z-score indicates a value less than the mean, and a Z-score of 0 indicates a value equal to the mean.

Table 1. General medical history questionnaire [35].

Answer Type	Question
(Multiple Choice/ Open Answer)	How old are you?
	How do you identify?
	What is your highest level of education?
	Are you currently employed or retired?
	What industry are/were you employed?
	Do you have a clinical diagnosis of any neurological conditions?
	If yes, have you been diagnosed with PD?
	If yes, in what year was your diagnosis?
	If yes, in what stage of Parkinson's Disease are you?
	If yes, please describe your first noticed symptoms? (e.g., shaky or smaller handwriting)
	If yes, when did your symptoms first become noticeable?
	Have you received a clinical diagnosis of any additional neurological condition? (e.g., dementia or stroke)
	If yes, what other condition(s)?
	If yes, when were you diagnosed?
	What is your medication schedule for your diagnosed condition(s)? (e.g., medication name, dosage, and timing for each listed condition)

Table 2. Questionnaire regarding symptom-specific effects of Parkinson's Disease [35].

Answer Type	Question (How often during the last month have you had...)
(Likert Scale 1–5) (1 = Never) (2 = Occasionally) (3 = Sometimes) (4 = Often) (5 = Always)	Issues and/or concerns with your Short Term Memory (e.g., what you had to eat for breakfast)?
	Issues and/or concerns with your Long Term Memory (e.g., the date of children's birthdays)?
	Issues and/or concerns with your Fine Motor Function (e.g., writing your name)?
	Issues and/or concerns with your Gross Motor Function (e.g., going from a sitting position to a standing position)?
	Issues and/or concerns with your Balance/Stability (e.g., standing still in an upright position without support)?
	Issues and/or concerns with your Word Finding (e.g., expressing words you want to say when you wish to say them)?
	Issues and/or concerns with your Attention (e.g., the ability to maintain focus on a specific thing)?
	Issues and/or concerns with your Judgment (e.g., the ability to make decisions considering many possible outcomes)?
	Issues and/or concerns with your Reasoning (e.g., the ability to consciously apply logic)?
	Issues and/or concerns with your Problem Solving (e.g., the ability to find solutions to complex problems)?
	Issues and/or concerns Following Conversations?
	Issues and/or concerns Reading (e.g., difficulty in following the information on the page)?
	Issues and/or concerns with your Speech (e.g., having quiet or effortful speech)?
	Poor Energy Levels (e.g., the ability to complete normal physical activities without being tired)?
	Poor Sleep Quality (e.g., restless, duration)?
	Bodily Pain (e.g., bodily aches, muscle or joint pain, headaches)?
	Issues and/or concerns in your Social Engagement (e.g., spending time with family and friends)?
	Issues and/or concerns with your Sensory Function(s) (e.g., touch, vision, hearing, taste, and/or smell)?
	Issues and/or concerns expressing your Emotions (e.g., your natural state of mind based on current circumstances, mood, and/or relationships)?

Table 3. Daily questionnaire regarding patient reported outcomes of sleep, autonomic function and activity.

Question	Function	Scale
How did you feel in general today?	Overall	(Scale of 0–10; 10 being the best)
What was the quality of your sleep last night?	Sleep	(Scale of 1–10; 10 being very high quality)
What affected your quality of sleep last night?	Sleep	(Mark all that apply)
What was your breathing capacity today?	Breathing	(Scale of 1–10; 10 being very high capacity)
What affected your breathing capacity today?	Breathing	(Mark all that apply)
What was your rate of perceived exertion today?	Heart Rate	(Borg Rating Scale of 0–10; 10 being maximal physical exertion)
What caused your rate of perceived exertion today?	Heart Rate	(Mark all that apply)
What was your activity level today?	Activity	(Scale of 1–10; 10 being very active)
How many active minutes did you have today?	Activity	Number of active minutes
What activities did you participate in today?	Activity	(Mark all that apply)

Following feature normalization both perceived and sensor-based aggregated scores were formed. Aggregated perceived functional scores were calculated from normalized response data from daily surveys found in Table 3. Aggregated sensor-based functional scores were calculated from normalized physiological parameters retrieved from Fitbit Charge 5 fitness tracker found in Table 4.

Table 4. Daily sensor-based smart tracker values from Fitbit Charge 5.

Smart Tracker Value	Function
Minutes Asleep	Sleep
Minutes Awake	Sleep
Time in Deep Sleep	Sleep
Count of Deep Sleep Intervals	Sleep
Time in Light Sleep	Sleep
Count of Light Sleep Intervals	Sleep
Time in REM Sleep	Sleep
Count of REM Sleep Intervals	Sleep
Average SPO2 Score	Breathing
Lower Bound SPO2 Score	Breathing
Upper Bound SPO2 Score	Breathing
Resting Heart Rate	Heart Rate
Time in Heart Rate Zones	Heart Rate
Daily Heart Rate	Heart Rate
Active Zone Minutes	Activity
Caloric Burn	Activity
Sedentary Minutes	Activity
Lightly Active Minutes	Activity
Moderately Active Minutes	Activity
Very Active Minutes	Activity
Step Count	Activity

3.4   Statistical Analysis

All normalized patient reported outcome measures and sensor-based scores were analyzed between groups using both ANOVAs and post hoc t-tests for statistical analysis.

4   Results

The depiction of perceived neurocognitive functionalities between PD populations and age-matched healthy control populations, is reported via normalized scores from the patient reported outcomes questionnaire for sleep, autonomic functions (e.g., breathing and heart rate), physical activity, in addition to how the individual feels in general. Average Z-scores for these perceived functional areas are shown in Fig. 1. This figure depicts that age-matched healthy controls have a higher average perceived functionality score across all functions (e.g., an individual's feeling in general, sleep, autonomic functions, and physical activity) compared to those with confirmed PD diagnosis.

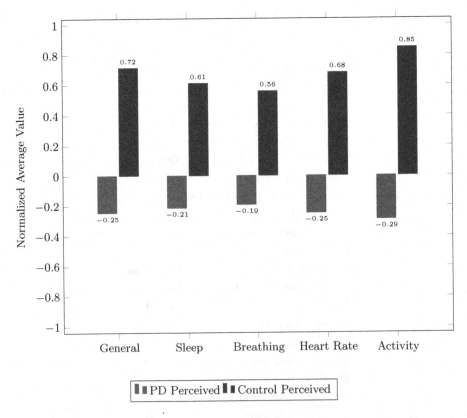

Fig. 1. Normalized perceived scores across overall functionality, sleep, autonomic function, and physical activity between healthy aging control populations and PD populations

Figure 2 presents both normalized perceived and sensor-based functional scores across sleep, autonomic functions, and physical activity between healthy aging control populations and PD populations. Figure 2 depicts that control populations have higher average scores for both perceived functionality and sensor-based features across all areas when compared to those with a confirmed PD diagnosis. Further, this figure shows that healthy age-matched populations perceive their functionality across all categories to be higher than sensor-based scores, whereas PD populations perceive their functionality to be worse than sensor-based scores for sleep, heart rate, and physical activity.

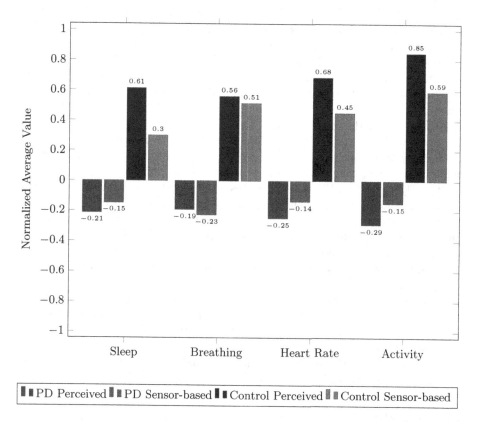

Fig. 2. Normalized perceived functionality and sensor-based scores across sleep, autonomic function, and physical activity between healthy aging control populations and PD populations

5   Discussion

Although PROs are commonly used to track a thoughts or opinions of the patient regarding short-term changes it is presumable that these thoughts and opinions have a high reliance on cognitive processes, memory of past exercise experiences, in addition to felt experiences in the body [9]. Further, it is noted that these patient reported outcomes may be negatively impacted in individuals with neurodegenerative diseases [7,8]. This concept is further depicted using the stereotype embodiment theory, which suggests that beliefs surrounding culture leads to self-definitions that may influence perceived functionality as it relates to health (e.g., such that if you are deemed 'healthy' you embody the perceived notion that you are comprehensively healthy, and vice versa) [14,15]. The stereotype embodiment theory perspective may be observed in Fig. 2 as the PD population's overall perceived scores for sleep quality, heart rate, and physical activity are significantly lower ($p = 0.018$, $p = 0.009$, and $p = 0.007$; respectively) than sensor-based normalized values. Conversely, the age matched healthy control population's overall perceived scores across all functions (e.g., sleep, breathing, heart rate, and physical activity) are higher than sensor-based normalized values; where sleep and heart rate are significantly higher ($p = 0.002$, and $p = 0.012$; respectively). It is noted that the PD population's overall perceived score for breathing is higher than sensor-based normalized values, as depicted in Fig. 2; however, it is also expressed that there is not a significant difference between these scores given this population.

Subsequently, Fig. 2 depicts the difference in objective measures between PD populations and healthy age-matched control populations. In this pilot study all functions (e.g., sleep, breathing, heart rate, and physical activity) differed significantly ($p << 0.01$) between groups. As individuals with neurodegenerative diseases may present with functional deficits across each of the following areas of neurocognition: motor, memory, speech, language, executive function, sensory, behavioral and psychological, sleep, and autonomic functions [6,36], the collection of accurate and sensor-based features using digital health technology is imperative for the assessment and monitoring of each functional area of neurocognition.

As there are significant differences in perceived functionalities and sensor-based normalized values across groups, the importance of using digital health technology (e.g., wearables) to increase the reliability and accuracy of patient reported outcome data is imperative [20,22]. The combination of PROs with objective digitally collected features should remain a main focus in the assessment and monitoring of health outcomes for all groups.

5.1   Limitations and Future Work

One of the main limitations of this pilot study results from the population size and breakdown. Future work should incorporate the collection of a larger dataset with respect to both diagnosed healthy control populations in addition to the inclusion of additional neurodegenerative diseases (e.g., amyotrophic lateral sclerosis, dementia, and Huntington's disease) and their stages. This would then allow for the separation of groups on the basis of disease presence and respective stages in a fine-grained classification approach. This is necessary for both the assessment of perceived functionality and sensor-based scores as they relate to representative aging populations. Further, this work only explores a subset of neurocognitive functions as they relate to digital health technologies (e.g., wearable devices and smartphones). Additional work with respect to wearable devices, utilizing electrodermal activity sensors for the assessment of stress and behavior [25, 37] would expand wearable monitoring efforts to include more functional areas of neurocognition. Expanding this work to include additional IoT devices, such as smartphones, would also allow for the expanded analysis of more functional areas of neurocognition [38]; via the comparison of PROs found in Tables 1 and 2 with objective, digitally collected features. Finally, the work presented in this pilot study should be extended to include the assessment of function-specific (e.g., autonomic function and sleep) benefits from a diverse set of clinically relevant therapeutics (e.g., pharmacological, medical, physical, speech, occupational, etc.).

Subsequently, with the collection of more digitally-collected, objective features across larger populations with respect to therapeutic protocols, machine learning methods could be used in the translation of this data into actionable knowledge [39, 40]. While previous research has focused on assessing different motor systems using a number of wearable sensors placed on different body parts [41, 42], advances in machine learning provide opportunities to measure motor symptoms using a smaller number of sensors (e.g., wearables worn on a wrist) [43]. Specifically, supervised machine learning for the purpose of prediction and classification of various diseases, and the provision of personalized healthcare decisions in response to prediction and classification (e.g., as they relate to a patient's ability to perform ADLs, the severity of symptoms, symptom progression, response to medication and other interventions, and their overall quality of life) is necessary for these aging populations given the increased susceptibility to neurodegenerative diseases (e.g., PD) [10, 44, 45]. However, future work regarding the development of robust machine learning models relies on an expanded dataset of adequate quality (e.g., one that comprehensively represents aging populations) [29, 46].

6 Conclusions

Although PROs are commonly utilized in practice for the monitoring of an individual's thoughts or opinions (e.g., with respect to short-term changes), the aim of digital health technology should be to increase both the reliability and accuracy of these PROs by combining it with objective digital outcome measures from mobile-based devices. This work utilized wearable devices to assess disparities between healthy aging populations and those with confirmed neurodegenerative diseases by comparing patient reported outcomes and sensor-based features across functional areas of neurocognition. As there were significant differences both between groups (e.g., healthy aging populations and those with confirmed neurodegenerative diseases) and between feature types (e.g., patient reported outcomes and sensor-based features) it is confirmed that mobile devices should be utilized in tandem with PROs for increased reliability and accuracy. As these wearables not only allow for the collection of objective features, both opportunistically and longitudinally, while requiring minimal interaction from the individual in the collection of vital health information, further advocacy for their use in these contexts should be seen. With the further integration of these wearable devices in neurocognitive digital health assessment systems, all future efforts should aim at improving the overall quality of life for aging populations by expanding personalized medicine.

References

1. Hansen, C., Sanchez-Ferro, A., Maetzler, W.: How mobile health technology and electronic health records will change care of patients with Parkinson's disease (2018)
2. Wiens, J., Shenoy, E.S.: Machine learning for healthcare: on the verge of a major shift in healthcare epidemiology. Clin. Infect. Dis. **66**, 149–153 (2018)
3. Vianello, A., Chittaro, L., Burigat, S., Budai, R.: MotorBrain: a mobile app for the assessment of users' motor performance in neurology. Comput. Methods Programs Biomed. **143**, 35–47 (2017)
4. Maguire, Á., Martin, J., Jarke, H., Ruggeri, K.: Psychological Services Getting Closer? Differences Remain in Neuropsychological Assessments Converted to Mobile Devices (2018)
5. Templeton, J.M., Poellabauer, C., Schneider, S.: The Case for Symptom-Specific Neurological Digital Biomarkers (2021)
6. Templeton, J.M., Poellabauer, C., Schneider, S.: Enhancement of neurocognitive assessments using smartphone capabilities: systematic review. JMIR mHealth uHealth **8**, e15517 (2020)
7. Vega, J., et al.: Back to Analogue: Self-reporting for Parkinson's Disease (2018)
8. Deshpande, P., Sudeepthi, B., Rajan, S., Abdul Nazir, C.: Patient-reported outcomes: a new era in clinical research. Perspect. Clin. Res. **2**(4), 137 (2011)
9. Bevan, A., Vidoni, E., Watts, A.: Rate of perceived exertion and cardiorespiratory fitness in older adults with and without Alzheimer's disease. Int. J. Exerc. Sci. **13**(3), 18 (2020)
10. Rodriguez, M., Rodriguez-Sabate, C., Morales, I., Sanchez, A., Sabate, M.: Parkinson's disease as a result of aging (2015)
11. Vo, A.: Usability in designing a mobile application for elderly users title of publication usability in designing a mobile application for elderly users case study: Dairo application. Technical report (2019)
12. Xiong, J., Muraki, S.: Effects of age, thumb length and screen size on thumb movement coverage on smartphone touchscreens. Int. J. Ind. Ergon. **53**, 140–148 (2016)
13. Zotz, N., Saft, S., Rosenlöhner, J., Böhm, P., Isemann, D.: Identification of age-specific usability problems of smartwatches. In: Miesenberger, K., Kouroupet-roglou, G. (eds.) ICCHP 2018. LNCS, vol. 10897, pp. 399–406. Springer, Cham (2018). https://doi.org/10.1007/978-3-319-94274-2_57
14. Levy, B.: Stereotype embodiment: a psychosocial approach to aging. Curr. Dir. Psychol. Sci. **18**, 332–336 (2009)
15. McGarrigle, C.A., Ward, M., Kenny, R.A.: Negative aging perceptions and cognitive and functional decline: are you as old as you feel? J. Am. Geriatrics Soc. (2021)

16. Goelema, M., Regis, M., Haakma, R., van den Heuvel, E., Markopoulos, P., Overeem, S.: Determinants of perceived sleep quality in normal sleepers. Behav. Sleep Med. **17**, 388–397 (2017). https://doi.org/10.1080/15402002.2017.1376205
17. Amara, A.W., Chahine, L., Seedorff, N., Caspell-Garcia, C.J., Coffey, C., Simuni, T.: Self-reported physical activity levels and clinical progression in early Parkinson's disease. Parkinsonism Relat. Disord. **61**, 118–125 (2019)
18. Chung, P.K., Zhao, Y., Liu, J.D., Quach, B.: A brief note on the validity and reliability of the rating of perceived exertion scale in monitoring exercise intensity among Chinese older adults in Hong Kong. Percept. Mot. Skills **121**, 805–809 (2015)
19. Nicolson, P.J., Hinman, R.S., Wrigley, T.V., Stratford, P.W., Bennell, K.L.: Self-reported home exercise adherence: a validity and reliability study using concealed accelerometers. J. Orthop. Sports Phys. Ther. **48**, 943–950 (2018)
20. Coravos, A., Khozin, S., Mandl, K.D.: Developing and adopting safe and effective digital biomarkers to improve patient outcomes (2019)
21. Reychav, I., Beeri, R., Balapour, A., Raban, D.R., Sabherwal, R., Azuri, J.: How reliable are self-assessments using mobile technology in healthcare? The effects of technology identity and self-efficacy. Comput. Hum. Behav. **91**, 52–61 (2019)
22. Prince, S.A., et al.: A comparison of self-reported and device measured sedentary behaviour in adults: a systematic review and meta-analysis (2020)
23. Park, K.H., Park, J., Lee, J.W.: An IoT system for remote monitoring of patients at home. Appl. Sci. (Switzerland) **7**(3) (2017)
24. Woo, M.W., Lee, J.W., Park, K.H.: A reliable IoT system for personal healthcare devices. Futur. Gener. Comput. Syst. **78**, 626–640 (2018)
25. Bent, B., et al.: The digital biomarker discovery pipeline: an open-source software platform for the development of digital biomarkers using mHealth and wearables data. J. Clin. Transl. Sci. **5**(1) (2021)
26. Majumder, S., Mondal, T., Deen, M., Majumder, S., Mondal, T., Deen, M.J.: Wearable sensors for remote health monitoring. Sensors **17**, 130 (2017)
27. Berryhill, S., et al.: Effect of wearables on sleep in healthy individuals: a randomized crossover trial and validation study. J. Clin. Sleep Med. **16**, 775–783 (2020)
28. Teixeira, E., et al.: Wearable devices for physical activity and healthcare monitoring in elderly people: a critical review. Geriatrics **6**, 38 (2021)
29. Rumsfeld, J.S., Joynt, K.E., Maddox, T.M.: Big data analytics to improve cardiovascular care: promise and challenges. Nat. Rev. Cardiol. **13**, 350–359 (2016)
30. Post, B., Van Den Heuvel, L., Van Prooije, T., Van Ruissen, X., Van De Warrenburg, B., Nonnekes, J.: Young Onset Parkinson's Disease: A Modern and Tailored Approach (2020)
31. Evenson, K.R., Goto, M.M., Furberg, R.D.: Systematic review of the validity and reliability of consumer-wearable activity trackers. Int. J. Behav. Nutr. Phys. Act. **12**, 1–22 (2015)
32. Straiton, N., et al.: The validity and reliability of consumer-grade activity trackers in older, community-dwelling adults: a systematic review. Maturitas **112**, 85–93 (2018)
33. Chan, A., Chan, D., Lee, H., Ng, C.C., Yeo, A.H.L.: Reporting adherence, validity and physical activity measures of wearable activity trackers in medical research: a systematic review. Int. J. Med. Inform. **160**, 104696 (2022)
34. Neff, C., Wang, M.C., Martel, H.: Using the PDQ-39 in routine care for Parkinson's disease. Parkinsonism Rel. Disord. **53**, 105–107 (2018)

35. Templeton, J.M., Poellabauer, C., Schneider, S.: Negative effects of COVID-19 stay-at-home mandates on physical intervention outcomes: a preliminary study. J. Parkinson's Dis. **11**, 1067–1077 (2021)

36. Zlokovic, B.V.: Neurovascular pathways to neurodegeneration in Alzheimer's disease and other disorders (2011)

37. Kourtis, L., Regele, O., Wright, J., Jones, G.: Digital biomarkers for Alzheimer's disease: the mobile/wearable devices opportunity. NPJ Digit. Med. **2**, 9 (2019)

38. Templeton, J.M., Poellabauer, C., Schneider, S.: Design of a mobile-based neurological assessment tool for aging populations. In: Ye, J., O'Grady, M.J., Civitarese, G., Yordanova, K. (eds.) MobiHealth 2020. LNICST, vol. 362, pp. 166–185. Springer, Cham (2021). https://doi.org/10.1007/978-3-030-70569-5_11

39. Mathan, K., Kumar, P.M., Panchatcharam, P., Manogaran, G., Varadharajan, R.: A novel Gini index decision tree data mining method with neural network classifiers for prediction of heart disease. Des. Autom. Embed. Syst. **22**(3), 225–242 (2018)

40. Waring, J., Lindvall, C., Umeton, R.: Automated machine learning: review of the state-of-the-art and opportunities for healthcare. Artif. Intell. Med. **104**, 101822 (2020)

41. Kotsavasiloglou, C., Kostikis, N., Hristu-Varsakelis, D., Arnaoutoglou, M.: Machine learning-based classification of simple drawing movements in Parkinson's disease. Biomed. Signal Process. Control **31**, 174–180 (2017)

42. Hossen, A., Muthuraman, M., Raethjen, J., Deuschl, G., Heute, U.: Discrimination of parkinsonian tremor from essential tremor by implementation of a wavelet-based soft-decision technique on EMG and accelerometer signals. Biomed. Signal Process. Control **5**, 181–188 (2010)

43. Thorp, J.E., Adamczyk, P.G., Ploeg, H.-K., Pickett, K.A.: Monitoring motor symptoms during activities of daily living in individuals with Parkinson's disease. Front. Neurol. **9**, 1036 (2018)

44. Ricciardi, C., et al.: Classifying different stages of Parkinson's disease through random forests. In: Henriques, J., Neves, N., de Carvalho, P. (eds.) MEDICON 2019. IP, vol. 76, pp. 1155–1162. Springer, Cham (2020). https://doi.org/10.1007/978-3-030-31635-8_140

45. Uddin, S., Khan, A., Hossain, M.E., Moni, M.A.: Comparing different supervised machine learning algorithms for disease prediction. BMC Med. Inform. Decis. Making **19**(1), 1–16 (2019)

46. Riley, R.D., et al.: Calculating the sample size required for developing a clinical prediction model. BMJ **368** (2020)

Author Index

© ICST Institute for Computer Sciences, Social Informatics and Telecommunications Engineering 2023
Published by Springer Nature Switzerland AG 2023. All Rights Reserved
A. Cunha et al. (Eds.): MobiHealth 2022, LNICST 484, pp. 375–376, 2023.
https://doi.org/10.1007/978-3-031-32029-3

Printed in the United States
by Baker & Taylor Publisher Services